RENAL, METABOLIC AND UROLOGIC DISORDERS

OVERACTIVE BLADDER (OAB)

PREVALENCE, RISK FACTORS AND MANAGEMENT

RENAL, METABOLIC AND UROLOGIC DISORDERS

Additional books in this series can be found on Nova's website under the Series tab.

Additional e-books in this series can be found on Nova's website under the eBooks tab.

RENAL, METABOLIC AND UROLOGIC DISORDERS

OVERACTIVE BLADDER (OAB)

PREVALENCE, RISK FACTORS AND MANAGEMENT

ELVIRA LARSON
EDITOR

NOVA BIOMEDICAL

New York

Library of Congress Cataloging-in-Publication Data

Library of Congress Control Number: 2016935304
ISBN: 978-1-63485-033-9

Published by Nova Science Publishers, Inc. † New York

CONTENTS

Preface		**vii**
Chapter 1	Overactive Bladder (OAB): Pathophysiology Epidemiology, and Treatment Options *Bárbara Padilla-Fernández, David Hernández-Hernández, Ruth D. Doherty and David M. Castro-Díaz*	**1**
Chapter 2	The Epidemiology of Lower Urinary Tract Symptoms and Urinary Incontinence: A Critical Review of the Literature *Megan Solomon, Bertha Chen and Lisa Rogo-Gupta*	**21**
Chapter 3	Overactive Bladder in the Pediatric Population *Sophie Ramsay, Anne-Sophie Blais, Geneviève Nadeau, Katherine Moore and Stéphane Bolduc*	**35**
Chapter 4	Current Updates on Overactive Bladder Management *Kirin K. Syed and Angelo E. Gousse*	**69**
Chapter 5	Investigational and Promising Novel Therapeutics for the Overactive Bladder and Urgency Urinary Incontinence *Emilio Sacco and Riccardo Bientinesi*	**95**
Chapter 6	Overactive Bladder (OAB): Is There a Place for Drugs Targeting the Purinergic Cascade? *M. Silva-Ramos, I. Silva, F. Ferreirinha, M. Faria and P. Correia-de-Sá*	**127**
Chapter 7	Mirabegron for the Treatment of Overactive Bladder *Federica Laraud, Simone Ferrero and Umberto Leone Roberti Maggiore*	**157**
Index		**171**

PREFACE

Overactive Bladder Syndrome (OAB) is a clinical entity characterised by urgency, with or without increased urinary frequency and/or urgency incontinence. It is a chronic condition with a high prevalence that increases with age, thus being a growing health problem especially in developed countries due to increased life expectancy. Patients with this disorder are often reluctant to seek advice due to embarassment, fear of social exclusion or the belief that symptoms are an expected consequence of ageing. Costs associated with treatments, use of pads/diapers and general economic burden are expected to increase in the future. OAB has a negative impact on quality of life (QoL) in varying degrees, depending upon the severity of symptoms and the presence of urgency incontinence. It has been linked to increased risk of fractures, institutionalization and depression in older populations particularly prone to the development of OAB. This books discusses the prevalence, risk factors and management options available for OAB.

Chapter 1 – Overactive Bladder Syndrome (OAB) is a clinical entity characterised by urgency, with or without increased urinary frequency and/or urgency incontinence. It is a chronic condition with a high prevalence that increases with age, thus being a growing health problem especially in developed countries due to increased life expectancy. Patients with this disorder are often reluctant to seek advice due to embarassment, fear of social exclusion or the belief that symptoms are an expected consequence of ageing. Costs associated with treatments, use of pads/diapers and general economic burden are expected to increase in the future.

OAB has a negative impact on quality of life (QoL) in varying degrees, depending upon the severity of symptoms and the presence of urgency incontinence. It has been linked to increased risk of fractures, institutionalization and depression in older populations particularly prone to the development of OAB.

Mechanisms underlying non-neurogenic OAB remain unclear. Its development may involve a combination of neurogenic (impaired afferent and efferent bladder innervation, c-fiber hypersensitivity), myogenic (detrusor muscle fibrosis, alterations in contractility) and vasculogenic (impaired blood flow) mechanisms. In both sexes, normal or physiological ageing is associated with a reduction in bladder contractility and total bladder capacity, with a slight increase in post-void residual urine. These changes, combined with the presence of concomitant diseases, polypharmacy and nocturnal polyuria are probably responsible for the high incidence of bothersome symptoms in the older population.

Diagnosis of OAB is clinical and one of exclusion. It is important to rule-out underlying pathology such as infection, urological cancer or urolithiasis. A general and neuro-urological assessment supported by questionnaires (QoL, OAB and urinary incontinence) is the recommended approach. Urodynamic studies are not universally available and are often reserved for patients who fail to respond to standard treatment.

Therapeutic intervention should start with general conservative measures that have proven efficacy such as weight loss, caffeine reduction, adequate fluid intake, bladder training and pelvic floor exercises. If conservative treatments fail, oral medication should be offered. Antimuscarinic drugs and, more recently, mirabegron (a new-class beta-3 adrenergic agonist) are the mainstay of treatment. A transdermal preperation of oxybutynin is also available. However, efficacy and adherence to these drugs have proven to be far from optimal. When oral drugs fail, Onabotulinum Toxin A and Sacral Root or Pudendal Neuromodulation is the next line of treatment available. These semi-invasive therapies result in varying degrees of success, so unfortunately, in some cases, more aggressive definitive procedures such as bladder augmentation may be required.

Chapter 2 – *Introduction.* Pelvic floor disorders (PFD) such as urinary incontinence (UI) and lower urinary tract symptoms (LUTS) represent chronic diseases that negatively impact adults on both individual and national levels. Several large epidemiologic studies on UI have been conducted worldwide over the past decade resulting in a large volume of publications. The authors' objective is to present a thorough comparison and critical evaluation of LUTS and UI epidemiologic literature focusing on databases involving large populations to identify common themes as well as inconsistencies that impact patient management and design of future epidemiologic studies.

Methods. Population-based studies and large epidemiologic clinical trials of PFD were identified using PubMed keywords urinary incontinence, pelvic floor disorders, and epidemiology. Given the evolving understanding about urinary symptoms, papers that were published from 2000-2014 were considered most recent and relevant. References of related studies were also hand searched. Publications using data obtained from these trials were reviewed independently by all authors for epidemiology, risk factors, and quality of life issues related to PFD.

Conclusion. Overall prevalence of LUTS ranged from 19-76% with studies demonstrating the most concordance in prevalence when analyzing female LUTS. There were also notable differences between the two genders. While the authors identified many similarities among epidemiologic studies of PFD such as similar age-related trends, rates of treatment seeking, and factors impacting symptoms, they also identified important inconsistencies.

The difficulty in reaching consensus is largely due to variations in the methods used to evaluate them. In the future the authors must look for consistent modifiable risk factors so that they may improve QOL due to urinary symptoms.

Chapter 3 – Overactive bladder (OAB) is a highly prevalent disorder in the pediatric population. This condition is especially troublesome for pediatric patients and their families when associated with incontinence since it negatively affects self-esteem and impairs children's development. From the patient's perspective, urgency and urge incontinence can have a significant impact, negatively affecting their quality of life. For a therapy to have true benefit, changes must not only be statistically significant, but must also be perceived as meaningful by the patient. A stepwise approach is favored to treat this pathology, starting with behavioral therapy, followed by medical management, and eventually more invasive procedures.

Antimuscarinic agents are the mainstay of medical treatment for OAB. Oxybutynin is the most commonly used antimuscarinic in the pediatric population. However, some patients have a suboptimal response to antimuscarinics and many experience bothersome side effects, which have been documented with all anticholinergics to a significantly higher degree than placebo. Although there have been reports about the use of tolterodine, fesoterodine, trospium, propiverine and solifenacin in children, to date, only oxybutynin has been officially approved for pediatric use by medical authorities in North America.

Oxybutynin use has been well documented in the pediatric population. However, patients with severe OAB symptoms seem not to always respond adequately to oxybutynin. Von Arendonk et al. found that in patients who have urinary incontinence on a daily basis, the likelihood that oxybutynin will be effective is only 20%. Moreover, the presence of muscarinic receptors in many organs apart from the bladder and the lack of specificity of oxybutynin for bladder receptors lead to troublesome side effects, which may lead to discontinuation of medication.

After failure with a first pharmacologic molecule, most practitioners will try a more specific anticholinergic. The authors have already studied various options to treat children with non-neurogenic refractory OAB, namely trying a different antimuscarinic (tolterodine, fesoterodine, or solifenacin) as well as combining two different anticholinergics. Despite favorable results with these options, they remain unapproved for pediatric use and other therapeutic avenues are therefore worth investigating. This is especially the case for molecules with different mechanisms of action and with favorable tolerability profiles.

Mirabegron, a new molecule with a distinct mechanism of action (β3-adrenoreceptor agonist), has recently been approved as monotherapy for idiopathic OAB in adults, but it has not been studied in the pediatric population. The authors recently concluded on two open-label studies to explore its efficacy and safety in children. Their studies allow us to support mirabegron as a new alternative for the treatment of refractory OAB in children. It appears as a safe and effective alternative for children with idiopathic OAB refractory to antimuscarinics, in monotherapy or in association with antimuscarinics (add-on dual therapy).

Invasive modalities such as botulinum toxin intra-detrusor injections and neuromodulation will also be covered in this chapter.

The different therapeutic alternatives reported could be included in a management algorithm for intractable OAB symptoms in children, but the need for prospective randomized controlled studies prior to official approbation is to be acknowledged.

Chapter 4 – The manuscript will provide the reader with a better understanding of the diagnosis and available treatment options for refractory non-neurogenic overactive bladder (OAB).

Non-neurogenic OAB is a symptom complex, which is defined by the International Continence Society (ICS) standardization committee as urgency, with or without urgency incontinence, usually with frequency and nocturia, in the absence of proven infection or other obvious pathology. It is diagnosed by patient symptomatology and does not rely on urodynamic findings and characteristics.

Previously published literature has estimated that approximately 16.5% of American adults have OAB and up to 37% of OAB patients have concomitant urinary incontinence

(OAB-wet). In fact, OAB is one the most common urologic disorders, accounting for more than 2 million physician office visits in the United States (2007).

To date, there is a paucity of validated instruments to define urinary urgency and therefore there is no consensus on an appropriate definition of “refractory” OAB. The diagnosis is based on clinical judgment and management is often at the discretion of the clinician due to a lack of standardized and established clinical care pathways to guide the clinician and the patient.

The current established approaches for refractory OAB has been on third line options as outlined by the most recent American Urologic Association and Society of Urodynamics, Female pelvic medicine and Urogenital reconstruction (AUA/SUFU) guidelines.

Of these options, the pharmacologic use of onabotulinumtoxinA (Botox®) has the strongest rating of “standard” (strength of evidence grade B) and was recently approved by the FDA in 2013 for use in patients with OAB who did not adequately respond to oral medications. Other third line options include neuromodulation with posterior tibial nerve stimulation and sacral nerve modulation. These modalities received a rating of “recommended” (strength of evidence grade C) and will be discussed in greater detail in this manuscript.

Chapter 5 – The increasing prevalence of overactive bladder (OAB) and the relevant limitations of current treatments urge the need for novel therapeutic approaches. To date, antimuscarinics dominate the first-line pharmacological treatment of OAB, together with β3-adrenergic agents, however side-effects and limited efficacy significantly affect patients compliance with these drugs. The growing knowledge of OAB pathophysiology fuelled a huge amount of basic and clinical research in this field of pharmacotherapy aiming to overcome these limitations. Several exiting hypothesis-driven pharmacological approaches for the future treatment of OAB have been suggested in the last few years and are shown in this chapter.

In particular, the exploratory agents alternative to available medications for OAB and that may ultimately prove to be therapeutically useful in the future management of OAB patients based on preclinical and early clinical data are presented. Many alternative pharmacological strategies have been discovered or are under investigation in disease-oriented studies. Several potential therapeutics are known for years but still find obstacles to pass the clinical stages of development, while other completely novel compounds, targeting new pharmacological targets, have been recently discovered and show a potential to translate into clinical therapeutic agents for idiopathic and neurogenic OAB syndrome.

Chapter 6 – It is widely accepted that purines, in particular ATP, are important regulators of urinary bladder functions in animals, as well as in humans. The nucleotide regulates both afferent and efferent signaling pathways. ATP (i) activates sensory nerves during bladder filling conveying both normal and abnormal sensations like urgency and pain, (ii) acts as a co-transmitter with acetylcholine (ACh) in the parasympathetic control of bladder contraction during voiding, and (iii) participates in the central control of bladder reflexes. Bladder ATP originates from both neuronal and non-neuronal sources, such as urothelial cells, interstitial cells, fibroblast-like cells and smooth muscle fibers. The mechanisms regulating the release of ATP in the urinary bladder are still a matter of debate, but may include vesicle exocytosis and translocation via pannexin-1 containing hemichannels among others.

The purinergic tone increases significantly with age and is responsible for up to 40% of nerve-evoked atropine-resistant bladder contractions in pathological conditions, including hypertrophic unstable bladder, overactive detrusor, neurogenic bladder and interstitial cystitis. Recent data showed that the release of ATP from urothelial cells and cholinergic nerves increases several fold in patients with overactive bladder (OAB). The greater purinergic tone may be partially related to the impairment of ecto-NTPDase1/CD39 activity, thus limiting the extracellular breakdown of ATP.

Excess of extracellular ATP released from the urothelium in response to stretch and chemical irritants may contribute to hyperexcitation of suburothelial nerve afferents via homomeric P2X3 and/or heteromeric P2X2/P2X3 receptors. In OAB patients, the increase in ATP release by the mucosa is associated with an increase in the expression of P2X3 receptors on nerves fibres, thus potentiating the sensory input. Although there is scant pharmacological data characterizing the P2 receptor involved in ATP-mediated detrusor contractions, quantitative mRNA studies and experiments with P2X1 knockout mice suggest that the P2X1 receptor might have a significant role. Few attempts have been made so far to investigate the pathophysiological role of P2Y and P1 receptors in the context of bladder overactivity, *vis-a-vis* the deficient formation of ATP metabolites, respectively ADP and adenosine.

The mechanisms underlying OAB are largely unknown, but these are usually divided into urothelial, myogenic and neurogenic. It thus, appears that ATP plays a chief role in all of these. Therefore, one may anticipate benefits in the treatment of OAB using a combination of drugs targeting the purinergic cascade, including ATP release sites, ectonuleotidases, and purinoceptors.

Chapter 7 – Mirabegron is used for the treatment of symptoms caused by overactive bladder (OAB) syndrome. It is a $ß_3$-adrenoreceptor agonist that relaxes the detrusor muscle, thus improving the urine storage during the filling phase. Several double-blind, randomized-controlled trials demonstrated the efficacy of mirabegron for the treatment of OAB. The majority of these trials compared various doses of mirabegron with placebo and/or tolterodine extended-release. Mirabegron improved the number of micturition per 24 hours and the number of incontinence episodes per 24 hours. Mirabegron is well tolerated; the most common adverse events observed with mirabegron in clinical trials were hypertension, nasopharyngitis, and urinary tract infection. The incidence of dry mouth was similar to placebo and was lower than for tolterodine extended release. Since dry mouth is the most common adverse event reported with antimuscarinics and one of the main causes of discontinuation of treatment, mirabegron may be a valuable treatment option for these patients. Future research should focus on the assessment of mirabegron concentrations in the central nervous system and on the evaluation of the potential of the combination of mirabegron with antimuscarinics.

In: Overactive Bladder (OAB)
Editor: Elvira Larson
ISBN: 978-1-63485-033-9

Chapter 1

Overactive Bladder (OAB): Pathophysiology Epidemiology, and Treatment Options

Bárbara Padilla-Fernández[1,*], David Hernández-Hernández[1], Ruth D. Doherty[2] and David M. Castro-Díaz[1]

[1]Department of Urology, University Hospital of the Canary Islands, Tenerife, Spain
[2]Department of Urology, The Queen Elizabeth Hospital, King's Lynn, UK

Abstract

Overactive Bladder Syndrome (OAB) is a clinical entity characterised by urgency, with or without increased urinary frequency and/or urgency incontinence. It is a chronic condition with a high prevalence that increases with age, thus being a growing health problem especially in developed countries due to increased life expectancy. Patients with this disorder are often reluctant to seek advice due to embarassment, fear of social exclusion or the belief that symptoms are an expected consequence of ageing. Costs associated with treatments, use of pads/diapers and general economic burden are expected to increase in the future.

OAB has a negative impact on quality of life (QoL) in varying degrees, depending upon the severity of symptoms and the presence of urgency incontinence. It has been linked to increased risk of fractures, institutionalization and depression in older populations particularly prone to the development of OAB.

Mechanisms underlying non-neurogenic OAB remain unclear. Its development may involve a combination of neurogenic (impaired afferent and efferent bladder innervation, c-fiber hypersensitivity), myogenic (detrusor muscle fibrosis, alterations in contractility) and vasculogenic (impaired blood flow) mechanisms. In both sexes, normal or physiological ageing is associated with a reduction in bladder contractility and total

* Corresponding author: Bárbara Padilla-Fernández. Department of Urology. University Hospital of the Canary Islands. Ctra. de Ofra, s/n. 38320 San Cristóbal de La Laguna, Santa Cruz de Tenerife (Spain). padillaf83@hotmail.com.

bladder capacity, with a slight increase in post-void residual urine. These changes, combined with the presence of concomitant diseases, polypharmacy and nocturnal polyuria are probably responsible for the high incidence of bothersome symptoms in the older population.

Diagnosis of OAB is clinical and one of exclusion. It is important to rule-out underlying pathology such as infection, urological cancer or urolithiasis. A general and neuro-urological assessment supported by questionnaires (QoL, OAB and urinary incontinence) is the recommended approach. Urodynamic studies are not universally available and are often reserved for patients who fail to respond to standard treatment.

Therapeutic intervention should start with general conservative measures that have proven efficacy such as weight loss, caffeine reduction, adequate fluid intake, bladder training and pelvic floor exercises. If conservative treatments fail, oral medication should be offered. Antimuscarinic drugs and, more recently, mirabegron (a new-class beta-3 adrenergic agonist) are the mainstay of treatment. A transdermal preperation of oxybutynin is also available. However, efficacy and adherence to these drugs have proven to be far from optimal. When oral drugs fail, Onabotulinum Toxin A and Sacral Root or Pudendal Neuromodulation is the next line of treatment available. These semi-invasive therapies result in varying degrees of success, so unfortunately, in some cases, more aggressive definitive procedures such as bladder augmentation may be required.

Keywords: overactive bladder, prevalence, management

DEFINITIONS

Overactive bladder syndrome (OAB) was defined in 2002 by the Standardisation Sub-Committee of the International Continence Society as urgency, with or without urge incontinence, usually with frequency and/or nocturia (P Abrams et al., 2002).

Urgency is defined as a complaint of the sudden compelling desire to pass urine, which is difficult to defer. This concept is different to *Detrusor overactivity* (DOA) which is defined as a urodynamic observation characterised by involuntary detrusor contractions during the filling phase which may be spontaneous or provoked (P Abrams et al., 2002) and which may not always have a clinical correlation. 10-45% of individuals have been reported to have asymptomatic unstable bladder contractions (Eckhardt, van Venrooij, & Boon, 2001).

Increased daytime urinary frequency has been traditionally considered as eight or more micturitions per day, while *nocturia* is the complaint of interruption of sleep one or more times per night due to the need to void. To be considered as nocturia it isimportant to note that each void must be preceded and followed by sleep.

Many patients with OAB also complain of *urge urinary incontinence* (UUI), which is the complaint of involuntary leakage of urine accompanied by or immediately preceded by urgency (P Abrams et al., 2002). This is also known as OAB "wet." We should always remember that the most important source of information is the patient himself, and therefore a detailed history is of paramount importance.

PREVALENCE AND CLINICAL IMPACT

There are many obstacles preventing certainty about the true prevalence of OAB. Firstly, patients are often ashamed, or accepting of OAB or urinary incontinence (UI) as an expected consequence of normal ageing. For these, amongst other reasons, patients do not seek medical advice, resulting in under-reporting of this disorder. Depending on the definition used, the demographics of the studied population and the population sampling method selected, the estimate of prevalence may differ (Lucas et al., 2015; Wennberg et al., 2009).

When reviewing the data reported by the European Association of Urology, the annual incidence of OAB is estimated to be 4% to 6%, with annual remission rates of OAB ranging from 2% to 3% (Lucas et al., 2015; Wennberg et al., 2009). The prevalence of OAB in adult males ranges from 10% to 26% and in adult females from 8% to 42% (Schröder et al., 2009). OAB increases with age, being present in 15% of people aged ≥ 65 years (Milsom & Irwin, 2007) and 30–40% of people aged ≥ 75 years (Stewart et al., 2003).

OAB is often associated with other lower urinary tract symptoms (LUTS) and also with many common chronic conditions, such as depression, constipation, neurological disorders and erectile dysfunction (Schröder et al., 2009).

OAB, in particular urgency incontinence, has a huge impact on QoL, affecting psychological, physical and sexual health. Fear of social exclusion, isolation, loneliness, change in daily activities, sleep disturbance and depression are all well-established associations. (K S Coyne et al., 2013; McGhan, 2001) Other co-existing disorders include fungal skin infections, cellulitis, urinary tract infections (UTI), increased body mass index, diabetes mellitus and even death (K S Coyne et al., 2013). A higher incidence of falls and fractures has also been reported (Brown, McGhan, & Chokroverty, 2000; Wagg et al., 2014). Not only patients, but also family caregivers experience powerlessness, helplessness, confusion, guilt and social isolation, resulting in physical and emotional burnout (Siu, 2015). The burden of OAB "wet" appears to be greater than that of stress urinary incontinence or OAB "dry" (K S Coyne et al., 2013).

Urinary incontinence is one of the main causes of premature institutionalization of elderly people (Viana Zulaica, Castiñeira Pérez, Costa Ribas, Fuentes Lema, & Sánchez Rodríguez-Losada, 2005). In addition, the supply of diapers/pads and the treatment of fractures and UTI's, combined with the loss of active working days and other direct and indirect costs were estimated at approximately $12 billion in the United States in 2000 (Erdem & Chu, 2006; Hu et al., 2003). A recent systematic review by Coyne et al. included seven articles exploring the economic burden of UUI in the United States. They reported an estimated total national cost of OAB with UUI in 2007 of $65.9 billion, expecting this figure to increase to $76.2 billion in 2015 and $82.6 billion in 2020 (Karin S Coyne et al., 2014).

PATHOPHYSIOLOGY AND RISK FACTORS

Many groups have studied the pathophysiology of OAB and UUI in both humans and animals, including electrical, morphologic and molecular aspects (W D Steers, 2002). We must remember that the bladder and the lower urinary tract do not work in isolation during the micturition cycle: dysfunction of the higher brain cortex, the pons, spinal cord, and the peripheral, autonomic, somatic, and sensory afferent innervation of the lower urinary tract may all contribute to the symptoms of OAB (Banakhar, Al-Shaiji, & Hassouna, 2012). It is hypothesised that the bladder has a limited repertoire of behaviours in response to disease, leading to variable pathologic mechanisms leading to similar symptoms. Conversely, some authors suggest that there are common factors underlying different disorders (Castro-Diaz et al., 2014).

Urothelial cells are presumed to act in a similar manner to sensory neurons (nociceptors/mechanoreceptors), involving diverse signal-transduction mechanisms to detect physiological stimuli and release of a number of signalling molecules. The urothelium is likely to play an important role by actively communicating with bladder afferent neurons, smooth muscle cells, lamina propia, interstitial cells and cells belonging to the immune and inflammatory systems (Birder, 2014).

Bladder afferent pathways (parasympathetic) comprise Aδ fibers which are myelinated and mechanosensitive and activated by both low and high intravesical pressures. C-fibers, which are unmyelinated are activated by cold, heat or chemical irritation of the bladder mucosa. They may have an important role in the neuroplasticity of the dorsal root ganglion cells due to enlargement and resulting increased electrical excitability (Andersson & Pehrson, 2003).

An enhanced spontaneous contractile activity has been shown in human bladder strips from obstructed unstable bladders (and also from neurourological patients), with a higher sensitivity to muscarinic agonists and potassium chloride (KCl) and reduced contractions upon nerve stimulation (Brading & Turner, 1994; GNA Sibley, 1984; GNA Sibley, 1997). In contrast, bladder strips from individuals with idiopathic instability show hypersensitivity to KCl but not to muscarinic drugs, and have a reduced contractile response to electrical stimulation (Mills, 1999). It has also been demonstrated that, compared to normal bladders, the unstable bladders have an enhanced coupling, allowing spontaneous electrical activity to propagate, synchronous uninhibited detrusor contractions to initiate, and tetanic contractions to occur (W D Steers, 2002).

There are characteristic structural changes in unstable human bladders such as patchy or complete denervation of the muscle bundles, with increased connective tissue mixed with normal fascicles. This may suggests the death of intrinsic bladder neurons, which could follow after severe obstruction with detrusor hypertrophy or peripheral vascular disease (Mills, 1999). Also, the presence of protrusion junctions and ultra-close abutments between myocytes has been reported (W D Steers, 2002).

The incidence of OAB increases with age. This has been hypothesised to be due to changes in neuronal and non-neuronal acetylcholine (Miller & Hoffman, 2006). Bladder outflow obstruction, more commonly seen in men, may lead to an increased production of nerve growth factor (NGF) and induced neuronal enlargement This may exert metabolic effects through the generation of free radicals and lipid peroxidises, and enhancement of the spinal micturition reflex (Banakhar et al., 2012; W D Steers, Creedon, & Tuttle, 1996; W D Steers & De Groat, 1988). NGF has also be found to be elevated in the bladder and urine of patients with bladder pain syndrome, and in models of bladder inflammation in animals (Dupont, Spitsbergen, Kim, Tuttle, & Steers, 2001; Vizzard, Erdman, & de Groat, 1996). Some authors have concluded that differences in neurotransmitter systems may be influenced by oestrogen and progesterone, especially 5-hydroxytryptamine (5-HT) which has been documented at reduced levels in women (Banakhar et al., 2012; W D Steers, 2002). Other authors suggest a relationship between depression, anxiety, attention deficit disorder, pain, irritable bowel syndrome, fibromyalgia and OAB following the same serotonin metabolic disturbances (W D Steers, 2002; Wolfe, Russell, Vipraio, Ross, & Anderson, 1997). Obesity and insulin-resistance have been associated with OAB in many studies spanning different populations (e.g., Caucasian, Asiatic) (Palma et al., 2014; Uzun, Yilmaz, Kemik, Zorba, & Kalkan, 2012; Wen et al., 2014).

DIAGNOSIS

Initial approach to a patient with suspected OAB should include a thorough medical history to assess concomitant disorders which may affect LUT function (*Australian Medicines Handbook Drug Choice Companion: Aged Care*, 2010; Movig, Leufkens, Belitser, Lenderink, & Egberts, 2002; Tsakiris, Oelke, & Michel, 2008). These include:

- Hypertension, diabetes and heart disease
- Neurological disease (Parkinsons Disease, Multiple Sclerosis, Cerebral infarction)
- Bowel dysfunction (constipation, altered bowel habit);
- Uro-gynaecological problems (birth history, menopause, pelvic irradiation, previous incontinence, prolapse or prostate surgery)
- Drugs (diuretics, systemic oestrogens, calcium channel blockers, valproic acid, baclofen, dantrolene, ketamine, clonazepam, tobacco, caffeine)
- Cognitive status, mobility and general health
- Dietary habits and fluid intake.

Regarding the OAB symptom complex, international practice guidelines on OAB and urinary incontinence recommend including questions about onset and duration of symptoms, severity, degree of bother and association with co-existing LUTS or POP symptoms (Gormley et al., 2015; Lucas et al., 2015; D. Staskin et al., 2009).

Sexual function should also be assessed in patients with suspected OAB for the association between sexual dysfunction in women and men and key OAB symptoms is now well established (Hansen, 2004; Irwin et al., 2008; Kim, Seo, & Yoon, 2005).

LUTS are an independent risk factor for erectile and ejaculatory dysfunction, decrease in libido and sexual activity, and overall impairment in sexual function in both women and men (Hansen, 2004; Temml, Haidinger, Schmidbauer, Schatzl, & Madersbacher, 2000).

Physical Examination

Physical examination in a patient with OAB symptoms aims to exclude and assess concomitant conditions that could mimic or exacerbate this chronic disease.

A complete physical examination including abdominal, pelvic and perineal assessment, genitalia and rectal examination is recommended. This should include abdominal palpation seeking scars from previous surgery, abdominal masses or an enlarged bladder to signifying chronic urinary retention. Sensation and reflexes in the urogenital area (bulbocavernous and anal reflexes), anal tone and pelvic floor muscle contraction should be assessed in order to exclude neurological diseases causing neurogenic bladder dysfunction. In men, genital examination should focus on penile skin, inspection of the external urethral meatus (balanitis xerotica obliterans, meatalstenosis) and digital rectal examination of the prostate gland to detect abnormalities such as an benign prostatic enlargement or a suspicious nodule.

In women it is crucial to assess oestrogen status as there is a clear associated with urinary incontinence and symptoms of OAB. Pelvic floor contraction through digital vaginal examination should be assessed, as well as the detection of pelvic organ prolapse, urethral hypermobility and urethral diverticula (Gormley et al., 2015; Lucas et al., 2015; D. Staskin et al., 2009).

Voiding Diaries and Questionnaires

Voiding diaries and/or frequency-volume charts are objective methods of quantifying the symptoms reported by the patient. They provide very useful information about micturition frequency and physiological bladder volume, fluid intake, daytime and nightime diuresis, incontinence, urgency episodes and use of pads. Repeated charts can be completed to objectively evaluate treatment response. High 24-hour voided volume may indicate excessive fluid intake which exacerbates urinary frequency. Small volume voids may indicate early sensation of urgency. Completion of at least three days of such voiding records are recommended.

Bladder diaries are widely used in clinical trials but uptake in clinical practice is generally poor. Nevertheless, they are a fantastic tool for symptom assessment, are widely available and very cheap. A combination of medical history and a three-day voiding diary is probably the most cost-effective approach to the assessment of a patient with idiopathic OAB (Jimenez-Cidre et al., 2016; López-Fando et al., 2015).

Although time-consuming, experts recommend using questionnaires and/or a form of patient-reported outcome measures (PROMs). For use in regular medical practise, questionnaires must be short, easy to understand and complete, and easy to score and interpret. Well established questionnaires include ICIQ-FLUTS and MLUTS (ICIQ-Female and Male LUTS), ICIQ-SF (ICIQ-Short Form, to evaluate urinary incontinence), IPSS in men (international prostate symptoms score), PPBC (patient-perception of bladder control) and B-SAQ (bladder self-assessment questionnaire) (Basra et al., 2007; K S Coyne, Matza, Kopp, & Abrams, 2006; Rosenberg & Dmochowski, 2005).

These tools allow both the clinician and the patient to gain insight into patient perception of symptoms, identify the most troublesome symptoms, and evaluate response of behavioural modifications and interventions.

Laboratory and Imaging

Microscopic urinalysis, or at least a simple dipstick urinalysis should be performed in all urological patients. These may identify UTI, haematuria, glycosuria or proteinuria requiring further assessment. In the context of OAB, urinalysis is largely used to rule out concomitant pathology such as UTI (positive test for leukocyte estearase and nitrites), diabetes (significant glucose in urine) and urothelial carcinoma of the bladder or urinary stones (positive test for erythrocytes)

A positive urine test should prompt further evaluation; in the case of suspected UTI with urine culture, and in the case of haematuria with other tests such as urinary tract imaging (CT urography, ultrasonography), urine cytology and/or cystoscopy.

The presence of significant glycosuria is a sign of poorly controlled or undiagnosed diabetes [excluding patients with type 2 diabetes mellitus receiving sodium-glucose cotransporter 2 (SGLT2) inhibitors], which is an established cause of LUTS and recurrent UTI.

Care must be taken not to automatically treat asymptomatic bacteriuria (without pyuria) in the presence of OAB symptoms, as this may be an incidental finding.

In conclusion, laboratory and imaging tests are used in the field of OAB diagnosis only to exclude underlying pathology and to confirm whether idiopathic OAB is the true cause of symptoms (Gerber & Brendler, 2002).

Novel urine biomarkers are being investigated for the diagnosis and management of OAB, such as nerve growth factor, brain-derived neurotropic factor, monocyte chemoattractant protein-1 or glycosaminoglycans. All these markers are found to be deranged in OAB patients, and their levels tend to reach normal values with treatment. But at present their utility remains within the field of research.

Urodynamics (UDS)

Free uroflowmetry (non-invasive UDS) or filling cystometry plus pressure-flow studies (invasive UDS) are not routinely indicated during the initial approach to OAB. Indications for free uroflowmetry and post-void residual urine measurement (PVR) remain unclear. In general, these should be used when patients complain of voiding symptoms (hesitancy, weak and/or interrupted stream, sensation of incomplete voiding) Due to the increase likelihood of bladder outlet obstruction in men, non-invasive UDS and PVR are much more frequently performed in men.

Although urodynamic investigation (invasive UDS) is the only method to objectively assess LUT function, there is a weak correlation between the main OAB-related urodynamic diagnosis of "detrusor overactivity," and the OAB syndrome. About 50% patients with OAB syndrome show no detrusor overactivity in a filling cystometry, while 50% of asymptomatic patients show detrusor overactivity in the urodynamic evaluation. Other findings include abnormal bladder sensitivity (first desire to void <100 mL), low bladder capacity (maximal cystometric capacity under 250-300 mL), low bladder compliance (<30 mL/cmH20) or incontinence. Urodynamic urgency incontinence or OAB "wet" is defined as the presence of urine leak associated with an uninhibited detrusor contraction. Urodynamic mixed urinary incontinence is diagnosed when the forementioned urodynamic findings are seen in combination with urinary leakage with Valsalva maneuver or cough.

Filling cystometry and pressure-flow studies are indicated when there is a suspicion of bladder outlet obstruction (high post-void residual urine in free uroflowmetry), after failure of conservative behavioural and pharmacologic treatment but before invasive therapies.

TREATMENT

Conservative Treatment

Following the recommendations of the National Institute for Health and Care Excellence (NICE) clinical guideline (CG) 171 addressing women with urge urinary incontinence, conservative treatment should be the first step in management. Drugs should be used in patients with OAB only when conservative treatment has failed (Hunjan & Smith, 2014; *NICE guidelines [CG171] - Urinary incontinence in women*, September 2013).

Weight loss (if overweight), management of constipation, reduced caffeine intake, bladder training, timed/prompted voiding, pelvic floor muscle exercises, and biofeedback are all intended to improve bladder function by modification of the patient's voiding habits and utilisation of techniques to preventing urine loss with the least risk of harm. This may be challenging to implement effectively in elderly patients with cognitive impairment, mobility disorders or other debilitating conditions (Erdem & Chu, 2006).

Treatment of existing comorbidities, particularly in the elderly, such as cardiac failure, chronic renal failure, neurologic diseases, obesity, etc. should be optimised. These conditions can lead to polyuria, nocturia, increased abdominal pressure and CNS disturbance. Treatment may therefore improve OAB symptoms (Lucas et al., 2015) or reduce the severity of such symptoms, although little evidence has been published in this field.

Antimuscarinics

Antimuscarinic (anticholinergic) drugs are considered the mainstay of treatment for OAB, these include many drugs which vary in their pharmacological profiles, pharmacokinetic properties and formulation. These drugs are mainly limited by their modest clinical benefit, high incidence of adverse effects - in particular moderate to severe dry mouth, constipation and blurred vision. These side effects lead to poor patient compliance and early treatment discontinuation (Castro et al., 2011; Gacci et al., 2015). High discontinuation rates have been reported for tolterodine and oxybutynin (68-95%) at 12 months (Lucas et al., 2014), most commonly due to poor efficacy, adverse effects and high cost. However, a study by Sears et al. reported that when patients do not fund their medication, only 35% did not collect a repeat prescription and a higher median medication possession ratio was observed (Sears, Lewis, Noel, Albright, & Fischer, 2010). Clinical guidelines recommend review of therapy four weeks after commencement of each OAB drug (through a telephone interview or face-to-face consultation) (Hunjan & Smith, 2014; *NICE guidelines [CG171] - Urinary incontinence in women*, September 2013).

Drug availability varies across continents, most notably between Europe, America and Asia. Oxybutynin and trospium chloride were the first medications used for the treatment of

OAB. Later, tolterodine was specifically developed for this indication. Since then, new drugs have been developed with the aim of decreasing adverse events improving efficacy and patient adherence to treatment. Such drugs include fesoterodine, solifenacin, darifenacin and imidafenacin (Padilla-Fernández, Hernández-Hernández, Morgenstern, Concepción-Masip, & Castro-Díaz, 2015).

Given the wide spectrum of antimuscarinic drugs available, several studies have been carried out in an attempt to evaluate safety, tolerability and efficacy. The STAR trial showed that flexible dosing with solifenacin (5 mg and 10 mg) was more effective in reducing OAB symptoms than tolterodine extended-release (ER) 4 mg, with statistically significant reductions in the number of episodes of urgency, UUI and overall incontinence. More patients in the tolterodine group withdrew from treatment, mainly stating lack of therapeutic effect, although side effects such as dry mouth and constipation were more common in the solifenacin group (C. R. Chapple et al., 2005).

A systematic review performed by Novara et al. in 2008 reported that tolterodine immediate-release (IR) had a more favorable profile of adverse events than oxybutynin IR, while the ER formulations of the two drugs had similar efficacy and safety profiles. Additionally, they concluded that more clinical studies are required to determine which drug should be used as first-, second-, or third-line treatment (Novara et al., 2008).

Extended-release drugs seem to be tolerated more favourably than immediate-release (Lucas et al., 2015). Oxybutynin is also available in a transdermal formulation, which avoids the hepatic first-pass mechanism. It may be utilised in patients who are unlikely to adhere to oral therapy or who dislike multiple-daily dose regimens. In clinical studies transdermal oxybutynin has been associated with a relatively low risk of side effects including a reduced rate of cognitive impairment. The most frequent adverse effect seems to be local application-site reactions which can be minimized by the application of topical corticosteroids or antihistamines (Dmochowski et al., 2003; Kay, Staskin, MacDiarmid, McIlwain, & Dahl, 2012). Phase 2 studies have already reported the safety and efficacy of an oxybutynin vaginal ring. These silicone rings, impregnated with oxybutynin, are placed in the vagina for 4 weeks, releasing oxybutynin 4 or 6 mg daily. Their use was studied in women with 10 or more UUI episodes per week and 8 or more micturitions per day, and demonstrated symptomatic benefit in patients receiving both oxybutynin 4 mg and 6 mg. The most frequent adverse events recorded were UTI, dry mouth and vaginal discharge, all of which were more common in the oxybutynin vaginal ring 6 mg daily group. Other common adverse events appearing in both groups were bleeding, soreness, candidal infection, local irritation, abrasions and bacterial vaginosis (Gittelman, Weiss, & Seidman, 2014).

A novel approach to the treatment of male LUTS is the combination of antimuscarinics and alpha-blockers. Antimuscarinics may theoretically decrease bladder contractility, and hence may lead to increased post-void residual urine (PVR) or urinary retention. In 2013 Van Kerrebroeck et al. published the results of a 12-week double-blind study comparing the combination of solifenacin and tamsulosin with tamsulosin monotherapy and placebo in 1334 men (mean age > 65 years) with both storage and voiding LUTS. Significant reductions in Total Urgency and Frequency Score (TUFS) were observed in the combination group compared with placebo and tamsulosin monotherapy. Furthermore, combination therapy was well tolerated with a low incidence of acute urinary retention (7 cases of drug-related AUR in total) and improved QoL measures (van Kerrebroeck et al., 2013). Even the EAU Guidelines now include a statement that short-term treatment with antimuscarinics are recommended in men with moderate-to-severe LUTS with storage LUTS. They may be used in patients with bladder outlet obstruction if care is taken to monitor patients for evidence of urinary retention (Gravas et al., 2015).

β-3 Adrenoceptor Agonist: Mirabegron

Mirabegron is the first β-3 adrenoceptor agonist approved for the treatment of OAB in Europe, USA, Canada, Australia and Japan. Mirabegron acts via stimulation of β-3 adrenoceptors located in the human detrusor muscle. This results in detrusor relaxation during the filling phase and thus a reduction in urinary frequency, urgency and incontinence episodes. In addition mean voided volume per micturition, number of nocturia episodes and patient reported outcome measures are all improved compared to placebo (Khullar et al., 2013; Nitti, Auerbach, et al., 2013). Furthermore, data from three 12-week, randomized, Phase III trials and from a further 1-year safety trial have evaluated mirabegron's efficacy and tolerability in elderly patients (≥65 and ≥75 years) (Wagg et al., 2014).

In 2014 Abrams et al. Released the results of a 12-week randomised, double-blind, trial based on data from 20 European countries evaluating the use of anticholinergic and beta-3 agonist combination treatment. Solifenacin with simultaneous mirabegron administration was compared with solifenacin monotherapy in 1306 male and female patients ≥18 years old with symptoms of OAB. They demonstrated that, in comparison to monotherapy, combination treatment with solifenacin and mirabegron led to significant improvement of OAB symptoms, mean voided volume per micturition (MVV), micturition frequency and urgency. This combination appeared to be safe, with minimal additional adverse events reported compared to monotherapy alone (Paul Abrams et al., 2015).

In July 2015, the European Medicines Agency recommended modification of the terms of the Marketing Authorization and the Summary of Product Characteristics of mirabegron based upon post-commercialization reports. Several cases of hypertensive crisis presumed to be linked to cerebrovascular and cardiac events occurring in patients taking mirabegron have been reported. Following these reports it is advised to avoid the use of mirabegron in patients with systolic blood pressure ≥180 mm Hg and/or diastolic blood pressure ≥110 mm Hg (*Mirabegron - Scientific conclusions and grounds recommending the variation to the terms of the marketing authorisation*, 23 July 2015). Several cases of urinary retention with a plausible temporal relationship to mirabegron treatment have also been reported with a frequency between 1/1,000-10,000. This is classified as a "rare" adverse effect. The frequency of other adverse effects such as insomnia are yet to be determined (European Medicines Agency, 2015).

There is no agreed consensus regarding the definition of "persistent" or "refractory" UUI, but patients who tend to fall into this category usually comprise of those who report inadequate symptom control after at least 2 first-line therapies. These should include 2 anticholinergic medications or 1 anticholinergic and mirabegron and at least 1 course of supervised behavioral therapy, physical therapy or biofeedback (Brubaker et al., 2008). Third-line treatment may also be recommended when bothersome adverse events or intolerance to medication occur.

Botulinum Toxin

Botulinum toxin is a potent neurotoxin derived from the bacterium *Clostridium botulinum* which blocks the release of acetylcholine at the neuromuscular junction, temporarily paralysing any muscle into which it is injected. It also blocks the release of other neuropeptides and neurotransmitters involved in afferent signalling. Two strains are available for clinical use. There are currently two preparations of toxin type A (BoNTA) licensed for the treatment of OAB with differing formulations and molecular structures.: Onabotulinum toxin A (BOTOX®, Allergan Ltd) and abobotulinum toxin A (Dysport®, Ipsen Ltd) (Mangera et al., 2014; *NICE guidelines [CG171] - Urinary incontinence in women*, September 2013). The injection of BoNTA directly into the detrusor muscle is performed with a rigid or flexible cystoscope. It is feasible to perform this procedure under local anaesthesia in the office on an outpatient basis. The efficacy of onabotulinum toxin A in idiopathic OAB has been demonstrated in two pivotal studies by Chapple et al. in Europe and Nitti et al. in the US. These included patients 18 years or older presenting with 3 or more UUI episodes recorded in a 3-day voiding diary and an average of 8 or more micturitions per day who reported inadequate response to anticholinergics. These patients were randomised 1:1 to placebo or BOTOX® 100 U with 20 intradetrusor injections of 0.5 ml each, avoiding the trigone. A significant decrease in the number of urgency and UI episodes, micturitions and nocturia episodes per 24-hour period was reported. An improvement in both patient health-related QoL and perception of change in their condition was also demonstrated (C. Chapple et al., 2013; Nitti, Dmochowski, et al., 2013) (Graph 1).

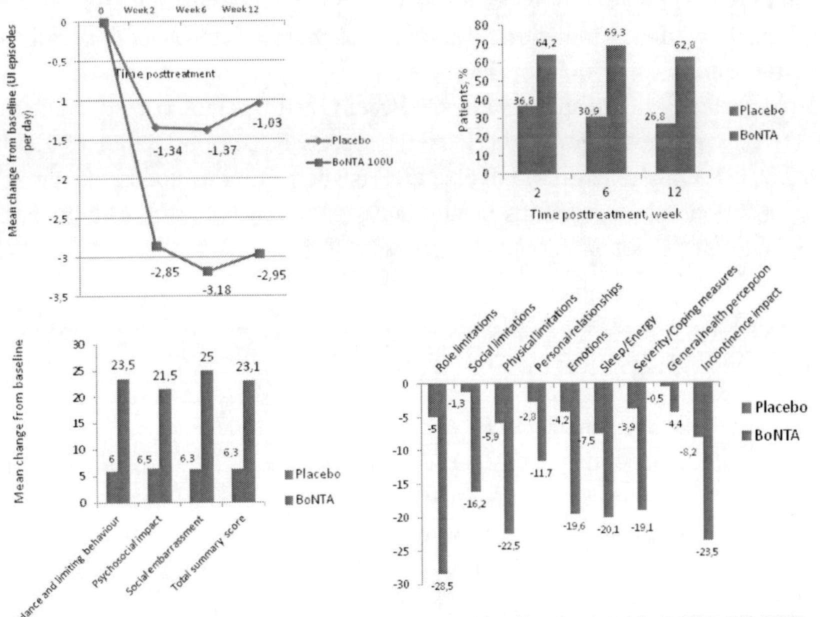

Adapted from Chapple et al, Eur Urol 2013; 64(2): 249-56

BoNTA leads to significant improvements in bladder diary parameters such as daily frequency (29%), daily urgency (38%), and daily incontinence (59%) and in urodynamic parameters such as maximum cystometric capacity (58%) and maximum detrusor pressure

(29%) (Mangera et al., 2014). Common adverse events include UTI, mild haematuria and transient rise in post-void residual urine which may necessitate temporary intermittent self-catheterisation (Lucas et al., 2015). A drawback of BoNTA is its duration of action, with each treatment lasting an average of 9 months. Repeated injections are usually required with sustained efficacy. A minimum interval of 3 months between treatments is recommended (Lucas et al., 2015).

BoNTA should not be used during pregnancy or lactation. It is contraindicated in patients with Myasthenia Gravis, Eaton-Lambert syndrome and other disorders of the neuromuscular junction.

Posterior Tibial Nerve Stimulation (PTNS)

Neuromodulation of the lower urinary tract via electrical stimulation of the posterior tibial nerve can be achieved percutaneously with a 34-gauge needle electrode inserted 3-5 cm above and posterior to the medial malleolus. Alternatively transcutaneous stimulation with a surface electrode can be utilised. Patients usually attend for weekly treatments lasting 30 minutes for 12 weeks, followed by occasional "top-up" treatments as required based on symptoms. Inhibition of DOA by PTNS in humans was first described in 1983 by McGuire et al. (McGuire, Zhang, Horwinski, & Lytton, 1983). It was approved by The Food and Drug Administration (FDA) in 2000 for the treatment of refractory OAB. It is also a valid option for non-obstructive urinary retention, chronic pelvic pain/painful bladder syndrome and functional bowel disorders.

The tibial nerve originates from spinal roots L4-S3. The therapeutic effects of PTNS can thus be explained by the modulation of reflex pathways at the sacral spinal cord level combined with central inhibition of motor neurons supplying the bladder. Two recent systematic reviews have shown success rates between 37-100% in non-responders to first line therapy of OAB, with no major complications reported (Burton, Sajja, & Latthe, 2012; Gaziev et al., 2013). Only temporary adverse effects such as mild-moderate pain or bleeding at the needle insertion site, leg cramps or numbness/pain involving the sole of the foot have been reported in around 8.5% of patients treated with PTNS.

Sacral Roots Neuromodulation (SRNM)

Implantation of a permanent sacral nerve root stimulator is designed to provide continuous direct stimulation of the S3 nerve roots,. Amongst other disorders, it is used as third-line treatment for refractory OAB, urge urinary incontinence and non-obstructive urinary retention. FDA-approval for urge urinary incontinence was granted in 1997, and in 1999 approval for use in patients with urgency-frequency syndrome and urinary retention followed.

The expense of this treatment ($26,269 for 3 years treatment) necessitates a two staged procedure. This ensures optimum patient selection for implantation of the permanent device (Watanabe et al., 2010). Patients first undergo a period of "test stimulation" utilizing either a temporary percutaneous nerve evaluation (PNE) system or implantation of a permanent tined lead which is connected to an *external* stimulation source. The initial test phase is of 2-3 weeks duration, during which time patients complete symptom diaries to allow objective assessment of improvement. Patients demonstrating a satisfactory response (50-70% improvement of symptoms) following the test-phase may then proceed to permanent implantation of the neurostimulator, most commonly situated in a subcutaneous position of the upper buttock (*NICE guidelines [CG171]-Urinary incontinence in women*, September 2013).

A study by Cameron et al. investigated the use of SNRM in two groups of patients – those who were privately funded and those eligible for government funding. They found that 45.8% of patients undergoing PNE and 35.4% of those undergoing the staged tined-lead technique in the government-funded group went on to receive permanent implantation. However, these numbers differed in the privately-funded group of patients, with 24.1% and 50.9% of patients receiving permanent implants respectively (Cameron, Anger, Madison, Saigal, & Clemens, 2011). In the long term, 80–90% of those patients receiving a permanent implant experience a satisfactory response with a significant decrease in episodes of incontinence per day and improved overall QoL (Kessler et al., 2011; Schmidt et al., 1999; D. R. Staskin, Peters, MacDiarmid, Shore, & de Groat, 2012).

Several studies have compared Botulinum toxin and SRNM, both considered as third-line treatments in OAB, in an attempt to ascertain which treatment may be the most cost-effective. During the first 2 years of treatment it has been suggested that BoNTA may be superior in terms of cost-effectiveness when compared to SRNM (Siddiqui, Amundsen, Visco, Myers, & Wu, 2009). One Italian National Health Service (INHS) Study compared ongoing costs of both treatment strategies. This study seemed to suggest that using SRNM in place of BoNTA may be cost-effective 3 years after implantation and onwards. This trend becomes clearer with time, with SRNM demonstrating increased efficacy and reduced costs by year 10. Cumulative costs are €32,975 for early SRNM and €33,309 for early BoNTA (Bertapelle et al., 2015). A Spanish research group has confirmed the incremental cost-effectiveness ratios (ICERs) observed with SRNM over time, estimating an extra €3775 compared to BoNTA and €3412 compared to standard medical treatment at 5 years. ICERs at 7 years, taking into account a replacement SRNM generator, are €9830 and €3433 compared to BoNTA and standard medical treatment respectively. However, at 10 years, cumulative costs were €29,166 for SNM, €29,458 for BoNTA, and €29,370 for standard medical treatment. This suggests that SNM may be the economically favourable treatment option over a 10-year time-frame (Arlandis et al., 2011).

Surgical Procedures

Invasive surgery including augmentation cystoplasty and diversion of urine either through the use of an indwelling catheter or via conduit formation are generally considered to be final options. These tend to be reserved for those patients with OAB who are refractory to semi-invasive therapies such as BoNTA injections and/or SRNM.

Clam cystoplasty was first described in the UK by Bramle in 1990 (Bramble, 1990) (Bramble, 1990). Diversion of urine through use of a permanent urethral or suprapubic catheter may be considered in order to reduce incontinence and incontinence-associated dermatitis. However, even this relatively simple option has considerable risks, including urinary tract infections, formation of bladder stones and even the development of bladder cancer following long-term use. It has been suggested that long-term supra-pubic catheters may be more favourable than long-term urethral catheters in male patients. Supra-pubic catheters allow male patients to retain sexual function and have been associated with a lower incidence of epididymo-orchitis and urethral trauma (Weld & Dmochowsky, 2000).

Surgical urinary diversion can be achieved through formation of a conduit, usually constructed from ileum. This option should be reserved for patients requesting a single definitive procedure. Candidates undergoing surgical diversion must accept a permanent stoma, and should be carefully consented regarding the long-term complications including pyocystis in the remnant bladder, stomal problems such as stenosis and hernias, uretero-ileal stenosis, upper urinary tract dilatation and renal dysfunction (Cody et al., 2012).

Augmentation cystoplasty (clam cystoplasty) is a well-established procedure with documented efficacy for storage LUTS and incontinence in patients with neurogenic detrusor overactivity. Augmentation of the bladder using a detubularized segment of segment leads to increased bladder capacity and restores urinary continence. Although alternative intestinal segments can be used, ileum is the preferred choice due to close proximity to the bladder and its ability to distend whilst maintaining compliance. This procedure, classically approached via an infra-umbilical laparotomy or Pfannenstiel incision has more recently been described via a laparoscopic approach (Núñez Mora, Cansino Alcaide, Alonso Gregorio, Martínez-Piñeiro, & De la Peña Barthel, 2007). Unfortunately its efficacy in patients with idiopathic OAB is slightly worse than patients with those with a neurogenic cause. Complete continence is achieved in around 50% of patients, while reports of "social continence" (use of 0 or 1 pad for confidence) varies from 70-75%. Following clam formation UTI is a frequent complication, though it is worth noting that asymptomatic bacteriuria is almost universal but may not require treatment. Patients must accept a possibility of the need for clean intermittent self-catheterization, indeed some authors advocate teaching patients to perform this prior surgery. Additional frequent complications include urinary tract stone formation and metabolic disturbance (most commonly hyperchloraemic acidosis). Less frequent complications include a change in bowel habit, bladder perforation and malignancy (Greenwell, Venn, & Mundy, 2001).

References

Abrams, P., Cardozo, L., Fall, M., Griffiths, D., Rosier, P., Ulmsten, U. & Society, S. S. c. o. t. I. C. (2002). The standardisation of terminology of lower urinary tract function: report from the Standardisation Sub-committee of the International Continence Society. *Neurourol Urodyn*, *21*(2), 167-178.

Abrams, P., Kelleher, C., Staskin, D., Rechberger, T., Kay, R., Martina, R. & Ridder, A. (2015). Combination Treatment with Mirabegron and Solifenacin in Patients with Overactive Bladder: Efficacy and Safety Results from a Randomised, Double-blind, Dose-ranging, Phase 2 Study (Symphony). *European Urology*, *67*(3), 577-588. doi: 10.1016/ j.eururo.2014.02.012.

Andersson, K. E. & Pehrson, R. (2003). CNS involvement in overactive bladder: pathophysiology and opportunities for pharmacological intervention. *Drugs*, *63*(23), 2595-2611.

Arlandis, S., Castro, D., Errando, C., Fernández, E., Jiménez, M., González, P. & Brosa, M. (2011). Cost-Effectiveness of Sacral Neuromodulation Compared to Botulinum Neurotoxin A or Continued Medical Management in Refractory Overactive Bladder. *Value in Health*, *14*(2), 219-228. doi: 10.1016/j.jval.2010.08.006.

Australian Medicines Handbook Drug Choice Companion: Aged Care. (2010). Adelaide, SA: Australian Medicines Handbook.

Banakhar, M. A., Al-Shaiji, T. F. & Hassouna, M. M. (2012). Pathophysiology of overactive bladder. *Int Urogynecol J*, *23*(8), 975-982. doi: 10.1007/s00192-012-1682-6.

Basra, R., Artibani, W., Cardozo, L., Castro-Diaz, D., Chapple, C., Cortés, E., & Kelleher, C. (2007). Design and Validation of a New Screening Instrument for Lower Urinary Tract Dysfunction: The Bladder Control Self-Assessment Questionnaire (B-SAQ). *Eur Urol*, *52*(1), 230-238. doi: 10.1016/j.eururo.2006.11.015.

Bertapelle, M. P., Vottero, M., del Popolo, G., Mencarini, M., Ostardo, E., Spinelli, M. … A, D. A. (2015). Sacral neuromodulation and Botulinum toxin A for refractory idiopathic overactive bladder: a cost-utility analysis in the perspective of Italian Healthcare System. *World J Urol*, *33*(8), 1109-1117. doi: 10.1007/s00345-014-1401-7.

Birder, L. A. (2014). Urinary Bladder, Cystitis and Nerve/Urothelial Interactions. *Auton Neurosci*, *182*, 89-94. doi: 10.1016/j.autneu. 2013. 12. 005.

Brading, A. F. & Turner, W. H. (1994). The unstable bladder: towards a common mechanism. *Br J Urol*, *73*(1), 3-8.

Bramble, F. J. (1990). The clam cystoplasty. *Br J Urol*, *66*(4), 337-341.

Brown, J. S., McGhan, W. F. & Chokroverty, S. (2000). Comorbidities associated with overactive bladder. *Am J Manag Care*, *6*(11 Suppl), S574-579.

Brubaker, L., Richter, H. E., Visco, A., Mahajan, S., Nygaard, I., Braun, T. M. & Wei, J. (2008). Refractory Idiopathic Urge Urinary Incontinence and Botulinum A Injection. *J Urol*, *180*(1), 217-222. doi: 10.1016/j.juro. 2008.03.028.

Burton, C., Sajja, A. & Latthe, P. M. (2012). Effectiveness of Percutaneous Posterior Tibial Nerve Stimulation for Overactive Bladder: A Systematic Review and Meta-Analysis. *Neurourol Urodyn*, *31*, 1206-1216.

Cameron, A. P., Anger, J. T., Madison, R., Saigal, C. S. & Clemens, J. Q. (2011). National trends in the usage and success of sacral nerve test stimulation. *J Urol*, *185*(3), 970-975. doi: 10.1016/j.juro.2010.10.060.

Castro-Diaz, D., Cardozo, L., Chapple, C. R., Espuña, M., Kelleher, C., Kirby, M. & Tubaro, A. (2014). Urgency and pain in patients with overactive bladder and bladder pain syndrome. What are the differences? *Int J Clin Pract*, *68*(3), 356-362. doi: 10.1111/ijcp.12317.

Castro, D., Miranda, P., Sánchez-Ballester, F., Arumi, D., Lizarraga, I. & Ebel, C. (2011). Assessment of reasons for overactive bladder treatment change. *Actas Urol Esp (English Edition)*, *35*(2), 73-79. doi: 10.1016/S2173-5786(11)70022-1.

Cody, J. D., Nabi, G., Dublin, N., McClinton, S., Neal, D. E., Pickard, R. & Yong, S. M. (2012). Urinary diversion and bladder reconstruction/ replacement using intestinal segments for intractable incontinence or following cystectomy. *Cochrane Database Syst Rev*, *2*, CD003306. doi: 10.1002/14651858.CD003306.pub2.

Coyne, K. S., Matza, L. S., Kopp, Z. & Abrams, P. (2006). The validation of the patient perception of bladder condition (PPBC): a single-item global measure for patients with overactive bladder. *Eur Urol*, *49*(6), 1079-1086. doi: 10.1016/j.eururo.2006.01.007.

Coyne, K. S., Wein, A., Nicholson, S., Kvasz, M., Chen, C. I. & Milsom, I. (2014). Economic Burden of Urgency Urinary Incontinence in the United States: A Systematic Review. *J Manag Care Pharm*, *20*(2), 130-140. doi: 10.18553/jmcp.2014.20.2.130.

Coyne, K. S., Wein, A., Nicholson, S., Kvasz, M., Chen, C. I. & Milsom, I. (2013). Comorbidities and personal burden of urgency urinary incontinence: a systematic review. *Int J Clin Pract*, *67*(10), 1015-1033. doi: 10.1111/ijcp.12164.

Chapple, C., Sievert, K. D., MacDiarmid, S., Khullar, V., Radziszewski, P., Nardo, C. & Haag-Molkenteller, C. (2013). OnabotulinumtoxinA 100 U significantly improves all idiopathic overactive bladder symptoms and quality of life in patients with overactive bladder and urinary incontinence: a randomised, double-blind, placebo-controlled trial. *Eur Urol*, *64*(2), 249-256. doi: 10.1016/j.eururo.2013.04.001.

Chapple, C. R., Martinez-Garcia, R., Selvaggi, L., Toozs-Hobson, P., Warnack, W., Drogendijk, T. & STAR study group. (2005). A comparison of the efficacy and tolerability of solifenacin succinate and extended release tolterodine at treating overactive bladder syndrome: results of the STAR trial. *Eur Urol*, *48*(9), 464-470. doi: 10.1016/j.eururo.2005.05.015.

Dmochowski, R. R., Sand, P. K., Zinner, N. R., Gittelman, M. C., Davila, G. W. & Sanders, S. W. (2003). Comparative efficacy and safety of transdermal oxybutynin and oral tolterodine versus placebo in previously treated patients with urge and mixed urinary incontinence. *Urology*, *62*(2), 237-242.

Dupont, M. C., Spitsbergen, J. M., Kim, K. B., Tuttle, J. B. & Steers, W. D. (2001). Histological and neurotrophic changes triggered by varying models of bladder inflammation. *J Urol*, *166*(3), 1111-1118.

Eckhardt, M. D., van Venrooij, G. E. & Boon, T. A. (2001). Symptoms, prostate volume, and urodynamic findings in elderly male volunteers without and with LUTS and in patients with LUTS suggestive of benign prostatic hyperplasia. *Urology*, *58*(6), 966-971. doi: 10.1016/S0090-4295(01)01413-3.

Erdem, N. & Chu, F. M. (2006). Management of Overactive Bladder and Urge Urinary Incontinence in the Elderly Patient. *Am J Med*, *119*(3A), 29S-36S.

European Medicines Agency. (2015). Betmiga: EPAR - Product Information. from http://www.ema.europa.eu/ema/index.jsp?curl=pages/medicines/human/medicines/002388/human_med_001605.jsp&mid=WC0b01ac058001d124.

Gacci, M., Sebastianelli, A., Salvi, M., Schiavina, R., Brunocilla, E., Novara, G. & Serni, S. (2015). Tolterodine in the Treatment of Male LUTS. *Curr Urol Rep*, *16*(9), 60. doi: 10.1007/s11934-015-0531-9.

Gaziev, G., Topazio, L., Iacovelli, V., Asimakopoulos, A., Di Santo, A., De Nunzio, C. & Finazzi-Agro, E. (2013). Percutaneous tibial nerve stimulation (PTNS) efficacy in the treatment of lower urinary tract dysfunctions: a systematic review. *BMC Urology*, *13*(1), 61. doi: 10.1186/1471-2490-13-61.

Gerber, G. S. & Brendler, C. B. (2002). Evaluation of the urologic patient: history, physical examination, and urinalysis. In P. C. Walsh (Ed.), *Campbell's Urology*, (8th ed., pp. 83-110). Philadelphia: Saunders.

Gittelman, M., Weiss, H. & Seidman, L. (2014). A phase 2, randomized, double-blind, efficacy and safety study of oxybutynin vaginal ring for alleviation of overactive bladder symptoms in women. *J Urol*, *191*(4), 1014-1021. doi: 10.1016/j.juro.2013.11.019.

Gormley, E. A., Lightner, D. J., Faraday, M., Vasavada, S. P., American Urological Association, & Society of Urodynamics and Female Pelvic Medicine. (2015). Diagnosis and treatment of overactive bladder (non-neurogenic) in adults: AUA/SUFU guideline amendment. *J Urol*, *193*(5), 1572-1580. doi: 10.1016/j.juro.2015.01.087.

Gravas, S., Bach, T., Bachmann, A., Drake, M., Gacci, M., Gratzke, C., . . . Tikkinen, K. A. O. (2015). *Guidelines on the Management of Non-Neurogenic Male Lower Urinary Tract Symptoms (LUTS), incl. Benign Prostatic Obstruction (BPO)*. European Association of Urology Retrieved from http://uroweb.org/wp-content/uploads/EAU-Guidelines-Non-Neurogenic-Male-LUTS-Guidelines-2015-v2.pdf.

Greenwell, T. J., Venn, S. N. & Mundy, A. R. (2001). Augmentation cystoplasty. *BJU Int*, *88*(6), 511-525. doi: 10.1046/j.1464-4096. 2001. 001206.

Hansen, B. L. (2004). Lower urinary tract symptoms (LUTS) and sexual function in both sexes. *Eur Urol*, *46*(2), 229-234. doi: 10.1016/j.eururo. 2004.04.005.

Hu, T. W., Wagner, T. H., Bentkover, J. D., LeBlanc, K., Piancentini, A., Stewart, W. F. & Hunt, T. L. (2003). Estimated economic costs of overactive bladder in the United States. *Urology*, *61*, 1123-1128. doi: 10.1016/S0090-4295(03)00009-8.

Hunjan, A. & Smith, K. (2014). B58. Drugs for urinary frequency, enuresis and incontinence 2.0. from http://www.prescqipp.info/resources/ viewcategory/224-urinary-incontinence.

Irwin, D. E., Milsom, I., Reilly, K., Hunskaar, S., Kopp, Z., Herschorn, S. & Abrams, P. (2008). Overactive bladder is associated with erectile dysfunction and reduced sexual quality of life in men. *J Sex Med*, *5*(12), 2904-2910. doi: 10.1111/j.1743-6109.2008.01000.x.

Jimenez-Cidre, M. A., López-Fando, L., Franco, A., Arlandis, S., Castro, D., Prieto, L. & Grupo de investigación en Resultados de Salud en Urología Funcional y Urodinámica, I. (2016). How should we address the diagnosis of overactive bladder in women? *Actas Urol Esp*, *40*(1), 29-36. doi: 10.1016/j.acuro.2015.08.007.

Kay, G. G., Staskin, D. R., MacDiarmid, S., McIlwain, M. & Dahl, N. V. (2012). Cognitive effects of oxybutynin chloride topical gel in older healthy subjects: a 1-week, randomized, double-blind, placebo- and active-controlled study. *Clin Drug Investig*, *32*(10), 707-714. doi: 10.2165/11636310-000000000-00000.

Kessler, T. M., Bachmann, L. M., Minder, C., Löhrer, D., Umbehr, M., Schünemann, H. J. & Kessels, A. G. (2011). Adverse event assessment of antimuscarinics for treating overactive bladder: a network metaanalytic approach. *PLoS One*, *6*(2), e16718. doi: 10.1371/journal.pone.0016718.

Khullar, V., Amarenco, G., Angulo, J. C., Cambronero, J., Høye, K., Milsom, I. & Chapple, C. (2013). Efficacy and Tolerability of Mirabegron, a β3-Adrenoceptor Agonist, in Patients with Overactive Bladder: Results from a Randomised European–Australian Phase 3 Trial. *European Urology*, *63*(2), 283-295. doi: 10.1016/j.eururo.2012.10.016.

Kim, Y. H., Seo, J. T. & Yoon, H. (2005). The effect of overactive bladder syndrome on the sexual quality of life in Korean young and middle aged women. *Int J Impot Res*, *17*(2), 158-163.

López-Fando, L., Carracedo, D., Jiménez, M., Gómez de Vicente, J. M., Martínez, L., Gómez Del Cañizo, C. & Burgos, F. J. (2015). Cost-effectiveness analysis of main diagnosis tools in women with overactive bladder. Clinical history, micturition diary and urodynamic study. *Actas Urol Esp*, *39*(1), 40-46. doi: 10.1016/j.acuro.2014.03.002.

Lucas, M. G., Bedretdinova, D., Berghmans, L. C., Bosch, J. L. H. R., Burkhard, F. C., Cruz, F. & Pickard, R. S. (2015). *Guidelines on Urinary Incontinence*. European Association of Urology Retrieved from http://uroweb.org/wp-content/uploads/EAU-Guidelines-Urinary-Incontinence-2015.pdf.

Lucas, M. G., Bedretdinova, D., Bosch, J. L. H. R., Burkhard, F. C., Cruz, F., Nambiar, A. K. & Pickard, R. S. (2014). Guidelines on Urinary Incontinence. from http://uroweb.org/wp-content/uploads/20-Urinary-Incontinence_LR.pdf.

Mangera, A., Apostolidis, A., Andersson, K. E., Dasgupta, P., Giannantoni, A., Roehrborn, C. & Chapple, C. (2014). An updated systematic review and statistical comparison of standardised mean outcomes for the use of botulinum toxin in the management of lower urinary tract disorders. *Eur Urol*, *65*(5), 981-990. doi: 10.1016/j.eururo.2013.10.033.

McGhan, W. F. (2001). Cost effectiveness and quality of life considerations in the treatment of patients with overactive bladder. *Am J Manag Care*, *7*(2 Suppl), S62-75.

McGuire, E., Zhang, S., Horwinski, E. & Lytton, B. (1983). Treatment of motor and sensory detrusor instability by electric stimulation. *J Urol*, *129*(1), 78-79.

Milsom, I. & Irwin, D. E. (2007). A cross-sectional, population-based, multinational study of the prevalence of overactive bladder and lower urinary tract symptoms: results from the EPIC study. *Eur Urol*, *6*(Suppl 1), 4-9.

Miller, J. & Hoffman, E. (2006). The causes and consequences of overactive bladder. *J Womens Health (Larchmt)*, *15*(3), 251-260.

Mills, I. W. (1999). *The Pathophysiology of Detrusor Instability and the Role of Bladder Ischemia in Its Etiology [DM thesis]*. Oxford University, Oxford, England.

Mirabegron - Scientific conclusions and grounds recommending the variation to the terms of the marketing authorisation. (23 July 2015). (EMA/CHMP/555332/2015). London, United Kingdom: European Medicines Agency.

Movig, K. L., Leufkens, H. G., Belitser, S. V., Lenderink, A. W. & Egberts, A. C. (2002). Selective serotonin reuptake inhibitor-induced urinary incontinence. *Pharmacoepidemiol Drug Saf*, *11*(4), 271-279. doi: 10.1002/pds.705.

NICE guidelines [CG171] - Urinary incontinence in women. (September 2013). London, UK: National Institute for Health and Care Excellence.

Nitti, V. W., Auerbach, S., Martin, N., Calhoun, A., Lee, M. & Herschorn, S. (2013). Results of a Randomized Phase III Trial of Mirabegron in Patients with Overactive Bladder. *J Urol*, *189*(4), 1388-1395. doi: 10.1016/j.juro. 2012.10.017.

Nitti, V. W., Dmochowski, R., Herschorn, S., Sand, P., Thompson, C., Nardo, C. & Haag-Molkenteller, C. (2013). OnabotulinumtoxinA for the Treatment of Patients with Overactive Bladder and Urinary Incontinence: Results of a Phase 3, Randomized, Placebo Controlled Trial. *The Journal of Urology*, *189*(6), 2186-2193. doi: 10.1016/j.juro.2012.12.022.

Novara, G., Galfano, A., Secco, S., D'Elia, C., Cavalleri, S., Ficarra, V. & Artibani, W. (2008). A Systematic Review and Meta-Analysis of Randomized Controlled Trials with Antimuscarinic Drugs for Overactive Bladder. *Eur Urol*, *54*(4), 740-763. doi: 10.1016/j.eururo.2008.06.080.

Núñez Mora, C., Cansino Alcaide, R., Alonso Gregorio, S., Martínez-Piñeiro, L. L. & De la Peña Barthel, J. (2007). Laparoscopic augmentation enterocystoplasty: Initial experience. *Actas Urol Esp*, *31*(1), 17-22.

Padilla-Fernández, B., Hernández-Hernández, D., Morgenstern, S. C., Concepción-Masip, T. & Castro-Díaz, D. M. (2015). Treatment of Overactive Bladder in Elderly Patients: Clinical Considerations. *Clinical Medicine Insights: Geriatrics*, *8*, 11-20. doi: 10.4137/CMGer.S10245.

Palma, T., Raimondi, M., Souto, S., Fozzatti, C., Palma, P. & Riccetto, C. (2014). Correlation between body mass index and overactive bladder symptoms in pre-menopausal women. *Rev Assoc Med Bras*, *60*(2), 111-117. doi: 10.1590/1806-9282.60.02.007.

Rosenberg, M. T. & Dmochowski, R. R. (2005). Overactive bladder: evaluation and management in primary care. *Cleve Clin J Med*, *72*, 149-156.

Schmidt, R. A., Jonas, U., Oleson, K. A., Janknegt, R. A., Hassouna, M. M., Siegel, S. W. & van Kerrebroeck, P. E. (1999). Sacral nerve stimulation for treatment of refractory urinary urge incontinence. *J Urol.*, *1999*, *162*, *352–7*, *162*(2), 352-357.

Schröder, A., Abrams, P., Andersson, K.-E., Artibani, W., Chapple, C. R., Drake, M. J. & Thüroff, J. W. (2009). EAU Guidelines on Urinary Incontinence. *EAU Guidelines.* from http://uroweb.org/wp-content/ uploads/EAU-Guidelines-Urinary-Incontinence-2009.pdf.

Sears, C. L., Lewis, C., Noel, K., Albright, T. S. & Fischer, J. R. (2010). Overactive bladder medication adherence when medication is free to patients. *J Urol*, *183*(3), 1077-1081. doi: 10.1016/j.juro.2009.11.026.

Sibley, G. (1984). *The Response of the Bladder to Lower Urinary Tract Obstruction [DM thesis].* Oxford University, Oxford, England.

Sibley, G. (1997). Developments in our understanding of detrusor instability. *Br J Urol*, *80* Suppl *1*, 54-61.

Siddiqui, N. Y., Amundsen, C. L., Visco, A. G., Myers, E. R. & Wu, J. M. (2009). Cost-effectiveness of sacral neuromodulation versus intravesical botulinum A toxin for treatment of refractory urge incontinence. *J Urol*, *182*(6), 2799-2804. doi: 10.1016/j.juro.2009.08.031.

Siu, J. Y. m. (2015). Coping with patients suffering from overactive bladder: experiences of family caregivers in Hong Kong. *Health Soc Care Community*, *[Epub ahead of print]*. doi: 10.1111/hsc.12278.

Staskin, D., Kelleher, C., Avery, K., Bosch, R., Cotterill, N., Coyne, K. & Kopp, Z. (2009). Committee 5 - Initial assessment of urinary and faecal incontinence in adult male and female patients. In International Continence Society (Ed.), *Incontinence: 4th International Consultation on Incontinence*. Paris, France: Health Publications.

Staskin, D. R., Peters, K. M., MacDiarmid, S., Shore, N. & de Groat, W. C. (2012). Percutaneous tibial nerve stimulation: a clinically and cost effective addition to the overactive bladder algorithm of care. *Curr Urol Rep*, *13*(5), 327-334. doi: 10.1007/s11934-012-0274-9.

Steers, W. D. (2002). Pathophysiology of overactive bladder and urge urinary incontinence. *Rev Urol*, *4 Suppl 4*, S7-S18.

Steers, W. D., Creedon, D. J. & Tuttle, J. B. (1996). Immunity to nerve growth factor prevents afferent plasticity following urinary bladder hypertrophy. *J Urol*, *155*(1), 379-385.

Steers, W. D. & De Groat, W. C. (1988). Effect of bladder outlet obstruction on micturition reflex pathways in the rat. *J Urol*, *140*(4), 864-871.

Stewart, W. F., Van Rooyen, J. B., Cundiff, G. W., Abrams, P., Herzog, A. R., Corey, R. & Wein, A. J. (2003). Prevalence and burden of overactive bladder in the United States. *World J Urol*, *20*(6), 327-336.

Temml, C., Haidinger, G., Schmidbauer, J., Schatzl, G. & Madersbacher, S. (2000). Urinary incontinence in both sexes: prevalence rates and impact on quality of life and sexual life. *Neurourol Urodyn*, *19*(3), 259-271. doi: 10.1002/(SICI)1520-6777(2000)19:3<259::AID-NAU7>3.0.CO;2-U.

Tsakiris, P., Oelke, M. & Michel, M. C. (2008). Drug-induced urinary incontinence. *Drugs Aging*, *25*(7), 541-549.

Uzun, H., Yilmaz, A., Kemik, A., Zorba, O. U. & Kalkan, M. (2012). Association of insulin resistance with overactive bladder in female patients. *Int Neurourol J*, *16*(4), 181-186. doi: 10.5213/inj.2012.16.4.181.

van Kerrebroeck, P., Chapple, C., Drogendijk, T., Klaver, M., Sokol, R., Speakman, M. & Drake, M. J. (2013). Combination Therapy with Solifenacin and Tamsulosin Oral Controlled Absorption System in a Single Tablet for Lower Urinary Tract Symptoms in Men: Efficacy and Safety Results from the Randomised Controlled NEPTUNE Trial. *European Urology*, *64*(6), 1003-1012. doi: 10.1016/j.eururo.2013.07.034.

Viana Zulaica, C., Castiñeira Pérez, C., Costa Ribas, C., Fuentes Lema, M. D. & Sánchez Rodríguez-Losada, J. (2005). Incontinencia urinaria. *FMC. Protocolos Formación Médica Continuada en Atención Primaria*, *12*(Protocolo_4), 1-34.

Vizzard, M. A., Erdman, S. L. & de Groat, W. C. (1996). Increased expression of neuronal nitric oxide synthase in bladder afferent pathways following chronic bladder irritation. *J Comp Neurol*, *370*(2), 191–202.

Wagg, A., Cardozo, L., Nitti, V. W., Castro-Diaz, D., Auerbach, S., Blauwet, M. B. & Siddiqui, E. (2014). The efficacy and tolerability of the β3-adrenoceptor agonist mirabegron for the treatment of symptoms of overactive bladder in older patients. *Age and Ageing*, *43*(5), 666-675. doi: 10.1093/ageing/afu017.

Watanabe, J. H., Campbell, J. D., Ravelo, A., Chancellor, M. B., Kowalski, J., & Sullivan, S. D. (2010). Cost analysis of interventions for antimuscarinic refractory patients with overactive bladder. *Urology*, *76*(4), 835-840. doi: 10.1016/j.urology.2010.01.080.

Weld, K. J. & Dmochowsky, R. R. (2000). Effect of bladder management on urological complications in spinal cord injured patients. *J Urol*, *163*(3), 768-772.

Wen, J. G., Li, J. S., Wang, Z. M., Huang, C. X., Shang, X. P., Su, Z. Q. & Heesakkers, J. P. (2014). The prevalence and risk factors of OAB in middle-aged and old people in China. *Neurourol Urodyn*, *33*(4), 387-391. doi: 10.1002/nau.22429.

Wennberg, A. L., Molander, U., Fall, M., Edlund, C., Peeker, R. & Milsom, I. (2009). A Longitudinal Population-based Survey of Urinary Incontinence, Overactive Bladder, and Other Lower Urinary Tract Symptoms in Women. *European Urology*, *55*(4), 783-791. doi: 10.1016/j.eururo. 2009. 01.007.

Wolfe, F., Russell, I. J., Vipraio, G., Ross, K. & Anderson, J. (1997). Serotonin levels, pain threshold, and fibromyalgia, symptoms in the general population. *J Rheumatol*, *24*(3), 555-559.

In: Overactive Bladder (OAB)
Editor: Elvira Larson
ISBN: 978-1-63485-033-9

Chapter 2

THE EPIDEMIOLOGY OF LOWER URINARY TRACT SYMPTOMS AND URINARY INCONTINENCE: A CRITICAL REVIEW OF THE LITERATURE

Megan Solomon[1,*]***, MD, Bertha Chen***[2,†]***, MD, and Lisa Rogo-Gupta***[3,‡]***, MD***
[1]Stanford University School of Medicine, Stanford, California, US
[2]Professor, Urogynecology and Pelvic Reconstructive Surgery, Stanford University School of Medicine, Stanford, California, US
[3]Clinical Assistant Professor, Urogynecology and Pelvic Reconstructive Surgery, Stanford University School of Medicine, Stanford, California, US

ABSTRACT

Introduction. Pelvic floor disorders (PFD) such as urinary incontinence (UI) and lower urinary tract symptoms (LUTS) represent chronic diseases that negatively impact adults on both individual and national levels. Several large epidemiologic studies on UI have been conducted worldwide over the past decade resulting in a large volume of publications. Our objective is to present a thorough comparison and critical evaluation of LUTS and UI epidemiologic literature focusing on databases involving large populations to identify common themes as well as inconsistencies that impact patient management and design of future epidemiologic studies.

Methods. Population-based studies and large epidemiologic clinical trials of PFD were identified using PubMed keywords urinary incontinence, pelvic floor disorders, and epidemiology. Given the evolving understanding about urinary symptoms, papers that

* E-mail: meganrs@stanford.edu.
† E-mail: bchen@stanford.edu.
‡ E-mail: lrgupta@stanford.edu.
The authors have no conflicts to disclose.

were published from 2000-2014 were considered most recent and relevant. References of related studies were also hand searched. Publications using data obtained from these trials were reviewed independently by all authors for epidemiology, risk factors, and quality of life issues related to PFD.

Conclusion. Overall prevalence of LUTS ranged from 19-76% with studies demonstrating the most concordance in prevalence when analyzing female LUTS. There were also notable differences between the two genders. While we identified many similarities among epidemiologic studies of PFD such as similar age-related trends, rates of treatment seeking, and factors impacting symptoms, we also identified important inconsistencies.

The difficulty in reaching consensus is largely due to variations in the methods used to evaluate them. In the future we must look for consistent modifiable risk factors so that we may improve QOL due to urinary symptoms.

INTRODUCTION

Pelvic floor disorders (PFD) such as urinary incontinence (UI) and lower urinary tract symptoms (LUTS) represent chronic diseases that negatively impact adults on both individual and national levels. The annual national economic impact in the US currently exceeds $76 billion for UI alone [1] and will climb as the population projections anticipate a shift towards a dominance of older adults, the group most heavily impacted by PFD [2, 3].

Several large epidemiologic studies on UI have been conducted worldwide over the past decade resulting in a large volume of publications. Our objective is to present a thorough comparison and critical evaluation of LUTS and UI epidemiologic literature focusing on databases involving large populations to identify common themes as well as inconsistencies that impact patient management and design of future epidemiologic studies.

METHODS

Population-based studies and large epidemiologic clinical trials of PFD were identified using PubMed. There was no specific time period outlined at the beginning of the search, however given the evolving understanding about urinary symptoms, papers that were published from 2000-2014 were considered most desirable with recent and relevant data. Keywords included urinary incontinence, pelvic floor disorders, and epidemiology. References of relevant studies were also hand searched.

Publications using data obtained from these trials were reviewed independently by all authors for epidemiology, risk factors, and quality of life issues related to PFD (See Table 1). These major studies have contributed significantly to the current understanding of PFD and their methods are described below.

BOSTON AREA COMMUNITY HEALTH SURVEY (BACH)

BACH is an epidemiologic evaluation of the prevalence and natural history of urologic disorders. A cross-sectional population-based survey of Boston area (US) residents was conducted from 2002-2005 using in-person interviews, examinations, and questionnaires collected from 5,503 white, black, and Hispanic adults ages 30-79 years old, 3,202 of which were women [4]. Participants then completed questionnaires at 5 years to evaluate the natural history of urologic disorders [5, 6].

Table 1. Included epidemiologic and population-based studies of LUTS and UI

	BACH	EPILUTS	NHANES	LIS
Epidemiology	[4-6]	[7, 8]	[9, 10, 15-18, 20]	[21-24]
Risk factors	[25-31]	[8, 13, 14]	[15-17, 32, 33]	[22, 23, 34, 35]
Quality of life	[5, 25]	[8, 12, 14, 36-38]	[10, 32]	[21]

LUTS were evaluated using validated questionnaires. The American Urologic Symptom Index (AUA-SI) evaluates the frequency of urologic symptoms over the preceding month, with a score of ≥8 indicating at least moderate symptoms. A participant was designated as having voiding symptoms if the AUA-SI was ≥5 in response to questions regarding intermittency, weak stream, hesitancy, or incomplete emptying. A participant was designated as having storage symptoms if the AUA-SI was ≥4 in response to questions regarding frequency, urgency, or nocturia. Post-micturition symptoms included inadequate emptying and dribbling. Symptom bother was measured using the Sandvik Severity Index (SSI) Scale for female UI combined with physical and metal quality of life scores from the Medical Outcomes Study Short Form (SF-12). A SSI score of ≥3 was considered positive for UI and correlates to moderate to severe symptoms, or leakage of more than a few drops occurring at least weekly over the preceding 12 months. Progression of LUTS was defined as an increase in score of ≥2 at five-year follow-up.

Epidemiology of Lower Urinary Tract Symptoms Survey (EpiLUTS)

EpiLUTS is a multi-national population-based evaluation of the epidemiology of LUTS conducted using an internet-based cross-sectional questionnaire of US, UK, and Swedish residents aged ≥40 years old. Thirty thousand participants completed the survey, 15, 861 of which were women and 20,000 of which were US residents (9,416 men and 10,584 women). Approximately 80% were white, with the remaining comprised of African American, Asian, Hispanic, and other races.

LUTS were evaluated using a 9-item questionnaire specific to the study. Respondents reported answers using a 5-point Likert scale for frequency and bother [7, 8]. Questions were asked regarding symptoms present in the preceding 4 weeks, while those regarding treatment seeking reflected the preceding 12 months. Participants were divided into those with more severe symptoms, reported at least ‘often,’ and those with less severe symptoms, reported at least ‘sometimes.’ Similarly, bother symptoms were divided into those with more severe bother, reported as at least ‘quite a bit,’ and those with less severe bother, reported at least 'somewhat.' OAB was defined as urinary urgency at least 'sometimes,' with or without urge UI.

National Health and Nutrition Examination Survey (NHANES)

NHANES is an annual population-based survey whose goal is to describe health status of US adults. The National Centers for Health Statistics Centers for Disease Control and Prevention have used a stratified cluster-design since the year 2000 to identify approximately 5,000 potential participants, approximately half of which are female. Eligible women undergo structured home interviews and mobile physical examinations. Race/ethnicity is categorized as non-Hispanic white, Mexican-American, and non-Hispanic black (http://www.cdc.gov/nchs/nhanes).

PFD were evaluated by patient responses to questions regarding the presence of bothersome symptoms while the subsequent data analyses used definitions created at the discretion of the publishing authors. This variation in PFD definitions is partly due to the changes in the NHANES questionnaires over time and explains discrepancies in results, such as UI prevalence ranging from 25-75%. For example, the 1999-2000 NHANES questionnaire cycle included a single question regarding UI 'with an activity like coughing' leaving investigators unable to categorize UI type [9]. In their analysis, the Pelvic Floor Disorders Network (PFDN) defined UI by converting participant responses into the SSI described above for the BACH survey. Participants described UI frequency as 'less than once per month,' 'a few times per month,' 'a few times a week,' or 'every day and/or night,' and amount of leakage as 'drops,' 'splashes,' or 'more.' A SSI score of ≥3 was similarly considered positive for UI and correlates to moderate to severe symptoms, or leakage of more than a few drops occurring at least weekly over the preceding 12 months.

AI was limited to fecal incontinence (FI). The same group calculated FI similarly to UI using patient-reported feces consistency and FI frequency and POP was considered present if participants answered affirmatively to a question derived from the validated Pelvic Floor Distress Inventory, 'Do you experience bulging or something falling out you can see or feel in the vaginal area?'

These PFD definitions can be compared to methods used by other groups. When examining a subset of NHANES data collected between 2001-2004, Dooley and colleagues defined SUI as a single positive response to leaking 'with an activity like coughing,' UUI as a single positive response to "an urge or pressure to urinate," and MUI as a positive response to both questions [10].

Leicestershire MRC Incontinence Study (LIS)

The Leicestershire MRC incontinence study is a single cross-sectional study whose aim was to establish the prevalence of urinary symptoms and needs in adults in the United Kingdom. A postal survey was completed of 15,904 community-dwelling adults age 40 years and above who were randomly selected by household from the Leicestershire Health

Authority Register. The survey included questions regarding demographic characteristics, general health, urinary and bowel symptoms, quality of life, and National Health Service use. A follow up survey was conducted annually up to year three in some subsets.

RESULTS

Epidemiology

BACH

Overall prevalence of LUTS in the BACH cohort was reported as 19%. Prevalence was similar across genders and ethnic groups, increasing with advancing age from 11% (30-39 years old) to 26% (≥50 years old). Gender differences in LUTS trends were found despite similar overall prevalence. Female LUTS prevalence remained overall stable across the postmenopausal years, while male LUTS peaked at 35% (60-69 years old) before returning to rates similar to females by 70 years old. Fewer than 3% reported the highest levels of symptom severity. Only 10% of men with LUTS were being treated compared to 7% of women, most of whom reported pelvic floor exercises as their current treatment plan.

Storage symptoms were more prevalent among women while voiding and post-micturition symptoms were more prevalent among men. Post-micturition symptoms were more often seen concurrently with voiding symptoms compared to storage symptoms (>50% and <50%, respectively). Thirty five percent of women reported storage symptoms, the majority of which reported urinary frequency (66%) and nocturia (52%). Voiding symptoms were present in 8%, mostly incomplete emptying (5%) and intermittency (4%). Female UI prevalence was 10%, with most suffering from mixed symptoms (57%) [11].

Progression was seen in 24% of women overall. De novo LUTS was reported in 14% of women compared to de novo UI in 9% [4].

EPILUTS

Overall prevalence of LUTS was 75% in the EPILUTS cohort with 52% reporting severe symptoms. LUTS prevalence remained relatively stable with advancing age. The presence of symptoms occurring at least sometimes increased over time from 37% (40-45 years old) to 51% (≥76 years old) [12]. Racial differences in OAB were identified. Asian women had the lowest prevalence of OAB (27%) compared to Hispanic (42%), Caucasian (43%), and African American women (46%) [13].

Nearly half of women reported the presence of more than one symptom type and 25% reported all three symptom types. Women also suffered from storage symptoms alone (22%), voiding symptoms alone (5%) or both storage and voiding symptoms (15%), while rarely reporting post-voiding symptoms alone (1%). OAB prevalence ranged from 33% (severe symptoms) to 43% (less severe symptoms). UI was reported in 68% of women. The most common UI types were SUI and MUI, impacting 23% and 21%, respectively. Those suffering from UUI tended to be older than those with SUI [14]. Similar trends were observed in participants in all countries.

NHANES

UI among NHANES participants increased over time from 38% (1999-2000) to 49% (2001-2004) and then remained relatively stable at 51% (2007-2008) [9, 15]. Thirty percent reported UI occurred at least weekly. SUI was the most common subtype among women (25-50%) followed by MUI (16-34%) and UUI (9-15%) [10, 16]. These results compared to analysis performed by the PFDN using the definitions described above which estimated an overall prevalence of PFD of 24% (2005-2006) with 16% reporting UI [17, 18].

The presence of UI increased with advancing age with variations depending on UI subtype. UUI was most prevalent amongst women ≥60 years old while SUI was most prevalent amongst women 40-59 years old [10]. Similar trends were described repeatedly but exact estimates varied by publication. Wu and colleagues described an increase in UI with advancing age from 4% (20-29 years old) to 22% (50-59 years old), peaking at 38% in those aged ≥ 80 (ref Wu 2014) and Anger and colleagues described a peak in UI at 44% among women 75-79 years old [19].

Reports of racial differences in UI prevalence were also inconsistent. While some reported no difference in UI [18], others reported non-Hispanic whites were the most symptomatic. Non-Hispanic whites reported the most SUI symptoms while non-Hispanic blacks reported the lowest UI rates overall but more UUI compared to other races [9, 17, 20].

LIS

The prevalence of symptoms increased with age, although men and women exhibited different patterns. UI in women peaked in the early 50s, declined in the 60s and then rose after the mid-70s. In men, the prevalence increased gradually with age. The prevalence of need also increased with age in both groups with men increasing steadily, while women's needs remained stable across age groups until 80s or more. The majority of participants with clinically significant symptoms did not find them bothersome or socially disabling, about a third of those with bothersome symptoms found them socially disabling. Those with extreme bother consisted of only 2% of the sample population [21].

In subsequent studies from this data set, prevalence of OAB in men was reported at baseline to be 9.4% and this increased with age (4.4% 40-49 years old, 7.2% 50-59 years old, 8.4% 60-69 years old, 16.7% 70-79 years old, and 24% for those 80 years and older). The incidence of OAB over one year was 5.3%. The incidence rate based on age group was: 2.7% 40-49 years old, 4.3% 50-59 years old, 5.9% 60-69 years old, 9.3% 70-79 years old, and 7.6% for those 80 years and older [22]. For women, SUI symptom severity varied in relation to age, with peaks in the 60s and 80s, and a trough in the 70s. In comparison, OAB symptom severity increased more progressively with age, in particular in the 60s. Baseline prevalence of pure SUI, pure OAB, and mixed incontinence were 7.7%, 7.7%, and 12.7%, respectively. The incidence rates over 1 year were 3.6%, 5.4%, and 4.5%, respectively [23]. Interestingly, remission rates for SUI and OAB appeared to be similar for all age groups with SUI ranging from 24.6-30.6% and OAB ranging from 28.3-35.2% [24].

Risk Factors

BACH

Medical history was linked to both prevalence and progression in the BACH cohort. Moderate to severe LUTS was correlated with the presence of depression, diabetes mellitus, heart disease, and hypertension in both genders [25]. LUTS prevalence was also highest in those who were less physically active. Factors associated with symptom progression included increased baseline abdominal circumference and history of gestational diabetes. Gynecologic history also played a role in symptom progression. A history of two vaginal deliveries or uterine prolapse increased LUTS progression significantly (odds ratio 2 and 3, respectively) [26].

Dietary factors were also found to impact the presence of LUTS. Dietary Vitamin C was inversely associated with urgency among both women and men, however supplemental Vitamin C had the opposite effect [27, 28]. Total energy intake was also associated with more frequent and severe UI (OR=3), and there may even be differing impacts depending on the quantity and type of fat intake [29]. Dietary factors impacted storage and voiding symptoms differently in men, the cause of which remains unclear [30]. Caffeine intake demonstrated different trends in women compared to men. Women who increased their caffeine intake by ≥2 cups per day had 64% higher odds of LUTS progression, independent of their baseline intake. This compared to men in whom baseline intake increased their odds of LUTS progression (OR=2) [31].

EPILUTS

Medical history was found to impact the prevalence of LUTS. Those suffering from all LUTS subtypes reported higher rates of arthritis, asthma, anxiety, depression, diabetes, hearth disease, irritable bowel syndrome, neurologic conditions, and sleep disorders. Women with depression and LUTS were most likely to report urgency, UI, and weak stream. Self-reported childhood bedwetting was more prevalent amongst those suffering from UUI compared to other UI types [14].

Weight was also linked to LUTS in women. Women who were overweight (BMI 25-29.9) or obese (BMI ≥ 30) were more likely to report UI than women of normal BMI [8]. BMI was also different amongst those with different types of UI. In women without UI, 46% reported normal BMI while 54% were overweight or obese. This compared to 31% and 69% of those with urge UI or SUI alone. Those with MUI were more most likely to be overweight.

Racial differences in comorbid conditions amongst those with OAB were identified, while race itself was not a risk factor for OAB. For example, African American women were more likely to have experienced childhood bedwetting overall compared to other races, while Asian women reported the lowest BMIs [13]. Similarly, white women were more likely to report arthritis, chronic anxiety, and IBS than women of other races. Hypertension, diabetes, and hysterectomy were more prevalent amongst African American women. Hispanic women were more likely to report recurrent urinary tract infections.

NHANES

Medical history also played a significant role in PFD among those in the NHANES cohort. Those with diabetes or impaired fasting glucose reported more frequent UI episodes consistent with previous reports of an association between UI and clinically severe diabetes mellitus (i.e., end-organ damage and increasing insulin requirements) [32]. Oral hormone therapy and hysterectomy were risk factors for UI among these women. Peripheral neuropathy secondary to diabetes was independently associated with UI. Women with diabetes or impaired fasting glucose also carried a threefold increase in UUI and a twofold increase of SUI compared to non-diabetic women. Among women with impaired fasting glucose, microalbuminuria, increasing age, increasing BMI, current oral estrogen use, and hysterectomy were all reported more frequently among those with weekly UI. One hypothesis for this association is that UI in these women results from microvascular complications such as neural injury in the genitourinary tract.

Women with UI were significantly more likely to report at least 2 comorbidities compared to those without UI [17]. Comorbidities associated with UI included hypertension, depression, diabetes, obesity, visual difficulties, angina, MI, emphysema, stroke, upper gastrointestinal problems, and osteoporosis. Women with these diagnoses often experience severe disability and limitations in their ability to live independently. However, UI was not independently associated with disability among these women, suggesting UI is not the isolated cause of disability in this cohort. It is essential to note that the NHANES cohort was a sample of community dwelling women, and associations between UI and performance of ADL has been repeatedly described in the literature amongst those in group living facilities. Medications were not solely responsible for UI among women with comorbidities. Anticholinesterase (ACE) inhibitors and angiotensin receptor blockers (ARB) for hypertension were not independently associated with SUI or UUI [15].

Dietary factors were also found to impact LUTS. High caffeine intake was associated with UI in women while poor diet was problematic in men [16, 33].

LIS

Independent predictors of OAB in this cohort included bowel urgency, imbalance, osteoporosis, ankle swelling, diabetes, DVT, cystitis, poor health and old age. Obesity was consistently associated with SUI [23]. Risk factors for development of SUI in women included higher intake of total fat, zinc and vitamin B12 [34] while OAB development in women was associated with vitamin D, protein, and potassium. Higher intake of these nutrients was significantly associated with decreased risk of onset of OAB in women [35]. In men, beer was found to have a protective role in the development of OAB [22].

Quality of Life

BACH

LUTS were found to negatively impact QOL within the BACH cohort. Patients often limited their daily activities due to their symptoms. Women, blacks, and older individuals were more bothered than men, non-blacks, and younger respondents [5, 25].

EPILUTS

LUTS were found to negatively impact QOL in the EPILUTS cohort. Not surprisingly, participants with all symptom types reported the most negative QOL and highest rates of anxiety (36-53%) and depression (30-38%) [36, 37]. Similarly, women with all symptom types also reported the highest rate of bother (89%), with 77% reporting the most severe bother. This compared to bother in 67% of those with storage and voiding symptoms, 11% with voiding symptoms alone, and 16% of those with post-micturition symptoms alone. When individual symptoms were examined, urinary urgency and UI were the most predictive of bother amongst women with LUTS. Of the 20% of women reporting OAB with UI, 82% were bothered at least quite a bit, while of the 7% reporting OAB without UI, 65% reported the same level of bother [12]. Increased bother was also demonstrated amongst African Americans, those with higher education levels, those with urinary tract infections or sleep apnea, and those who had undergone menopause. Those without symptoms reported the best QOL and overall health [37].

LUTS also negatively impacted work performance. Women without UI were more likely to be working full-time and have higher education compared to those with UI. Twelve percent of participants with OAB and UI reported their symptoms negatively impacted their work performance, compared to lesser numbers of those without UI and those without LUTS [38]. As expected many women (36%) reported constant worry about proximity to and frequent use of restroom facilities, and fear of resultant leakage. Some (15%) allowed these concern to impact their choice of work, the stress of which might have additional impact on work output that is difficult to quantify. That being said, the age group most impacted by LUTS is also the most likely to be retired. Urge UI is more closely associated with negative quality of life scores than any other type of UI and 38-39% of women with urge UI reported it caused significant life problems [14]. Treatment seeking behavior was multifactorial. Most commonly reported reasons to seek treatment included urinary frequency, urgency and nocturia. Women with MUI were more likely to seek treatment than those suffering from SUI or UUI alone and were more likely to report having used coping strategies for their symptoms [8]. While bother was the greatest amongst those reporting all three LUTS types, only 28% of these women reported seeking treatment. Women who sought treatment for LUTS were more likely to be Hispanic, have higher education levels, have more frequent physician contact or history of infections or uterine prolapse. Age alone did not impact treatment seeking amongst women.

NHANES

Bother due to urinary symptoms and impact on QOL was also described for women of the NHANES cohort. Bother was significantly associated with UI type. Women with MUI reported nearly twice the amount of bother compared to those with either SUI or UUI alone [10]. Age also played a role in UI bother, as women ages 40-59 years were most bothered by any type of UI. Bother due to urinary symptoms was similar across racial groups.

Medical comorbidities were an important risk factor for negative impact of urinary symptoms upon QOL. For example, diabetics were more likely to be bothered by their UI than non-diabetics and those with normal glucose levels reported the least impact of UI upon their daily lives [32]. Bother also tended to increase with increasing BMI, among current smokers, and among those who reported lower levels of leisure time activities.

LIS

The majority of participants with clinically significant symptoms did not find them bothersome or socially disabling. Of the 34% reporting clinically significant symptoms, only 2% reported that these were socially disabling [21].

CONCLUSION

The epidemiology of PFD is complex and there remains no clear consensus on many aspects despite multiple large-scale trials. However, the larger studies reviewed here do provide us with estimates of LUTS in the US and regions of Europe (See Table 2). Overall prevalence of LUTS ranged from 19-76% with studies demonstrating the most concordance in prevalence when analyzing female LUTS. There were also notable differences between the two genders. For example among men, black and Hispanic participants were twice as likely to develop LUTS compared with white men; the racial and ethnic differences were not statistically significant among the women [4].

While we identified many similarities among epidemiologic studies of PFD such as similar age-related trends, rates of treatment seeking, and factors impacting symptoms (See Table 3) we also identified important inconsistencies. For example, publications related to the BACH cohort described a 19% prevalence of LUTS compared to 70-75% among participants of EpiLUTS. Female UI was noted in 68% women when the EpiLUTS cohort was used compared to 17-51% of NHANES participants.

Epidemiologic studies have limitations inherent to their study design. First, there is no standard method for evaluating PFD. This is mostly due to the inherent evolution in our understanding of PFD. Most of these studies were initiated in the early days of a shift from a specialty-based approach towards the interdisciplinary approach of Female Pelvic Medicine and Pelvic Reconstructive Surgery. Recent focus has shifted from a predominance of objective measures, such as number of episodes over a defined time period, towards subjective measures, such as bother scores or impact on activities of daily living.

Table 2. Prevalence and incidence of LUTS and UI

	BACH	EPILUTS	NHANES	LIS
Prevalence				
LUTS	19%	70-75%		
UI (male)	5%		12-14%	
SUI	10%		13%	
UUI	16%		49%	
MUI	15%		15%	
UI (female)	10%	68%	16-51%	
SUI	26%	23%	25-50%	8%
UUI	10%	21%	9-15%	8%
MUI	57%		16-34%	13%
Incidence				
LUTS	11%	14%		5%
UI (overall)		9%		

Table 3. Factors associated with an increased prevalence of LUTS

	BACH	EPILUTS	NHANES	LIS
Weight	Increased abdominal circumference	BMI Weight	BMI	BMI
Medical Conditions	Depression Diabetes Gestational Diabetes Heart Disease Hypertension	Arthritis Asthma Anxiety Depression Diabetes Heart Disease Inflammatory Bowel Disease Neurologic conditions Sleep disorders	Angina Depression Diabetes Emphysema Hypertension Impaired fasting glucose Myocardial infarction Osteoporosis Peripheral neuropathy Stroke	Ankle edema Bowel urgency Cystitis Diabetes Deep Vein Thrombosis Imbalance Osteoporosis Poor health
Gynecologic History	Uterine prolapse Vaginal delivery		Hormone therapy Hysterectomy Vaginal delivery	
Diet	Caffeine Fat intake Supplemental Vitamin C Total energy intake		Caffeine Dairy Dietary variety Poor intake Protein	Fat intake Vitamin C Zinc
Physical Activity	Little activity		Little activity	

Many use multiple measures and there are multiple validated questionnaires available to investigators. In addition, each provides their own definitions making it difficult to compare studies to one other. For example, one might consider a patient reporting any UI symptoms as meeting criteria while others define leakage only in the presence of moderate to severe symptoms. Second, demographic factors impact epidemiologic estimates. Some PFD such as SUI preferentially impact women with risk factors such as vaginal delivery and menopause, while others such as OAB appear to equally impact both genders. PFD prevalence increases overall with advancing age, however some tend to wax and wane over time while others are slowly progressing. For these reasons cohorts comprised of different genders and age distributions cannot be combined. Lastly, genetics plays a role in connective tissue quality, muscle strength, and likely other ways not yet identified, making international comparisons risky and large-scale data collection challenging.

Great insight can be gained from review of epidemiologic studies of PFD. EpiLUTS reveals a disturbing trend of high rates of symptom bother coupled with low rates of treatment seeking behavior and identifies a clear area for improvement in the care of women suffering from PFD. This low rate of treatment seeking provides insight into what symptoms patients are willing to accept and consider 'normal' versus what symptoms ought to be treated. For example, storage symptoms were often associated with treatment seeking and women with activity-related SUI were more likely to seek treatment compared to those with laugh, sneeze, cough-related SUI. There was also a low rate of treatment seeking among UK women, suggesting this is a cultural issue that spans across nations.

In conclusion, upon review of the significant recent epidemiological studies of PFD it is clear that the difficulty in reaching consensus is largely due to variations in the methods used to evaluate them. Comparison cannot be made between different cohorts and readers should proceed cautiously when interpreting epidemiologic data. We interpret these findings through the current lens of Female Pelvic Medicine and Reconstructive Surgery, which encourages us to examine the natural history of PFD as well as the overall impact of these chronic conditions on quality of life. We must look for modifiable risk factors so that we may improve QOL due to urinary symptoms in the future.

References

[1] Coyne, K. S., et al., Economic burden of urgency urinary incontinence in the United States: a systematic review. *J. Manag. Care Pharm.*, 2014. 20(2): p. 130-40.

[2] Gorina, Y., et al., Prevalence of incontinence among older americans. *Vital Health Stat.*, 3, 2014(36): p. 1-33.

[3] Hu, T. W., et al., Costs of urinary incontinence and overactive bladder in the United States: a comparative study. *Urology,* 2004. 63(3): p. 461-5.

[4] Maserejian, N. N., et al., Incidence of lower urinary tract symptoms in a population-based study of men and women. *Urology,* 2013. 82(3): p. 560-4.

[5] Kupelian, V., et al., Prevalence of lower urinary tract symptoms and effect on quality of life in a racially and ethnically diverse random sample: the Boston Area Community Health (BACH) Survey. *Arch. Intern. Med.*, 2006. 166(21): p. 2381-7.

[6] McKinlay, J. B. and C. L. Link, Measuring the urologic iceberg: design and implementation of the Boston Area Community Health (BACH) Survey. *Eur. Urol.*, 2007. 52(2): p. 389-96.

[7] Sexton, C. C., et al., The overlap of storage, voiding and postmicturition symptoms and implications for treatment seeking in the USA, UK and Sweden: EpiLUTS. *BJU Int.,* 2009. 103 Suppl. 3: p. 12-23.

[8] Khullar, V., et al., The relationship between BMI and urinary incontinence subgroups: results from EpiLUTS. *Neurourol. Urodyn.,* 2014. 33(4): p. 392-9.

[9] Anger, J. T., et al., The prevalence of urinary incontinence among community dwelling adult women: results from the National Health and Nutrition Examination Survey. *J. Urol.,* 2006. 175(2): p. 601-4.

[10] Dooley, Y., et al., Urinary incontinence prevalence: results from the National Health and Nutrition Examination Survey. *J. Urol.,* 2008. 179(2): p. 656-61.

[11] Tennstedt, S. L., et al., Prevalence of and risk factors for urine leakage in a racially and ethnically diverse population of adults: the Boston Area Community Health (BACH) Survey. *Am. J. Epidemiol.*, 2008. 167(4): p. 390-9.

[12] Coyne, K. S., et al., National community prevalence of overactive bladder in the United States stratified by sex and age. *Urology,* 2011. 77(5): p. 1081-7.

[13] Coyne, K. S., et al., Racial differences in the prevalence of overactive bladder in the United States from the epidemiology of LUTS (EpiLUTS) study. *Urology*, 2012. 79(1): p. 95-101.

[14] Coyne, K. S., et al., Urinary incontinence and its relationship to mental health and health-related quality of life in men and women in Sweden, the United Kingdom, and the United States. *Eur. Urol.*, 2012. 61(1): p. 88-95.

[15] Elliott, C. S. and C. V. Comiter, The effect of angiotensin inhibition on urinary incontinence: data from the National Health and Nutrition Examination Survey (2001-2008). *Neurourol. Urodyn.*, 2014. 33(8): p. 1178-81.

[16] Gleason, J. L., et al., Caffeine and urinary incontinence in US women. *Int. Urogynecol. J.*, 2013. 24(2): p. 295-302.

[17] Wu, J. M., et al., Lifetime risk of stress urinary incontinence or pelvic organ prolapse surgery. *Obstet. Gynecol.*, 2014. 123(6): p. 1201-6.

[18] Nygaard, I., et al., Prevalence of symptomatic pelvic floor disorders in US women. *JAMA,* 2008. 300(11): p. 1311-6.

[19] Anger, J. T., et al., True prevalence of urinary incontinence among female nursing home residents. *Urology,* 2006. 67(2): p. 281-7.

[20] Markland, A. D., et al., Prevalence and trends of urinary incontinence in adults in the United States, 2001 to 2008. *J. Urol.,* 2011. 186(2): p. 589-93.

[21] Perry, S., et al., An epidemiological study to establish the prevalence of urinary symptoms and felt need in the community: the Leicestershire MRC Incontinence Study. Leicestershire MRC Incontinence Study Team. *J. Public Health Med.*, 2000. 22(3): p. 427-34.

[22] Dallosso, H. M., et al., The association of diet and other lifestyle factors with the onset of overactive bladder: a longitudinal study in men. *Public Health Nutr.*, 2004. 7(7): p. 885-91.

[23] McGrother, C. W., et al., Urinary storage symptoms and comorbidities: a prospective population cohort study in middle-aged and older women. *Age Ageing,* 2006. 35(1): p. 16-24.

[24] Donaldson, M. M., et al., The natural history of overactive bladder and stress urinary incontinence in older women in the community: a 3-year prospective cohort study. *Neurourol. Urodyn.*, 2006. 25(7): p. 709-16.

[25] Maserejian, N. N., et al., Prevalence of post-micturition symptoms in association with lower urinary tract symptoms and health-related quality of life in men and women. *BJU Int.*, 2011. 108(9): p. 1452-8.

[26] Maserejian, N. N., et al., Reproductive history and progression of lower urinary tract symptoms in women: results from a population-based cohort study. *Urology,* 2014. 83(4): p. 788-94.

[27] Curto, T. M., et al., Associations between supplemental or dietary intake of vitamin C and severity of lower urinary tract symptoms. *BJU Int.,* 2015. 115(1): p. 134-42.

[28] Maserejian, N. N., et al., Dietary, but not supplemental, intakes of carotenoids and vitamin C are associated with decreased odds of lower urinary tract symptoms in men. *J. Nutr.,* 2011. 141(2): p. 267-73.

[29] Maserejian, N. N., et al., Dietary macronutrient and energy intake and urinary incontinence in women. *Am. J. Epidemiol.*, 2010. 171(10): p. 1116-25.

[30] Maserejian, N. N., E. L. Giovannucci, and J. B. McKinlay, Dietary macronutrients, cholesterol, and sodium and lower urinary tract symptoms in men. *Eur. Urol.*, 2009. 55(5): p. 1179-89.

[31] Maserejian, N. N., et al., Intake of caffeinated, carbonated, or citrus beverage types and development of lower urinary tract symptoms in men and women. *Am. J. Epidemiol.,* 2013. 177(12): p. 1399-410.

[32] Brown, J. S., et al., Lifestyle intervention is associated with lower prevalence of urinary incontinence: the Diabetes Prevention Program. *Diabetes Care,* 2006. 29(2): p. 385-90.

[33] Erickson, B. A., et al., Lower urinary tract symptoms and diet quality: findings from the 2000-2001 National Health and Nutrition Examination Survey. *Urology*, 2012. 79(6): p. 1262-7.

[34] Dallosso, H., et al., Diet as a risk factor for the development of stress urinary incontinence: a longitudinal study in women. *Eur. J. Clin. Nutr.,* 2004. 58(6): p. 920-6.

[35] Dallosso, H. M., et al., Nutrient composition of the diet and the development of overactive bladder: a longitudinal study in women. *Neurourol. Urodyn.*, 2004. 23(3): p. 204-10.

[36] Coyne, K. S., et al., The burden of lower urinary tract symptoms: evaluating the effect of LUTS on health-related quality of life, anxiety and depression: EpiLUTS. *BJU Int.,* 2009. 103 Suppl. 3: p. 4-11.

[37] Milsom, I., et al., Effect of bothersome overactive bladder symptoms on health-related quality of life, anxiety, depression, and treatment seeking in the United States: results from EpiLUTS. *Urology*, 2012. 80(1): p.90-6.

[38] Sexton, C. C., et al., Impact of overactive bladder on work productivity in the United States: results from EpiLUTS. *Am. J. Manag. Care*, 2009. 15(4 Suppl): p. S98-S107.

In: Overactive Bladder (OAB)
Editor: Elvira Larson
ISBN: 978-1-63485-033-9

Chapter 3

Overactive Bladder in the Pediatric Population

Sophie Ramsay, Anne-Sophie Blais, Geneviève Nadeau, Katherine Moore and Stéphane Bolduc*
Division of Urology, CHU de Québec-Université Laval,
Québec, Canada

Abstract

Overactive bladder (OAB) is a highly prevalent disorder in the pediatric population. This condition is especially troublesome for pediatric patients and their families when associated with incontinence since it negatively affects self-esteem and impairs children's development. From the patient's perspective, urgency and urge incontinence can have a significant impact, negatively affecting their quality of life. For a therapy to have true benefit, changes must not only be statistically significant, but must also be perceived as meaningful by the patient. A stepwise approach is favored to treat this pathology, starting with behavioral therapy, followed by medical management, and eventually more invasive procedures.

Antimuscarinic agents are the mainstay of medical treatment for OAB. Oxybutynin is the most commonly used antimuscarinic in the pediatric population. However, some patients have a suboptimal response to antimuscarinics and many experience bothersome side effects, which have been documented with all anticholinergics to a significantly higher degree than placebo. Although there have been reports about the use of tolterodine, fesoterodine, trospium, propiverine and solifenacin in children, to date, only oxybutynin has been officially approved for pediatric use by medical authorities in North America.

Oxybutynin use has been well documented in the pediatric population. However, patients with severe OAB symptoms seem not to always respond adequately to oxybutynin. Von Arendonk et al. found that in patients who have urinary incontinence on a daily basis, the likelihood that oxybutynin will be effective is only 20%. Moreover, the presence of muscarinic receptors in many organs apart from the bladder and the lack of

* Corresponding author: Email: stephane.bolduc@fmed.ulaval.ca.

specificity of oxybutynin for bladder receptors lead to troublesome side effects, which may lead to discontinuation of medication.

After failure with a first pharmacologic molecule, most practitioners will try a more specific anticholinergic. We have already studied various options to treat children with non-neurogenic refractory OAB, namely trying a different antimuscarinic (tolterodine, fesoterodine, or solifenacin) as well as combining two different anticholinergics. Despite favorable results with these options, they remain unapproved for pediatric use and other therapeutic avenues are therefore worth investigating. This is especially the case for molecules with different mechanisms of action and with favorable tolerability profiles.

Mirabegron, a new molecule with a distinct mechanism of action (β3-adrenoreceptor agonist), has recently been approved as monotherapy for idiopathic OAB in adults, but it has not been studied in the pediatric population. We recently concluded on two open-label studies to explore its efficacy and safety in children. Our studies allow us to support mirabegron as a new alternative for the treatment of refractory OAB in children. It appears as a safe and effective alternative for children with idiopathic OAB refractory to antimuscarinics, in monotherapy or in association with antimuscarinics (add-on dual therapy).

Invasive modalities such as botulinum toxin intra-detrusor injections and neuromodulation will also be covered in this chapter.

The different therapeutic alternatives reported could be included in a management algorithm for intractable OAB symptoms in children, but the need for prospective randomized controlled studies prior to official approbation is to be acknowledged.

Keywords: overactive bladder, children, anticholinergics, mirabegron, botulinum toxin, neuromodulation

INTRODUCTION

As described by the International Children's Continence Society (ICCS), overactive bladder (OAB) is "urinary urgency, usually accompanied by frequency and nocturia, with or without urinary incontinence, in the absence of urinary tract infection or other obvious pathology" [1], and it is the most common voiding dysfunction in children [2]. OAB represents a major economic burden with billions of dollars spent on its investigation and treatment every year in the United States [3, 4]. Healthcare expenses for OAB have actually exponentially increased in the last few decades in the US [5].

There is presently scarce data on the prevalence of OAB in the pediatric population. A 6,917-patient Japanese study from 2006 reported a 17.8% prevalence rate in children [6] while a 19,240-patient Korean study from 2008 reported a similar rate of 16.6% (27% wet OAB vs. 73% dry OAB) [7]. Although it has generally been thought and reported that OAB is more common in girls than in boys [8], these two large-scale studies reported a higher prevalence in boys than in girls (19.1 vs. 16.6%, and 17.4 vs. 15.8%, respectively), which is what we have also noted in our own clinical practice. There seems to be a decrease in the frequency and severity of urinary symptoms as children aged with reports of prevalence of daytime incontinence of 2.5%, 0.6%, and 0.3% in children of 7, 11 to 13, and 15 to 17 years old, respectively [9, 10]. Similarly, Chung et al. reported a decreasing prevalence of OAB with age, from 23.0% at 5 years old down to 12.2% at 13 years old [7].

OAB most likely has a multifactorial etiology with probable organic and psychological contributing factors. There is a well-known association between constipation and OAB. Chung et al. have identified factors that could potentially be associated with the development of OAB in children [7]. Indeed, compared to children without symptoms, they noted that those with OAB had a greater prevalence of nocturnal enuresis, constipation, fecal incontinence, history of urinary tract infections (UTIs), delayed bladder control, and poor toilet facilities. It has also been proven that voiding problems are more common in children with attention deficit hyperactivity disorder [11].

OAB has been shown to have a harmful impact on quality of life [12-16], as well as a detrimental influence on social, emotional, and behavioral well-being [17]. Enhancement of quality of life is of course a chief goal in the treatment of OAB, which can often be challenging and might possibly mandate a multidisciplinary approach in difficult cases.

There is ongoing questioning as whether OAB in children and adults represent the same condition. In a 2012 article, Salvatore et al. reported a debate on the subject that took place at the International Consultation on Incontinence Research Society meeting in 2010 [18]. Their conclusion was clear; there is abundant literature demonstrating the existence of a strong epidemiological and genetic link between OAB occurring in childhood and adulthood, although there is no confirmation that the early and late OAB are in fact part of the same disease. It is possible that OAB in children is simply a predisposing factor for the occurrence of OAB in adults. Regardless of the truth, families should not be merely told that their child will outgrow his symptoms as he enters puberty or adulthood, as this might not always be the case. Fascinatingly, a locus for urinary incontinence has been found in a genetic study [19].

In this chapter, we will review the clinical evaluation of the child with lower urinary symptoms and conservative therapy for idiopathic OAB. Medications approved for use in the pediatric population will be discussed as well as more recent molecules not currently approved for children by medical authorities. More invasive treatment modalities, which are usually reserved for severe or refractory cases of OAB, will also be reviewed.

Diagnostic Workup

The clinical history is the most important component in the evaluation of the child with incontinence or urinary frequency complaints [20]. Detailed and structured questionnaire is critical in defining the causes and impacts of urinary symptoms, to minimize unnecessary invasive evaluation, and to direct treatment. Careful history and physical exam permit to distinguish or eliminate most anatomical and neurogenic etiologies of incontinence. A routine checklist will identify the frequency, severity, and causes of incontinence.

Global history needs to be cautiously performed. Personal, developmental, and familial medical history should be reviewed. Particular attention should be given to history of UTIs and previous evaluation of the urinary tract. The questionnaire should address the pattern of voiding as well as the pattern of incontinence. The history helps categorizing the incontinence as primary or secondary, and characterizing it as a continuous dribbling or occasional leaking (large or small volumes) with dry intervals, stress or urge, pre-void or post-void, and nocturnal or diurnal. It should establish the duration of symptoms, the urinary frequency and urgency, the timing of incontinence and its relation to voiding, the amount of leakage and use of protection products, the voiding position, the triggering factors, and the circumstances in which the symptoms occur. The voiding and drinking habits should be carefully reviewed through the questionnaire as well as in a three-day voiding diary. Indeed, this useful tool allows objectively differentiating the urgency perceived by the infrequent voider who leaks on large volumes of urine with the child with OAB who leaks well under his estimated bladder capacity. The parents and the child are invited to comment on the frequency of micturition, urgency, quality of the stream, sensation of emptiness, and presence of straining or holding manoeuvers.

Scoring systems for pediatric incontinence are not popular among pediatric urologists, despite the fact that scoring systems in general provide a more standardized assessment of voiding pathologies. They can help the clinician to evaluate the child and to monitor treatment, but only a few addressing specifically OAB symptomatology have yet been validated for the pediatric population [21-24]. Evaluation of bowel movement routine is as essential as the voiding history [25]. The Bristol stool scale is a simple and convenient tool that can be used in children [26]. The frequency and the consistency of stools must be evaluated, as failure to diagnose and treat constipation may compromise the success of management of the urinary condition.

Specific physical evaluation of the abdomen, genitalia, back, and feet is imperative for the assessment of the child with OAB symptoms. Abdominal palpation can reveal a distended bladder or stool impaction despite child and parents' denial. Evidence of lower back anomalies, such as skin discoloration, dimple, hair patches, subcutaneous lipoma, spine defect, or asymmetry of the buttocks or gluteal cleft, may suggest the presence of an underlying spinal dysraphism. In presence of these findings, strong consideration must be given to obtain a magnetic resonance imaging (MRI). Imaging the spinal cord should also be contemplated if the neurologic evaluation of the lower extremities is abnormal or the expected goals of treatment are not reached. In the event of secondary incontinence, MRI should also be considered to eliminate a tethered cord phenomenon. Examination of the external genitalia may occasionally reveal the origin of the symptomatology. In girls, labial fusion, ureterocele, ectopic ureter, urogenital sinus, hypospadias, and epispadias are anatomical anomalies explaining incontinence while in boys with lower urinary tract symptoms (LUTS), meatal stenosis is often discovered. As part of the standard physical exam, a post-void residual (PVR) volume should always be measured. To be reliable, the PVR measurement should be done immediately after voiding. As per the ICCS, a repetitive PVR of more than 20 mL or more than 10% of bladder capacity is considered to be significantly increased in children aged 4 to 6 years [1]. Rectal exam is not mandatory, but allows the evaluation of anal tone, pelvic sensation, and presence of impacted stools, and confirmation of the presence of the sacrum.

The non-consecutive three-day voiding diary is an essential tool in the evaluation of the child complaining of frequency and/or incontinence. Time of voiding, voided volumes, sensation of urgency, and leaks are recorded, and they provide an objective assessment of the situation. Indeed, it gives concrete data to families and helps them realize the amplitude of the problem. Some families will easily understand the causes and find specific solutions, especially in the case of the infrequent voider who uses the bathroom two or three times per day and wets himself after reaching volumes over his estimated bladder capacity. Sometimes, the voiding diary will show that a child with high urinary frequency has a rather normal voiding pattern that is simply related to high fluid intake. The voiding diary is also important to monitor treatment. The pad test has not been demonstrated reliable in the pediatric population.

During the first assessment of the child, urinalysis and urine culture are performed to eliminate infection, proteinuria, and glycosuria, and to evaluate the specific gravity. Blood samples are not routinely collected except if specific anomalies are suspected after history and physical exam. Uroflowmetry with simultaneous pelvic floor electromyography (EMG) tracing is another non-invasive test used in the evaluation of the incontinent child. Uroflowmetry consists of measurement of urine flow during voiding and is described in terms of volume voided, rate, and pattern. It evaluates the urinary stream during the emptying phase, gives an idea about bladder function and outlet function, and quantifies the volume of fluid expelled through the urethra per unit of time. The coordination between contraction of the bladder and relaxation of the pelvic floor can also be assessed. Non-invasive uroflow/EMG is useful not only for diagnosing specific LUTS conditions, but also in objectively monitoring treatment efficacy. Subjective improvement on targeted therapy correlates well with objective improvement in uroflow/EMG parameters, lending validation to this simplified approach to diagnosis [27]. The full (video)urodynamic evaluation with urethral and anal catheters is reserved for cases refractory to standard treatment or for evaluation and follow-up of neurogenic bladder. Its intrusive characteristics sometimes make it difficult to perform in the pediatric population. An 85% concordance was found between the diagnosis of OAB obtained by anamnesis and noninvasive exams (ultrasound and uroflowmetry) and the diagnosis of detrusor overactivity obtained by urodynamic study [8].

Bladder ultrasound can be obtained to measure the PVR, bladder wall thickness, and rectal diameter. The ultrasonographic evaluation of the upper tract is mandated by history findings of febrile UTIs, continuous incontinence suggesting ectopic ureter, or failure of conventional treatment. Voiding cystourethrogram (VCUG) should be reserved for patients with febrile UTIs, abnormal urinary upper tract on ultrasound, neurogenic bladder, and suspected urethral anomalies. Videourodynamic study allows combination of VCUG and urodynamics, and decreases the number of urethral catheterizations.

Starting with a non-invasive diagnostic approach in children with OAB symptoms will lead to judicious selection of the children requiring more invasive assessment in order to provide adequate treatment and to prevent long-term damage to the urinary tact.

Conservative Management

The first steps for successful treatment are for the child and his family to have motivation and realistic goals in terms of treatment efficacy. Teaching is imperative for them to understand the mechanisms of micturition and the circumstances in which incontinence occurs. Indeed, changes are more easily made if the pathology and its underlying causes are well understood.

Fluid intake should be regular throughout the day, but it should be decreased when getting close to bedtime. Clear urine is a good indicator of adequate fluid intake. Caffeine, chocolate, and carbonated and citrus beverages can trigger urgency and frequency symptoms, and should therefore be avoided. Urotherapy combines cognitive, behavioral, and physical therapy with the goal of normalizing the pattern of micturition. Timed voiding every two to three hours should initially be established during the day even in the absence of urges [28]. A multi-alarm watch may help the busy, overactive, or inattentive child to remember to use the bathroom. Parents and school collaboration is essential in the establishment of the new voiding routine. Positive reinforcement with rewards may increase self-confidence and help keeping the child motivated and willing to continue putting effort to improve his condition. Adequate and dedicated periods of time should be given to the child for voiding to ensure sufficient time to relax the pelvic floor and achieve complete emptying. The toilet should have an adequate height, or a footstool should be available, in order for the child's heals to touch the ground. In addition, children should void with their legs well spread apart. Wiener et al. reported a 50% long-term improvement of frequency and urgency symptoms in children with daytime incontinence after simple behavioral therapy without any particular bowel management program [29].

Aggressive bowel evaluation and management should be undertaken early in the treatment of pediatric patients with urgency and/or incontinence. Until proven otherwise, all patients with bladder disorders are constipated [30]. It is not sufficient to ask parents' opinion concerning their child's bowel function. As children are gaining independence, parents are no longer supervising their bowel movements and are often mistaken about their state of constipation. Therefore, children must be asked directly about their bowel habits, and in different ways, to ensure that there is no underlying constipation causing their urinary symptoms. Using the Bristol stool scale often makes the difference in the interpretation of vague answers. Indeed, a picture is always worth a thousand words. Successful treatment of constipation results in resolution of daytime incontinence in 50 to 90% of patients [31, 32]. Increased fluid intake and high-fiber diet are the first steps of a bowel management program. Proper timing and positioning are also important. Laxatives may be necessary to make stools softer and easier to pass. An initial bowel clean-out may be necessary followed by a maintenance regimen.

Biofeedback therapy is an objective tool that allows better understanding and perception of the work of the pelvic musculature. It leads to enhanced control of the pelvic floor since explanations are better assimilated than with standard counseling. The goal of therapy might be to learn to reinforce or relax the pelvic floor muscles. Although sessions may be time-consuming for the children and their families, great improvement can be expected not only for dysfunctional voiding, but also for OAB symptoms [33-35]. Biofeedback should be used in conjunction with behavioral modifications to maximize the chance of success. However, medication may eventually be necessary, especially if functional bladder capacity is less than 60% of the expected bladder capacity for age [36]. In the event that a medication needs to be initiated, urotherapy should be continued throughout the treatment.

Pharmacologic Treatment Options

Oxybutynin

Oxybutynin chloride is a non-selective tertiary amine with anticholinergic properties and has been approved for the treatment of OAB in adults for decades, but its approval for the pediatric population dates only to the beginning of the twenty-first century. It is currently the only antimuscarinic agent officially approved by medical authorities in North America for the treatment of OAB symptoms in children. It comes in various formulations and routes of administration, but oral immediate release (IR) oxybutynin (Ditropan®) and extended release (ER) oxybutynin (Ditropan XL®) are the only agents presently accepted for use in children less than eighteen years of age [37]. Other formulations of oxybutynin include a transdermal patch (Oxytrol®) and a topical gel (Gelnique®). Intravesical instillations of oxybutynin have also been reported.

Immediate Release

Although IR oxybutynin is the antimuscarinic agent that has been used for the longest time for the treatment of OAB in children, there is no published article evaluating it compared to placebo. However, small observational studies showing its efficacy have been reported. For instance, in 2006, Van Arendonk et al. reported on 81 children with daytime incontinence treated with oxybutynin for at least three months. After an average follow up of 1.2 years, 38.3% of children were dry, 30.9% were significantly improved, 23.5% were slightly improved, and 7.4% experienced no changes in their symptoms [38].

IR oxybutynin is available as a 5-mg tablet and as a 1-mg/mL suspension. The recommended daily dose is 0.3 to 0.6 mg/kg/day with a maximum total dose of 15 mg/day, and it should be titrated in progressively increasing doses to reduce the occurrence of side effects [37]. For children over 5 years of age, starting with a twice-daily dose of 5 mg and increasing to 5 mg three times a day if symptoms do not resolve and if the medication is well tolerated is an adequate management.

Disadvantages of the IR form are its administration schedule and its side effect profile. Side effects are common and include dry mouth, dry eyes, dry skin, constipation and other gastrointestinal abnormalities, flushing, blurred vision, dizziness, and sleep disturbances. In children, these can occasionally be severe enough to warrant decreasing the dose or discontinuing the medication [39-42]. Fortunately, other formulations of the drug have been developed.

Extended Release

ER oxybutynin has a more favorable pharmacokinetic profile than the IR form because it bypasses the first pass metabolism in the liver [43, 44]. Preliminary studies have reported less frequent side effects with the ER formulation [45, 46], but the incidence of side effects between IR and ER oxybutynin was similar in other studies [43]. The ER formulation also has the advantage of being a once daily medication, which could be associated with an increase adherence, although this has not been demonstrated yet in the pediatric population with OAB.

In 2002, Youdim and Kogan published the first study to evaluate safety and efficacy of ER oxybutynin in children. All of the 25 patients evaluated in their retrospective study experienced improvement in incontinence or voiding dysfunction while on ER oxybutynin, and 48% of the patients experienced no side effects. The side effects reported in 13 patients were dry mouth, constipation, heat intolerance, and drowsiness. They concluded that ER oxybutynin is safe and efficacious in children [46]. Compared to the IR form, the ER form has been shown to be superior in various studies [43, 46, 47]. For example, Van Arendonk et al. reported that 48% of children in their 27-patient study became dry or had significant improvement in the frequency of wetting episodes after switching from the IR to the ER form.

They also noted significant objective improvements in voided volume and total bladder capacity [43].

ER oxybutynin is available as a 5-, 10-, and 15-mg tablet. For children over 5 years of age, it is recommended to start with a 5-mg tablet once daily and to increase the dose in 5-mg increments up to a maximum of 20 mg/day.

A notable disadvantage of ER oxybutynin is that it requires the child to be able to swallow an intact tablet. To circumvent this difficulty, other routes of delivery have been investigated, but are not yet accepted for use in children.

Transdermal Patch

Similarly to the ER formulation, the oxybutynin transdermal delivery system circumvents the first pass metabolism in the liver, which possibly decreases side effects [48]. The transdermal system removes the need for the child to be able to swallow a tablet and necessitates infrequent administration. The oxybutynin transdermal patch comes at a single dose of 3.9 mg/day and needs to be changed twice weekly. It should be applied to dry, intact skin on the abdomen, hips, or buttocks and reapplication to the same area should be avoided within a one-week period [48]. If the dose needs to be increased, a second complete or partial patch could be applied.

There is currently scarce data on the use of the oxybutynin patch for the treatment of non-neuropathic OAB in children, but the Toronto group reported their experience in 2014. In a retrospective review of 35 patients, among which 69% had prior exposure to an oral formulation of oxybutynin, subjective improvement in OAB symptoms was noted in 96% of patients. Bladder capacity also significantly increased. The main side effect noted was skin irritation in 35% of patients, which led to discontinuation of the patch in 20% of the group. They concluded that the oxybutynin patch is an option to be considered in children who do not tolerate other formulations of oxybutynin [48].

Topical Gel

In the adult population with urge urinary incontinence, two large, randomized, double-blind, placebo controlled studies have been published. Both studies demonstrated that the oxybutynin gel significantly decreases the number of urge urinary incontinence and the daily urinary frequency, and significantly increases voided volumes, while causing no serious adverse events [49, 50]. However, there is no data yet available concerning the efficacy or safety of the oxybutynin gel for children with OAB.

Intravesical Instillations

Intravesical instillations of oxybutynin, which are usually prepared by crushing and dissolving a 5-mg oxybutynin tablet in 30 mL of distilled water, is a viable alternative for patients who are refractory to other routes of administration or who cannot tolerate side effects [51].

In various non-comparative trials, the intravesical administration of a single 5-mg dose or multiple doses of oxybutynin led to subjective improvement of voiding symptoms in the adult population [39, 40, 52-57]. Moreover, intravesical oxybutynin appeared to be associated with no significant adverse effects in multiple studies [40, 58-60]. For example, Weese et al. reported a significant improvement in 55% of their patients with no evidence of side effects

[56], and Enzelsberger et al. reported a subjective improvement in 82% of their population with only 13% experiencing minor side effects after two weeks of treatment [52]. Improvements in children with neurogenic bladder have also been noted [39, 60, 61], but no study to date has evaluated intravesical oxybutynin in the neurology intact children. The main limitation with this population is that the great majority of children with OAB symptoms have a sensate urethra and do not require frequent clean intermittent catheterization (CIC) as it is the case with neurogenic patients. Therefore, the need for urethral catheterization in this group of sensate patients might be a painful and traumatizing experience. Thus, the intravesical route should be reserved for refractory patients and highly motivated patients and families.

Investigational Drugs

Other Anticholinergic Agents

Oxybutynin is the only antimuscarinic agent officially approved for pediatric use in North America. Even though it is currently the most commonly used antimuscarinic in the pediatric population, it is occasionally associated with a suboptimal response and/or bothersome side effects, limiting its clinical usefulness. Therefore, original researches have led to the introduction of newer antimuscarinics in the treatment of OAB in pediatrics. So far, there have been reports in children about the off-label use of tolterodine (Detrol®), fesoterodine (Toviaz®), solifenacin (Vesicare®), trospium (Sanctura®, Trosec®), and propiverine.

Because of its high selectivity for bladder muscarinic receptors, tolterodine, a tertiary amine, has been of great interest for its use in detrusor overactivity. It is available as long-acting or intermediate-release formulations. Goessl et al. first investigated the urodynamic effects and adverse effects of tolterodine in a cohort of 22 children with detrusor hyperreflexia [62]. They showed a significant increase in bladder capacity (+44%) and compliance (+55%) in anticholinergic-naive patients at a dose of 0.1 mg/kg daily. Only one out of 22 patients experienced side effects, but the study was limited to three months of follow-up. Since this first publication, many authors have investigated the efficacy and tolerability of tolterodine in children. These studies have supported the fact that tolterodine is effective in children with OAB [63-65]. Literature on the efficacy of tolterodine compared to oxybutynin in children is minimal. Reinberg et al. have demonstrated that ER oxybutynin was more effective than immediate and long acting tolterodine for control of daytime urinary incontinence and urinary frequency [47]. On the other hand, a review has suggested that tolterodine was as effective as oxybutynin, but with fewer side effects [66]. Moreover, tolterodine has been shown to be a possible alternative treatment for children who do not tolerate oxybutynin by Bolduc et al. [63]. In this study, 77% of patients who were started on tolterodine because they could not tolerate oxybutynin, continued their treatment with no significant side effects for a median of 11.5 months. Finally, a placebo-controlled study has confirmed the favorable long-term safety profile of tolterodine for its use in children [67].

Fesoterodine is an anticholinergic agent available as an extended-release formulation. Following administration, fesoterodine is converted to 5-hydroxy-methyltolterodine (5-HMT), the same active metabolite as seen with tolterodine. However, it has been shown that fesoterodine has less pharmacokinetic variability than tolterodine [68]. Malhotra et al. studied the pharmacokinetics, safety, and tolerability of fesoterodine in 21 pediatric patients with

OAB [69]. The children were given a dose-escalating regimen of fesoterodine for a total of eight weeks, and endpoints were evaluated mostly through physical examinations, PVR volumes, bladder diaries, and plasma concentrations of 5-HMT in blood samples. The results showed that administrating a 4 or 8 mg dose of fesoterodine once daily to pediatric patients weighing over 25 kilograms produced 5-HMT plasmatic concentrations similar to those in adults. The medication was well tolerated by the patients. Trials evaluating the efficacy of fesoterodine are worthwhile. Currently, two studies registered on clinicaltrials.gov are recruiting patients. One is a randomized, single-blind, crossover study (two arms of treatment, 8 weeks each) comparing the efficacy and tolerability of fesoterodine and ER oxybutynin in children with OAB and aims at recruiting 50 children. The second is an extension study of the first one and aims at evaluating the safety and efficacy of fesoterodine in children with OAB for an additional 12 months.

Solifenacin is a tertiary amine that has been approved by the FDA for the treatment of OAB in adults since 2005. It has an excellent bioavailability, a long half-life, and selectivity for the M3 over the M2 receptors. Scarce data is available for its use in the pediatric population. Hoebeke et al. performed a retrospective study on 138 children treated with solifenacin for an average of 23 months [70]. They found an overall 85% response rate, a full response in more than 50% of patients, and side effects in only 6.5% of their cohort. This study was followed by a prospective, open-label study by Bolduc et al. that evaluated 72 children who were receiving solifenacin for an average of 15.6 months [71]. Continence improved in all patients. Fifteen and three patients had mild and moderate side effects, respectively, but four patients had intolerable side effects and withdrew from the protocol. The tolerability was judged acceptable. More recently, Nadeau et al. reported on the long-term results of this open-label study on 191 OAB patients followed for a mean of 21 months. They showed benefits in overall satisfaction and continence rates after the introduction of solifenacin, and an overall success rate of 94%, with greater benefits observed with higher doses [72].

A randomized trial of interest was recently presented at the 2015 European Society for Paediatric Urology (ESPU) Congress. Newgreen et al. randomized 189 pediatric patients to 12 weeks of either solifenacin or placebo [73]. Both groups were also undergoing standard urotherapy. Children on solifenacin had a greater increase in mean voided volume compared to those on placebo. Moreover, there was a significant reduction in micturition frequency with solifenacin when analyses were adjusted for change in fluid intake. A 40-week extension of this trial was then presented by Bosman et al. [74]. Solifenacin still appeared to be effective and well tolerated in this long-term trial. More details about these trials are expected in future publications.

Trospium is a quaternary amine and it is associated with less central nervous system (CNS) side effects than other antimuscarinic agents, as it does not cross the blood-brain barrier. It is hydrophilic, minimally metabolized, and not highly protein-bound. There is a paucity of data about its use in children as only a few trials have been specifically dedicated to this population. Even if early trials have demonstrated promising results, no new publications have emerged since 2006 [45, 75, 76]. At the 2015 ESPU Congress, Wright et al. presented a retrospective review of 13 children with OAB treated with trospium [77]. Most patients of the cohort had a history of CNS adverse effects while using other anticholinergics or an emotional behavioral disorder. Only one out of 13 patients experienced CNS side effects with trospium. This highlights the possible use of trospium as an alternative option for children with a history of emotional behavioral disorder or CNS adverse effects. Detailed analysis and publication are pending.

Propiverine is a benzilic acid derivative that has antimuscarinic and calcium antagonistic properties [78]. Moreover, recent literature has shown that propiverine also has alpha-blockade effects [79]. Propiverine is available in IR and ER formulas. Literature on the use of propiverine in children and adolescents provides evidence that it may be a promising treatment option. A multicenter, controlled, double-blind study conducted over eight weeks compared the efficacy of propiverine and placebo in 171 children aged 5 to 10 years [80]. Significant improvement in urinary frequency with propiverine, the primary endpoint, was reached at the end of the study. Incontinence episodes and mean voided volume were also significantly improved with the medication compared to placebo.

A retrospective review of 68 children with OAB treated with propiverine for a median duration of 7.5 weeks was also conducted [81]. In this study, median daytime voiding frequency decreased from 14.0 to 8.5, and median functional bladder capacity improved from 140 to 150 mL. The overall response rate after propiverine treatment was 86.8%. The medication was well tolerated. Finally, the efficacy and safety of propiverine were compared to oxybutynin in a retrospective, multicenter, observational cohort study involving 621 children [42]. Continence was achieved in 61.6% compared to 58.7% of patients taking propiverine and oxybutynin, respectively. Moreover, improvement in incontinence episodes per week and voiding frequency per day were not significantly different between the two groups. The authors concluded that propiverine was at least as effective as oxybutynin. Propiverine had a favorable tolerability profile compared to oxybutynin. However, few concerns have been raised regarding this study and possible biases [45]. Lack of standard conservative treatment before initiation of medical treatment, choice of medication in regards to physician's preference, and low prescribed dose of propiverine have been pointed out as possible sources of bias.

Mirabegron

Recently, a new molecule for the medical treatment of OAB has entered the market. Mirabegron (Myrbetriq®), a novel first-in-class therapy, has a different target than antimuscarinics and acts as a selective agonist on β3-adrenergic receptors found in the detrusor muscle. It induces smooth muscle relaxation during the storage phase, thus enhancing bladder compliance and capacity, without affecting voiding pressure or PVR [82, 83]. Available since 2011 in Japan, mirabegron 25 and 50 mg once daily has been approved as monotherapy for adults with idiopathic OAB. Its efficacy, tolerability and durability of effect have been established in five large-scale phase III multinational randomized controlled trials [84-88]. With regards to efficacy, it decreases the mean number of incontinence episodes, urgency incontinence episodes, and urgency episodes per 24 hours compared with placebo. In a post hoc subgroup analysis, the benefit of mirabegron was also observed in both antimuscarinic-naive and antimuscarinic-refractory patients [89]. However, the BEYOND trial failed to demonstrate that mirabegron was noninferior to solifenacin in antimuscarinic non-responders [90]. In the SYMPHONY (phase II) and BESIDE (phase IIIb, add-on) trials, combination therapy (mirabegron with an antimuscarinic) achieved its primary efficacy endpoints with good tolerability [91, 92]. Ongoing large phase III studies (SYNERGY, SYNERGY II) by the manufacturer are estimated to be reported in the next few months to better assess the efficacy and innocuity of combination therapy [93, 94].

Side effects commonly reported with antimuscarinics have not been observed more often with mirabegron than with placebo (headache 2.9%, dry mouth 2.0%, constipation 1.6%) [95]. Despite a favorable tolerability profile, the most common adverse events reported with mirabegron have been hypertension, UTIs, headache, and nasopharyngitis [96]. Caution is warranted regarding some susceptible drug interactions since mirabegron is metabolized by the CYP450 enzymes [97].

Despite high specificity of mirabegron for the β3-adrenoreceptor, concerns have been raised regarding its cardiovascular (CV) safety profile. In a systematic review, Rosa et al. concluded that the slight pulse rate and blood pressure changes (increase of ~1 beat/minute and of 1 mm Hg, respectively) seen with mirabegron did not result in more CV adverse events and that those changes were reversible on treatment discontinuation [98]. Nevertheless, caution should be exercised and periodic monitoring of blood pressure is warranted for patients with CV morbidities treated with this agent [96, 99].

Our group conducted a prospective study with an open-label design on a cohort of 58 pediatric patients with refractory idiopathic OAB treated with 25 or 50 mg of mirabegron over almost a year. Statistically significant improvements in mean bladder capacity, subjective continence, and patient perception of bladder condition (PPBC) scores were seen in all patients with no worrisome toxicity. Mild or moderate side effects were observed for eight (14%) patients [100]. Moreover, similar results of efficacy and innocuity were obtained with mirabegron add-on therapy with an antimuscarinic for 32 children with refractory idiopathic OAB followed over 12 months [101].

In our opinion, mirabegron appears as a safe alternative for children with idiopathic OAB since it improves symptoms in patients refractory to antimuscarinics. Despite encouraging preliminary data, pediatric usage of mirabegron to treat OAB is currently off-label as no recommendations have been issued by the manufacturer nor medical regulatory bodies.

Dual Therapy

Pediatric patients experiencing intractable symptoms of OAB might be challenging to treat. Some patients will undergo dose-escalation of their anticholinergic medication to achieve symptom relief. However, in up to 30% of patients, a single anticholinergic agent will not be sufficient to completely cure severe OAB symptoms. Moreover, the maximal anticholinergic dose might sometimes not be attainable due to side effects. Optimizing the medical therapy by combining two different anticholinergic agents in pediatric patients has first been addressed by Bolduc et al. in 2009 [102]. Thirty-three patients with refractory OAB and incontinence were enrolled and given two anticholinergic medications simultaneously (oxybutynin, tolterodine, and/or solifenacin). After a median combination therapy of 18.4 months, continence was improved in all patients, including 52% being completely dry. Mild or moderate side effects were reported in 63% of patients. However, these side effects were not severe enough to warrant discontinuation of the medication. These results show that a combination of two antimuscarinics can improve incontinence with acceptable side effects.

The long-term extension of this open-label study was then published in 2014 [103]. Fifty-six patients took a combination of two anticholinergic agents for a mean duration of 36 months. At the end of follow-up, 41% of patients were dry and 32% improved significantly. Mean voided volumes, cystometric bladder capacity, and maximum pressure of detrusor contractions all improved significantly with treatment. Twenty-eight patients reported mild or moderate side effects, and two patients required a change of regimen due to bothersome side effects. The authors concluded that a double anticholinergic regimen is a safe and efficient treatment in children refractory to anticholinergic monotherapy, even with long-term use.

Recently, two adult studies have shown a significant improvement in OAB symptoms with combination therapy of mirabegron and solifenacin [91, 104]. With this in mind, we conducted a study at our center to optimize pharmacotherapy in children with OAB refractory to anticholinergic monotherapy, by adding-on mirabegron to an anticholinergic agent [101]. Preliminary results are promising with improvement of continence in all of the 32 patients included in the study and overall improvement of bladder capacity. So far, this combination therapy has generally been well tolerated. No major adverse events have been reported, and only one patient required change of regimen due to bothersome side effects. Mild side effects have been reported in four patients, with constipation being the most frequent. This study was recently presented at the 2015 Northeastern Section of the American Urological Association annual meeting by Morin et al. and will be the subject of a future publication. As of now, combination therapy of mirabegron and an anticholinergic agent remains an off-label treatment.

Medication Adherence and Persistence

It is well recognized that OAB is a chronic condition necessitating long-term therapy. Adherence and persistence to medication are fundamental to ensure treatment success. On a day-to-day basis, poor adherence to medication represents a major challenge in the management of any disease. Adherence has been demonstrated to be dismal in adults taking antimuscarinic medications. For instance, in 2013, Sicras-Mainar et al. reported adherence rates at 12 months of 35.8%, 31.9%, and 30.9% for fesoterodine, solifenacin, and tolterodine, respectively [105]. Likewise, other studies have reported that solely 14% [106] and 30% [107] of their population were more than 80%-adherent to their antimuscarinic medication. Balkrishnan et al. reported a medication possession ratio (MPR) of their population across three years of 42% [108].

There is presently no published data available on adherence to antimuscarinics in children with OAB, but our group conducted an observational study on 72 children to assess their adherence to medication as well as possible influencing factors. We noticed a self-reported adherence rate of 93% compared to a MPR ≥ 80% in only 64% of patients. Six months after children were recruited in the study and had to fill a questionnaire, a MPR ≥ 80% was seen in 71% of them. It therefore appears that the recruitment visit and administration of a questionnaire might have had a positive impact on medication adherence. No factors significantly affecting adherence were identified. This study was recently presented by Fortin et al. at the 2015 ESPU Congress and will be the subject of an upcoming publication [109].

Although our study showed that adherence to antimuscarinics in children with OAB is higher than in adults, it is still unsatisfactory. Poor medication adherence leads to sub-optimal treatment efficacy and therefore lessens the improvement in quality of life associated with treatment success. Strategies are thus necessary to increase adherence to medication. Using a questionnaire assessing adherence might be a possible approach, but this has to be carefully reviewed.

Persistence to antimuscarinic medications has been assessed in adults with OAB and the treatment discontinuation rate has been noticed to be high. For example, Kelleher et al. noted a persistence rate of 18.2% in women with OAB at six months after initial prescription [110]. Likewise, Wagg et al. showed that only 14 to 35% of patients remained on their initial therapy at 12 months [111].

Similarly to adherence, persistence to antimuscarinics for the treatment of OAB has not been commented on in the pediatric literature. We retrospectively evaluated a group of 374 children on antimuscarinic therapy over a four-year period. In our study, patients refilled their index prescription for an average of 429 days and solifenacin had the highest mean duration of index therapy (765 days). At the end of the follow-up period, only 11.8% of patients were still taking their antimuscarinic medication. This study was presented by Blais et al. at the 2015 ESPU Congress and has recently been accepted for publication [112].

This persistence rate to antimuscarinic therapy in children is comparable to what has been reported in adult patients with OAB. However, children seemed to persist on medications for a longer duration before persistence rates started declining. Solutions are needed to improve persistence of antimuscarinics in children with OAB.

INVASIVE TREATMENT OPTIONS

Botulinum Toxin Injections

For OAB refractory to lifestyle modifications and pharmacotherapy, intradetrusor injections of botulinum toxin A (BoNTA) are an alternative. Approved by the medical regulatory bodies for the treatment of neurogenic and idiopathic OAB in adults since 2011 and 2013, respectively, the use of botulinum toxin for pediatric incontinence has been pioneered by Schulte-Baukloh et al. in 2002 but remains off-label [113]. By selectively blocking acetylcholine release at the neuromuscular junction, the botulinum toxin temporarily prevents contraction of the targeted muscle [114]. Serotypes A and B are commercially available forms for clinical use. Several formulations exist, the three most common being onabotulinumtoxinA (Botox®, 100-unit vials, Allergan, Irvine, CA), abobotulinumtoxinA (Dysport®, 500-unit vials, Ipsen, Boston, MA), and incobotulinumtoxinA (Xeomin®, 100-unit vials, Merz Pharmaceuticals UK Ltd, Herts, UK), with most of the literature pertaining to the former [115]. The conversion ratio between preparations is still debated and formulations are not interchangeable [116].

In pediatric urology, BoNTA is mostly used as a second-line treatment for neurogenic or idiopathic OAB (including low bladder compliance). Criteria to determine first-line failure vary widely, but usually include unsatisfactory efficacy to more than one medication or bothersome side effects [117]. The use of BoNTA has also been described for detrusor sphincter dyssynergia, and occasionally, one may inject the external urethral sphincter at the same time as the bladder [118]. Contraindications to BoNTA injections include pregnancy, peripheral motor neuropathic diseases (e.g., amyotrophic lateral sclerosis), neuromuscular junction disorders (e.g., myasthenia gravis), active untreated UTI, and uncorrected coagulopathy [119].

For this minimally invasive procedure, prior workup with voiding diary, urine culture, and systematic urodynamics are advocated by most experts [120]. Periprocedural antibioprophylaxis is mandatory. In our institution, we follow the French recommendations and administer antibiotics 1 to 3 days prior to treatment, on the day of treatment, and 1 to 3 days following treatment [120]. Aminoglycosides should be avoided as they may potentiate the effect of BoNTA [119]. Children and their parents should be warned about the potential risk for partial or complete urinary retention and need to be able and willing to perform CIC should it happen.

The technique has not been standardized. Under general, spinal, or local anesthesia, using a rigid or flexible cystoscope, suburothelial or intramuscular injections of 0.5 to 1 mL-aliquots of diluted toxin (10 units/mL with normal saline) at 10 to 30 sites, including or not the trigone, are performed with the bladder moderately full [121]. The effect may appear as early as 24 to 72 hours later [122] and lasts on average 5 to 12 months, similar as in adults, with no apparent tachyphylaxis [123-127]. Adjuvant antimuscarinic agents may be discontinued or dosage reduced in most patients [128]. Injections may be repeated after a minimum of 12 weeks [120]. Minimum age reported for treatment is 1.5 years [129], but 3 years old is the suggested threshold (grade of recommendation C) [118].

For onabotulinumtoxinA, recommended dosage varies between 5 and 10 units per kilogram of body weight [118]. For idiopathic OAB, dose will usually vary from 50 to 100 units (up to 200 units has been reported) [125, 130], while for neurogenic OAB, higher doses are usually required, up to a maximum of 200 to 300 units. The estimated lethal dose is unknown but estimated around 40 units per kilogram [131].

Side effects might occur in up to 20% of patients, but most are procedure-related transient pain, UTIs, autonomic dysreflexia, and mild hematuria [124]. Detrusor underactivity with increased PVR or complete urinary retention requiring CIC might occur in about 2 to 9% of patients with idiopathic OAB [125, 132-134], very similar to what has been reported across adult studies [135]. Systemic absorption of the toxin can lead to dysphagia, diplopia, blurred vision, dysarthria, etc. [136]. Ultimately and exceptionally, generalized muscle weakness or hyposthenia leading to respiratory depression and need for mechanical ventilation might happen. In 2009, the FDA issued a warning based on reports of life-threatening systemic toxicity from local BoNTA injections, which may have been related to a toxin overdose [119]. Therefore, practitioners should be particularly cautious when treating children with OAB, especially those with spasticity who may receive BoNTA at other concomitant sites, and adjust treatments appropriately (decrease dosage, delay repeat injections).

Monitoring of PVR 4 to 6 weeks after the first set of injections is crucial in those not performing CIC [137]. The decision to initiate or not CIC should take into account, apart from the absolute value of the PVR, the ratio between the PVR and the bladder capacity, and the patient tolerance [120]. For all patients, follow-up within three months is recommended to assess treatment efficacy and determine if subsequent dosage adjustment is warranted based on the benefit-risk ratio [138]. Follow-up cystometry is optional.

Concerns about bladder wall scarring from repeated punctures have been invalidated by Pascali et al. who observed decreased fibrosis and wall trabeculation after multiple injections in 40 children with neurogenic bladder [139].

Due to the antigenicity of the neurotoxin, patients may develop neutralizing antibodies, hypothetically explaining some therapeutic failures. Among children with a neurogenic bladder, up to 71% of patients have positive serum titers, but their presence has not been systematically correlated to BoNTA clinical resistance [140, 141]. To date, no study has observed a blunted response over time and the longest follow-up available in the pediatric population goes up to 7 to 10 years [142].

Several studies have reported improvements in various clinical and urodynamic parameters with durability of effect over time in the pediatric population. Overall, for neurogenic OAB in children, 14 studies have reported favorable outcomes (complete response or improvement) in 53 to 87% of patients, including two level 2 studies, both for abobotulinumtoxinA [115]. For idiopathic OAB in children, five studies, all level 3, have reported response rates of 44 to 95% [125, 130, 132, 133, 143].

In a systematic review of children with neurogenic OAB treated with BoNTA, maximum detrusor pressure decreased on average by 25 cm H_2O, maximum cystometric capacity increased by a mean of 113 mL, and bladder volume at first uninhibited detrusor contraction increased by 101 mL [124].

Treatment goals may be slightly different for each group of patients. Indeed, alleviating symptoms to maintain social continence is highly sought after among idiopathic OAB children, while lowering intravesical pressure and preventing upper tract deterioration is the primary objective with neurogenic bladder patients [137]. Despite a growing body of evidence, there is still a need for larger and controlled studies.

Injections of BoNTA to treat neurogenic and idiopathic OAB in children have shown long-lasting improvement in symptoms and urodynamic parameters, with a favorable benefit-risk ratio over the last decade. As part of an escalated treatment regimen, they remain an effective, off-label, second-line treatment option for selected patients, despite the need for anesthesia and cystoscopy, to prevent or at least delay the need for bladder augmentation or urinary diversion.

Neuromodulation

Neuromodulation has emerged as an alternative treatment option for cases of refractory OAB and other urological conditions, and has gained widespread recognition since its approval for use in adults in urology. There used to be a paucity of literature addressing the efficacy and safety of neuromodulation in children, but the last decade has seen a plethora of studies reporting on the subject. Various nerve stimulation techniques exist and most have now been studied in children with OAB.

Intravesical Electrical Stimulation

Intravesical electrical stimulation (IVES) consists of using stimulation between a catheter electrode inserted in the bladder and another electrode placed on the skin of the suprapubic area to treat urinary symptoms. Two papers published in the 1970s and 1980s and evaluating children with neurogenic bladder using IVES showed reasonable outcomes in terms of efficacy (26% cure rates, 33-80% improvement rates), but an obvious shortcoming to this method was the need for multiple sessions, possibly up to a few hundred times [144, 145]. A randomized, blinded, sham-controlled trial done in children in the early 1990s did not demonstrate significant differences between the IVES and sham groups [146]. Two more recent studies supported IVES in a population of children with nonobstructive urinary retention and neurogenic bladder, but this might have been attributable to very careful patient selection [147, 148].

Functional Electrical Nerve Stimulation

Functional electrical nerve stimulation (FES) involves stimulation of the afferent pudendal nerves through vaginal, anal, clitoral, or penile electrodes. In 1996, Trsinar and Kralj reported a 75% improvement rate in micturition problems in a group of girls using an anal stimulator compared to a 14% rate in girls in a sham group [149]. Similarly, another sham-controlled study more recently described favorable results for the FES group [150]. Although outcomes appeared promising with FES, stimulation of the anal and genital regions is invasive and definitely not an ideal solution, especially in children.

Transcutaneous Electrical Nerve Stimulation

In transcutaneous electrical nerve stimulation (TENS), surface electrodes are applied to the skin of the sacral area for varying durations of time depending on the study (from as infrequently as twenty minutes three times per week [151] to as often as two hours every day [152, 153]). Foster et al. have demonstrated that there is no significant difference in response rate and complications between two different frequencies [154], but the optimal frequency for TENS is not currently known. There is a fair amount of pediatric literature on TENS. Earlier, uncontrolled studies showed promising results with improvement and cure rates of OAB or lower urinary tract dysfunction ranging from 56 to 100% [153, 155-157]. Two sham-controlled studies demonstrated similar results. In 2009, Hagstroem et al. reported a significant decrease in incontinence in between their treatment (sacral TENS two hours every day) and sham groups (61% and 17%, respectively) [152], and in 2010, Lordêlo et al. reported a 62% cure rate in their treatment group (sacral TENS 20 minutes three times per week) compared to 0% in their sham group [151]. A 2015 uncontrolled study including children with OAB and dysfunctional voiding reported a complete response rate of 70% and a partial response rate of 22% [158]. Two very recent papers evaluated TENS compared to currently approved treatment for OAB in children. Sillén et al. conducted a randomized trial comparing urotherapy alone to urotherapy and TENS and saw no significant differences in the overall treatment response [159]. Likewise, Quintiliano et al. evaluated oxybutynin against TENS and concluded that they were both as effective to treat OAB in children [160]. No significant side effects have been noted with TENS [149]. A recent cost-effectiveness analysis has favored TENS over antimuscarinic medications for the treatment of children with OAB [161]. Another study has identified enuresis as the only predictor of failure of TENS [162]. Although TENS does not appear to be better than already approved treatment options for pediatric OAB, it is a non-invasive approach that might be appealing for children unable to tolerate antimuscarinic medications or if the use of a daily medication wants to be avoided.

Percutaneous Tibial Nerve Stimulation

In percutaneous tibial nerve stimulation (PTNS), a needle electrode is inserted in the lower leg, near the medial malleolus, and a surface electrode is applied over the calcaneum of the same leg. Uncontrolled studies have shown encouraging results with this technique for the treatment of children with OAB [163-165], but at least one study has noted a less significant response in the neurogenic population compared to children with idiopathic OAB [163]. In 2015, two groups published randomized, sham-controlled trials, and interestingly, they both used a transcutaneous approach (i.e., applying a surface electrode over the medial malleolus) rather than the previously described percutaneous needle approach. Patidar et al. evaluated 40 children with non-neuropathic OAB. Children were subjected to 30 minutes of treatment per week during 12 weeks. In the treatment group, two-thirds of children were cured and 24% were improved, compared to 0% and 6%, respectively, in the sham group [166]. Using a resembling regimen of treatment (30 minutes twice a week for 12 weeks), Boudaoud et al. reported a similar clinical efficacy between their two groups [167]. Few side effects have been reported with the transcutaneous approach, the most common being skin reaction under the adhesive electrodes [168]. PTNS appears like a reasonable alternative for the treatment of OAB in children, but the transcutaneous approach should be favored because of its non-invasive nature.

Sacral Neuromodulation with an Implantable Device

Sacral neuromodulation with an implantable device, such as InterStim®, has been approved for use in adults with urological issues for almost two decades. The main disadvantage of this technique is the requirement for surgical implantation of a neurostimulator and lead. There is limited data on the effectiveness of this treatment in children with OAB. Groen et al. retrospectively evaluated 16 children with lower urinary tract dysfunction who underwent sacral neurmodulation with an implantable device, only four of which had idiopathic OAB [169]. They noted a short-term response of 78% and a long-term response of 73%. However, 27% of the devices had to be explanted because of failure, and eight patients had to be reoperated for either infectious complications, displacement of the device, or lost of therapeutic effect. In 2015, Schober et al. assessed a group of 23 children with OAB who underwent a staged procedure with initial lead insertion followed by permanent neurostimulator placement if improvement was noted with the test lead [170]. They reported significant improvement in voiding dysfunction scores and in urodynamic parameters. Complications such as infection, pain at the surgical site, lower extremity pain, and need for device removal were noted. Another 2015 study by Schober et al. evaluated eight children with attention deficit hyperactivity disorder and refractory lower urinary tract dysfunction treated with a sacral neurostimulator. They noted a significant improvement in urinary incontinence and urinary frequency voiding scores, but no significant changes in urodynamic parameters [171]. All in all, sacral neuromodulation with an implantable device might be an option for carefully selected children with OAB who have failed other forms of therapy.

CONCLUSION

In conclusion, with a 15 to 20% prevalence rate in the pediatric population, OAB represents a substantial clinical challenge for physicians. Mastering the basic diagnostic workup for children with lower urinary tract symptoms is essential, and one should not fail to recognize easily correctable contributing factors, such as constipation. Voiding diaries and PVR measurement are two simple tools that are fundamental to follow up. Conservative treatment measures are to be initiated promptly in the evaluation of a child with urinary symptoms, and should be maintained throughout the course of therapy whether or not they are curative. Patient and family education is key to treatment success and might have an impact on medication adherence and persistence. Likewise, setting realistic expectations of treatment efficacy is crucial.

Oxybutynin is the only medical treatment currently approved in North America for the treatment of idiopathic OAB in children. However, there is a growing body of evidence that different oxybutynin formulations, other anticholinergic agents, as well as the more recent mirabegron, might be appropriate alternatives for this population. Dual therapy with a combination of anticholinergics and/or mirabegron is an interesting avenue that needs to be further explored. Botulinum toxin injections and different neuromodulation techniques have shown promising results and appear to be appropriate choices in select cases.

Finally, the treatment armamentarium for children suffering from idiopathic OAB is vast, and although regulatory bodies have not yet formally approved most treatment options available, our approach is mirroring more and more the management algorithm used for adults with intractable OAB symptoms. Nonetheless, more prospective, randomized, controlled studies are needed prior to official approbation.

REFERENCES

[1] Austin, PF; Bauer, SB; Bower, W; Chase, J; Franco, I; Hoebeke, P; et al. The standardization of terminology of lower urinary tract function in children and adolescents: Update report from the standardization committee of the International Children's Continence Society. *Neurourology and urodynamics.*, 2015.

[2] Franco, I. Overactive bladder in children. Part 1: Pathophysiology. *The Journal of urology.*, 2007, 178(3 Pt 1), 761-8, discussion 8.

[3] Wagner, TH; Hu, TW. Economic costs of urinary incontinence. *International urogynecology journal and pelvic floor dysfunction.*, 1998, 9(3), 127-8.

[4] Wagner, TH; Hu, TW. Economic costs of urinary incontinence in 1995. *Urology.*, 1998, 51(3), 355-61.

[5] Currie, CJ; McEwan, P; Poole, CD; Odeyemi, IA; Datta, SN; Morgan, CL. The impact of the overactive bladder on health-related utility and quality of life. *BJU international.*, 2006, 97(6), 1267-72.

[6] Kajiwara, M; Inoue, K; Kato, M; Usui, A; Kurihara, M; Usui, T. Nocturnal enuresis and overactive bladder in children: an epidemiological study. *International journal of urology: official journal of the Japanese Urological Association.*, 2006, 13(1), 36-41.

[7] Chung, JM; Lee, SD; Kang, DI; Kwon, DD; Kim, KS; Kim, SY; et al. Prevalence and associated factors of overactive bladder in Korean children 5-13 years old: a nationwide multicenter study. *Urology.*, 2009, 73(1), 63-7, discussion 8-9.

[8] Lebl, A; Fagundes, SN; Koch, VH. Clinical course of a cohort of children with non-neurogenic daytime urinary incontinence symptoms followed at a tertiary center. *Jornal de pediatria.*, 2015.

[9] Hellstrom, A; Hanson, E; Hansson, S; Hjalmas, K; Jodal, U. Micturition habits and incontinence at age 17--reinvestigation ofa cohort studied at age 7. *British journal of urology.*, 1995, 76(2), 231-4.

[10] Swithinbank, LV; Carr, JC; Abrams, PH. Longitudinal study of urinary symptoms in children. Longitudinal study of urinary symptoms and incontinence in local

schoolchildren. *Scandinavian journal of urology and nephrology Supplementum*., 1994, 163, 67-73.

[11] Burgu, B; Aydogdu, O; Gurkan, K; Uslu, R; Soygur, T. Lower urinary tract conditions in children with attention deficit hyperactivity disorder: correlation of symptoms based on validated scoring systems. *The Journal of urology*., 2011, 185(2), 663-8.

[12] Abrams, P; Kelleher, CJ; Kerr, LA; Rogers, RG. Overactive bladder significantly affects quality of life. *The American journal of managed care*., 2000, 6(11 Suppl), S580-90.

[13] Bartoli, S; Aguzzi, G; Tarricone, R. Impact on quality of life of urinary incontinence and overactive bladder: a systematic literature review. *Urology*., 2010, 75(3), 491-500.

[14] Martinez Agullo, E; Ruiz Cerda, JL; Gomez Perez, L; Rebollo, P; Perez, M; Chaves, J. [Impact of urinary incontinence and overactive bladder syndrome on health-related quality of life of working middle-aged patients and institutionalized elderly patients]. *Actas urologicas espanolas*., 2010, 34(3), 242-50.

[15] Stewart, WF; Van Rooyen, JB; Cundiff, GW; Abrams, P; Herzog, AR; Corey, R; et al. Prevalence and burden of overactive bladder in the United States. *World journal of urology*., 2003, 20(6), 327-36.

[16] Vaughan, CP; Johnson, TM; 2nd, Ala-Lipasti, MA; Cartwright, R; Tammela, TL; Taari, K; et al. The prevalence of clinically meaningful overactive bladder: bother and quality of life results from the population-based FINNO study. *European urology*., 2011, 59(4), 629-36.

[17] Landgraf, JM; Abidari, J; Cilento, BG; Jr. Cooper, CS; Schulman, SL; Ortenberg, J. Coping, commitment, and attitude: quantifying the everyday burden of enuresis on children and their families. *Pediatrics*., 2004, 113(2), 334-44.

[18] Salvatore, S; Serati, M; Origoni, M; Candiani, M. Is overactive bladder in children and adults the same condition? ICI-RS 2011. *Neurourology and urodynamics*., 2012, 31(3), 349-51.

[19] Eiberg, H; Shaumburg, HL; Von Gontard, A; Rittig, S. Linkage study of a large Danish 4-generation family with urge incontinence and nocturnal enuresis. *The Journal of urology*., 2001, 166(6), 2401-3.

[20] Hoebeke, P; Bower, W; Combs, A; De Jong, T; Yang, S. Diagnostic evaluation of children with daytime incontinence. *The Journal of urology*., 2010, 183(2), 699-703.

[21] Farhat, W; Bagli, DJ; Capolicchio, G; O'Reilly, S; Merguerian, PA; Khoury, A; et al. The dysfunctional voiding scoring system: quantitative standardization of dysfunctional voiding symptoms in children. *The Journal of urology*., 2000, 164(3 Pt 2), 1011-5.

[22] Sureshkumar, P; Craig, JC; Roy, LP; Knight, JF. A reproducible pediatric daytime urinary incontinence questionnaire. *The Journal of urology*., 2001, 165(2), 569-73.

[23] Akbal, C; Sahan, A; Sener, TE; Sahin, B; Tinay, I; Tarcan, T; et al. Diagnostic value of the pediatric lower urinary tract symptom score in children with overactive bladder. *World journal of urology*., 2014, 32(1), 201-8.

[24] Afshar, K; Mirbagheri, A; Scott, H; MacNeily, AE. Development of a symptom score for dysfunctional elimination syndrome. *The Journal of urology*., 2009, 182(4 Suppl), 1939-43.

[25] Combs, AJ; Van Batavia, JP; Chan, J; Glassberg, KI. Dysfunctional elimination syndromes--how closely linked are constipation and encopresis with specific lower urinary tract conditions? *The Journal of urology*., 2013, 190(3), 1015-20.

[26] Heaton, KW; Radvan, J; Cripps, H; Mountford, RA; Braddon, FE; Hughes, AO. Defecation frequency and timing, and stool form in the general population: a prospective study. *Gut.*, 1992, 33(6), 818-24.

[27] Van Batavia, JP; Combs, AJ; Fast, AM; Glassberg, KI. Use of non-invasive uroflowmetry with simultaneous electromyography to monitor patient response to treatment for lower urinary tract conditions. *Journal of pediatric urology.*, 2014, 10(3), 532-7.

[28] Allen, HA; Austin, JC; Boyt, MA; Hawtrey, CE; Cooper, CS. Initial trial of timed voiding is warranted for all children with daytime incontinence. *Urology.*, 2007, 69(5), 962-5.

[29] Wiener, JS; Scales, MT; Hampton, J; King, LR; Surwit, R; Edwards, CL. Long-term efficacy of simple behavioral therapy for daytime wetting in children. *The Journal of urology.*, 2000, 164(3 Pt 1), 786-90.

[30] Queiroz Machado, V; Monteiro, A; Pecanha, A; Garcez da Fonseca, E. Slow transit constipation and lower urinary tract dysfunction. *Journal of pediatric urology.*, 2015, 11(6), 357 e1-5.

[31] Loening-Baucke, V. Urinary incontinence and urinary tract infection and their resolution with treatment of chronic constipation of childhood. *Pediatrics.*, 1997, 100(2 Pt 1), 228-32.

[32] Bush, NC; Shah, A; Barber, T; Yang, M; Bernstein, I; Snodgrass, W. Randomized, double-blind, placebo-controlled trial of polyethylene glycol (MiraLAX(R)) for urinary urge symptoms. *Journal of pediatric urology.*, 2013, 9(5), 597-604.

[33] Tugtepe, H; Thomas, DT; Ergun, R; Abdullayev, T; Kastarli, C; Kaynak, A; et al. Comparison of biofeedback therapy in children with treatment-refractory dysfunctional voiding and overactive bladder. *Urology.*, 2015, 85(4), 900-4.

[34] Yagci, S; Kibar, Y; Akay, O; Kilic, S; Erdemir, F; Gok, F; et al. The effect of biofeedback treatment on voiding and urodynamic parameters in children with voiding dysfunction. *The Journal of urology.*, 2005, 174(5), 1994-7, discussion 7-8.

[35] Yamanishi, T; Yasuda, K; Murayama, N; Sakakibara, R; Uchiyama, T; Ito H. Biofeedback training for detrusor overactivity in children. *The Journal of urology.*, 2000, 164(5), 1686-90.

[36] Herndon, CD; Decambre, M; McKenna, PH. Interactive computer games for treatment of pelvic floor dysfunction. *The Journal of urology.*, 2001, 166(5), 1893-8.

[37] Chang, SJ; Van Laecke, E; Bauer, SB; von Gontard, A; Bagli, D; Bower, WF; et al. Treatment of daytime urinary incontinence: A standardization document from the International Children's Continence Society. *Neurourology and urodynamics.*, 2015.

[38] Van Arendonk, KJ; Austin, JC; Boyt, MA; Cooper, CS. Frequency of wetting is predictive of response to anticholinergic treatment in children with overactive bladder. *Urology.*, 2006, 67(5), 1049-53, discussion 53-4.

[39] Greenfield, SP; Fera, M. The use of intravesical oxybutynin chloride in children with neurogenic bladder. *The Journal of urology.*, 1991, 146(2 (Pt 2)), 532-4.

[40] Massad, CA; Kogan, BA; Trigo-Rocha, FE. The pharmacokinetics of intravesical and oral oxybutynin chloride. *The Journal of urology.*, 1992, 148(2 Pt 2), 595-7.

[41] Kasabian, NG; Vlachiotis, JD; Lais, A; Klumpp, B; Kelly, MD; Siroky, MB; et al. The use of intravesical oxybutynin chloride in patients with detrusor hypertonicity and detrusor hyperreflexia. *The Journal of urology.*, 1994, 151(4), 944-5.

[42] Alloussi, S; Murtz, G; Braun, R; Gerhardt, U; Heinrich, M; Hellmis, E; et al. Efficacy, tolerability and safety of propiverine hydrochloride in comparison to oxybutynin in children with urge incontinence due to overactive bladder: Results of a multicentre observational cohort study. *BJU international.*, 2010, 106(4), 550-6.

[43] Van Arendonk, KJ; Knudson, MJ; Austin, JC; Cooper, CS. Improved efficacy of extended release oxybutynin in children with persistent daytime urinary incontinence converted from regular oxybutynin. *Urology.*, 2006, 68(4), 862-5.

[44] Swithinbank, LV; Heron, J; von Gontard, A; Abrams, P. The natural history of daytime urinary incontinence in children: a large British cohort. *Acta paediatrica.*, 2010, 99(7), 1031-6.

[45] Schroder, A; Thuroff. JW. New strategies for medical management of overactive bladder in children. *Current opinion in urology.*, 2010, 20(4), 313-7.

[46] Youdim, K; Kogan, BA. Preliminary study of the safety and efficacy of extended-release oxybutynin in children. *Urology.*, 2002, 59(3), 428-32.

[47] Reinberg, Y; Crocker, J; Wolpert, J; Vandersteen, D. Therapeutic efficacy of extended release oxybutynin chloride, and immediate release and long acting tolterodine tartrate in children with diurnal urinary incontinence. *The Journal of urology.*, 2003, 169(1), 317-9.

[48] Gleason, JM; Daniels, C; Williams, K; Varghese, A; Koyle, MA; Bagli, DJ; et al. Single center experience with oxybutynin transdermal system (patch) for management of symptoms related to non-neuropathic overactive bladder in children: an attractive, well tolerated alternative form of administration. *Journal of pediatric urology.*, 2014, 10(4), 753-7.

[49] Goldfischer, ER; Sand, PK; Thomas, H; Peters-Gee, J. Efficacy and safety of oxybutynin topical gel 3% in patients with urgency and/or mixed urinary incontinence: a randomized, double-blind, placebo-controlled study. *Neurourology and urodynamics.*, 2015, 34(1), 37-43.

[50] Staskin, DR; Dmochowski, RR; Sand, PK; Macdiarmid, SA; Caramelli, KE; Thomas, H; et al. Efficacy and safety of oxybutynin chloride topical gel for overactive bladder: a randomized, double-blind, placebo controlled, multicenter study. *The Journal of urology.*, 2009, 181(4), 1764-72.

[51] Frohlich, G; Burmeister, S; Wiedemann, A; Bulitta, M. [Intravesical instillation of trospium chloride, oxybutynin and verapamil for relaxation of the bladder detrusor muscle. A placebo controlled, randomized clinical test]. *Arzneimittel-Forschung.*, 1998, 48(5), 486-91.

[52] Enzelsberger, H; Helmer, H; Kurz, C. Intravesical instillation of oxybutynin in women with idiopathic detrusor instability: a randomised trial. *British journal of obstetrics and gynaecology.*, 1995, 102(11), 929-30.

[53] Yarker, YE; Goa, KL; Fitton, A. Oxybutynin. A review of its pharmacodynamic and pharmacokinetic properties, and its therapeutic use in detrusor instability. *Drugs & aging.*, 1995, 6(3), 243-62.

[54] Brendler, CB; Radebaugh, LC; Mohler, JL. Topical oxybutynin chloride for relaxation of dysfunctional bladders. *The Journal of urology.*, 1989, 141(6), 1350-2.

[55] Madersbacher, H; Jilg, G. Control of detrusor hyperreflexia by the intravesical instillation of oxybutynine hydrochloride. *Paraplegia.*, 1991, 29(2), 84-90.

[56] Weese, DL; Roskamp, DA; Leach, GE; Zimmern, PE. Intravesical oxybutynin chloride: experience with 42 patients. *Urology.*, 1993, 41(6), 527-30.

[57] O'Flynn, KJ; Thomas, DG. Intravesical instillation of oxybutynin hydrochloride for detrusor hyper-reflexia. *British journal of urology.*, 1993, 72(5 Pt 1), 566-70.

[58] Prasad, KV; Vaidyanathan, S. Intravesical oxybutynin chloride and clean intermittent catheterisation in patients with neurogenic vesical dysfunction and decreased bladder capacity. *British journal of urology.*, 1993, 72(5 Pt 2), 719-22.

[59] Mizunaga, M; Miyata, M; Kaneko, S; Yachiku, S; Chiba, K. Intravesical instillation of oxybutynin hydrochloride therapy for patients with a neuropathic bladder. *Paraplegia.*, 1994, 32(1), 25-9.

[60] Holland, AJ; King, PA; Chauvel, PJ; O'Neill, MK; McKnight, DL; Barker, AP. Intravesical therapy for the treatment of neurogenic bladder in children. *The Australian and New Zealand journal of surgery.*, 1997, 67(10), 731-3.

[61] Amark, P; Bussman, G; Eksborg, S. Follow-up of long-time treatment with intravesical oxybutynin for neurogenic bladder in children. *European urology.*, 1998, 34(2), 148-53.

[62] Goessl, C; Sauter, T; Michael, T; Berge, B; Staehler, M; Miller, K. Efficacy and tolerability of tolterodine in children with detrusor hyperreflexia. *Urology.*, 2000, 55(3), 414-8.

[63] Bolduc, S; Upadhyay, J; Payton, J; Bagli, DJ; McLorie, GA; Khoury, AE; et al. The use of tolterodine in children after oxybutynin failure. *BJU international.*, 2003, 91(4), 398-401.

[64] Munding, M; Wessells, H; Thornberry, B; Riden, D. Use of tolterodine in children with dysfunctional voiding: an initial report. *The Journal of urology.*, 2001, 165(3), 926-8.

[65] Hjalmas, K; Hellstrom, AL; Mogren, K; Lackgren, G; Stenberg, A. The overactive bladder in children: a potential future indication for tolterodine. *BJU international.*, 2001, 87(6), 569-74.

[66] Medhi, B; Mittal, N; Bansal, D; Prakash, A; Sarangi, SC; Nirthi, B. Comparison of tolterodine with standard treatment in pediatric patients with non-neurogenic dysfunctional voiding/over active bladder: a systematic review. *Indian journal of physiology and pharmacology.*, 2013, 57(4), 343-53.

[67] Nijman, RJ; Borgstein, NG; Ellsworth, P; Siggaard, C. Long-term tolerability of tolterodine extended release in children 5-11 years of age: results from a 12-month, open-label study. *European urology.*, 2007, 52(5), 1511-6.

[68] Malhotra, B; Darsey, E; Crownover, P; Fang, J; Glue, P. Comparison of pharmacokinetic variability of fesoterodine vs. tolterodine extended release in cytochrome P450 2D6 extensive and poor metabolizers. *British journal of clinical pharmacology.*, 2011, 72(2), 226-34.

[69] Malhotra, B; El-Tahtawy, A; Wang, EQ; Darekar, A; Cossons, N; Crook, TJ; et al. Dose-escalating study of the pharmacokinetics and tolerability of fesoterodine in children with overactive bladder. *Journal of pediatric urology.*, 2012, 8(4), 336-42.

[70] Hoebeke, P; De Pooter, J; De Caestecker, K; Raes, A; Dehoorne, J; Van Laecke, E; et al. Solifenacin for therapy resistant overactive bladder. *The Journal of urology.*, 2009, 182(4 Suppl), 2040-4.

[71] Bolduc, S; Moore, K; Nadeau, G; Lebel, S; Lamontagne, P; Hamel, M. Prospective open label study of solifenacin for overactive bladder in children. *The Journal of urology.*, 2010, 184(4 Suppl), 1668-73.

[72] Nadeau, G; Schroder, A; Moore, K; Genois, L; Lamontagne, P; Hamel, M; et al. Long-term use of solifenacin in pediatric patients with overactive bladder: Extension of a prospective open-label study. *Canadian Urological Association journal = Journal de l'Association des urologues du Canada*., 2014, 8(3-4), 118-23.

[73] Newgreen, D; Bosman, B; Sawyer, W; Hollestein-Havelaar, A; Besuyen, R; Dahler, E; et al. Solifenacin in children and adolescents with overactive bladder: results of a phase 3 clinical trial. *26th European Society for Paediatric Urology Congress; Prague, Czech Republic*, 2015.

[74] Bosman, B; Newgreen, D; Sawyer, W; Hollestein-Havelaar, A; Dahler, E; Bolduc, S; et al. Solifenacin in children and adolescents with overactive bladder: results of an open-label, long-term clinical trial. *26th European Society for Paediatric Urology Congress; Prague, Czech Republic*, 2015.

[75] Humphreys, MR; Reinberg, YE. Contemporary and emerging drug treatments for urinary incontinence in children. *Paediatric drugs*., 2005, 7(3), 151-62.

[76] Madersbacher, H; Rovner, E. Trospium chloride: the European experience. *Expert opinion on pharmacotherapy*., 2006, 7(10), 1373-80.

[77] Wright, A; Clothier, J. Trospium: a useful alternative anticholinergic in children with emotional behavioural disorders. *26th European Society for Paediatric Urology Congress; Prague, Czech Republic*, 2015.

[78] McKeage, K. Propiverine: a review of its use in the treatment of adults and children with overactive bladder associated with idiopathic or neurogenic detrusor overactivity, and in men with lower urinary tract symptoms. *Clinical drug investigation*., 2013, 33(1), 71-91.

[79] Wuest, M; Witte, LP; Michel-Reher, MB; Propping, S; Braeter, M; Strugala, GJ; et al. The muscarinic receptor antagonist propiverine exhibits alpha(1)-adrenoceptor antagonism in human prostate and porcine trigonum. *World journal of urology*., 2011, 29(2), 149-55.

[80] Marschall-Kehrel, D; Feustel, C; Persson de Geeter, C; Stehr, M; Radmayr, C; Sillen, U; et al. Treatment with propiverine in children suffering from nonneurogenic overactive bladder and urinary incontinence: results of a randomized placebo-controlled phase 3 clinical trial. *European urology*., 2009, 55(3), 729-36.

[81] Kim, WJ; Lee, DG; Lee, SW; Lee, YK; Lee, JS; Park, KH; et al. Efficacy and safety of propiverine in children with overactive bladder. *Korean journal of urology*., 2012, 53(4), 275-9.

[82] Sacco, E; Bientinesi, R. Mirabegron: a review of recent data and its prospects in the management of overactive bladder. *Ther Adv Urol*., 2012, 4(6), 315-24.

[83] Takasu, T; Ukai M, Sato S, Matsui T, Nagase I, Maruyama T, et al. Effect of (R)-2-(2-aminothiazol-4-yl)-4'-{2-[(2-hydroxy-2-phenylethyl) amino]ethyl} acetanilide (YM178), a novel selective beta3-adrenoceptor agonist, on bladder function. *J Pharmacol Exp Ther*., 2007, 321(2), 642-7.

[84] Chapple, CR; Kaplan, SA; Mitcheson, D; Klecka, J; Cummings, J; Drogendijk, T; et al. Randomized double-blind, active-controlled phase 3 study to assess 12-month safety and efficacy of mirabegron, a beta(3)-adrenoceptor agonist, in overactive bladder. *European urology*., 2013, 63(2), 296-305.

[85] Herschorn, S; Barkin, J; Castro-Diaz, D; Frankel, JM; Espuna-Pons, M; Gousse, AE; et al. A phase III, randomized, double-blind, parallel-group, placebo-controlled,

multicentre study to assess the efficacy and safety of the beta(3) adrenoceptor agonist, mirabegron, in patients with symptoms of overactive bladder. *Urology*., 2013, 82(2), 313-20.

[86] Khullar, V; Amarenco, G; Angulo, JC; Cambronero, J; Hoye, K; Milsom, I; et al. Efficacy and tolerability of mirabegron, a beta(3)-adrenoceptor agonist, in patients with overactive bladder: results from a randomised European-Australian phase 3 trial. *European urology*., 2013, 63(2), 283-95.

[87] Kuo, HC; Lee, KS; Na, Y; Sood, R; Nakaji, S; Kubota, Y; et al. Results of a randomized, double-blind, parallel-group, placebo- and active-controlled, multicenter study of mirabegron, a beta3-adrenoceptor agonist, in patients with overactive bladder in Asia. *Neurourology and urodynamics*., 2015, 34(7), 685-92.

[88] Nitti, VW; Auerbach, S; Martin, N; Calhoun, A; Lee, M; Herschorn, S. Results of a randomized phase III trial of mirabegron in patients with overactive bladder. *The Journal of urology*., 2013, 189(4), 1388-95.

[89] Khullar, V; Cambronero, J; Angulo, JC; Wooning, M; Blauwet, MB; Dorrepaal, C; et al. Efficacy of mirabegron in patients with and without prior antimuscarinic therapy for overactive bladder: a post hoc analysis of a randomized European-Australian Phase 3 trial. *BMC Urol*., 2013, 13, 45.

[90] Batista, JE; Kolbl, H; Herschorn, S; Rechberger, T; Cambronero, J; Halaska, M; et al. The efficacy and safety of mirabegron compared with solifenacin in overactive bladder patients dissatisfied with previous antimuscarinic treatment due to lack of efficacy: results of a noninferiority, randomized, phase IIIb trial. *Ther Adv Urol*., 2015, 7(4), 167-79.

[91] Abrams, P; Kelleher, C; Staskin, D; Rechberger, T; Kay, R; Martina, R; et al. Combination treatment with mirabegron and solifenacin in patients with overactive bladder: efficacy and safety results from a randomised, double-blind, dose-ranging, phase 2 study (Symphony). *European urology*., 2015, 67(3), 577-88.

[92] Drake, M; Esen, A; Athanasiou, S; Herholdt, C; Baronio, R; Saleem, T; et al. Efficacy and safety of mirabegron add-on treatment to solifenacin in incontinent OAB subjects with an inadequate response to initial 4-week solifenacin monotherapy. *2015 American Urological Association Annual Meeting; New Orleans, United States*, 2015.

[93] A randomized, double-blind, parallel-group, placebo- and active-controlled, nulti-center study to evaluate the efficacy, safety and tolerability of combinations of solifenacin succinate and mirabegron compared to solifenacin succinate and mirabegron monotherapy in the treatment of overactive bladder: Astellas Pharma Europe B.V.; 2016 [2016/01/10]. Available from: https://clinicaltrials.gov/ct2/show/NCT01972841?term=mirabegron+synergy&rank=1.

[94] A randomized, double-blind, parallel-group, active-controlled, multi-center study to evaluate the long-term safety and efficacy of combination of solifenacin succinate with mirabegron compared to solifenacin succinate and mirabegron monotherapy in subjects with overactive bladder: Astellas Pharma Europe B.V.; 2016 [2016/01/10]. Available from:https://clinicaltrials.gov/ct2/show/NCT02045862?term=mirabegron+synergy&rank=2.

[95] Nitti, VW; Khullar, V; van Kerrebroeck, P; Herschorn, S; Cambronero, J; Angulo, JC; et al. Mirabegron for the treatment of overactive bladder: a prespecified pooled efficacy

analysis and pooled safety analysis of three randomised, double-blind, placebo-controlled, phase III studies. *Int J Clin Pract*., 2013, 67(7), 619-32.

[96] Myrbetriq canadian approved product monograph: Astellas Pharma Canada I; 2013 [2016/01/10]. Available from: http://www.cmsastellas. ca/uploads/pdf/131-2013-03-04-myrbetriq PM-Approved.pdf.

[97] Krauwinkel, W; Dickinson, J; Schaddelee, M; Meijer, J; Tretter, R; van de Wetering, J; et al. The effect of mirabegron, a potent and selective beta3-adrenoceptor agonist, on the pharmacokinetics of CYP2D6 substrates desipramine and metoprolol. *Eur J Drug Metab Pharmacokinet*., 2014, 39(1), 43-52.

[98] Rosa, G; Ferrero, S; Nitti, VW; Wagg, A; Saleem, T; Chapple, C. Cardiovascular safety of β3-adrenoceptor agonists for the treatment of patients with overactive bladder syndrome. *European urology*., 2016, 69(2), 311-23.

[99] Herschorn, S; Kowey, P; Nitti, VW; Milsom, I; Auerbach, S; Blauwet, MB. Cardiovascular (CV) assessments in short- and long-term Phase 3 mirabegron trials in patients with overactive bladder (OAB). *Eur urol Suppl*., 2013, 12(1), 739-40.

[100] Blais, A; Nadeau, G; Moore, K; Genois, L; Bolduc, S. Prospective pilot study of mirabegron in pediatric patients with overactive bladder. *European urology*., 2016. In revision.

[101] Morin, F; Blais, A; Nadeau, G; Moore, K; Bolduc, S. Dual therapy for refractory overactive bladder in children: a prospective open-label study. *67th Northeastern Section of the American Urological Association Annual Meeting;* Quebec City, Canada, 2015.

[102] Bolduc, S; Moore, K; Lebel, S; Lamontagne, P; Hamel, M. Double anticholinergic therapy for refractory overactive bladder. *The Journal of urology*., 2009, 182(4 Suppl), 2033-8.

[103] Nadeau, G; Schroder, A; Moore, K; Genois, L; Lamontagne, P; Hamel, M; et al. Double anticholinergic therapy for refractory neurogenic and nonneurogenic detrusor overactivity in children: Long-term results of a prospective open-label study. *Canadian Urological Association journal = Journal de l'Association des urologues du Canada*., 2014, 8(5-6), 175-80.

[104] Yamaguchi, O; Kakizaki, H; Homma, Y; Igawa, Y; Takeda, M; Nishizawa, O; et al. Safety and efficacy of mirabegron as 'add-on' therapy in patients with overactive bladder treated with solifenacin: a post-marketing, open-label study in Japan (MILAI study). *BJU international*., 2015, 116(4), 612-22.

[105] Sicras-Mainar, A; Rejas, J; Navarro-Artieda, R; Aguado-Jodar, A; Ruiz-Torrejon, A; Ibanez-Nolla, J; et al. Antimuscarinic persistence patterns in newly treated patients with overactive bladder: a retrospective comparative analysis. *International urogynecology journal*., 2014, 25(4), 485-92.

[106] Pelletier, EM; Vats, V; Clemens, JQ. Pharmacotherapy adherence and costs versus nonpharmacologic management in overactive bladder. *The American journal of managed care*., 2009, 15(4 Suppl), S108-14.

[107] D'Souza, AO; Smith, MJ; Miller, LA; Doyle, J; Ariely, R. Persistence, adherence, and switch rates among extended-release and immediate-release overactive bladder medications in a regional managed care plan. *Journal of managed care pharmacy: JMCP*., 2008, 14(3), 291-301.

[108] Balkrishnan, R; Bhosle, MJ; Camacho, FT; Anderson, RT. Predictors of medication adherence and associated health care costs in an older population with overactive bladder syndrome: a longitudinal cohort study. *The Journal of urology.*, 2006, 175(3 Pt 1), 1067-71, discussion 71-2.

[109] Fortin, A; Morin, V; Ramsay, S; Bolduc, S. Compliance to antimuscarinics in children with overactive bladder. *26th European Society for Paediatric Urology Congress; Prague, Czech Republic*, 2015.

[110] Kelleher, CJ; Cardozo, LD; Khullar, V; Salvatore, S. A medium-term analysis of the subjective efficacy of treatment for women with detrusor instability and low bladder compliance. *British journal of obstetrics and gynaecology.*, 1997, 104(9), 988-93.

[111] Wagg, A; Compion, G; Fahey, A; Siddiqui, E. Persistence with prescribed antimuscarinic therapy for overactive bladder: a UK experience. *BJU international.*, 2012, 110(11), 1767-74.

[112] Blais, A; Bergeron, M; Nadeau, G; Ramsay, S; Bolduc, S. Anticholinergic use in children: persistence and patterns of therapy. *Canadian Urological Association journal = Journal de l'Association des urologues du Canada.*, 2016. In press.

[113] Schulte-Baukloh, H; Knispel, HH; Michael, T. Botulinum-A toxin in the treatment of neurogenic bladder in children. *Pediatrics.*, 2002, 110(2 Pt 1), 420-1.

[114] Smith, CP; Chancellor, MB. Emerging role of botulinum toxin in the management of voiding dysfunction. *The Journal of urology.*, 2004, 171(6 Pt 1), 2128-37.

[115] Mangera, A; Andersson, KE; Apostolidis, A; Chapple, C; Dasgupta, P; Giannantoni, A; et al. Contemporary management of lower urinary tract disease with botulinum toxin A: a systematic review of botox (onabotulinumtoxinA) and dysport (abobotulinumtoxinA). *European urology.*, 2011, 60(4), 784-95.

[116] Ravenni, R; De Grandis, D; Mazza, A. Conversion ratio between Dysport and Botox in clinical practice: an overview of available evidence. *Neurological sciences: official journal of the Italian Neurological Society and of the Italian Society of Clinical Neurophysiology.*, 2013, 34(7), 1043-8.

[117] Carmel, M; Goldman, H. Management of overactive bladder. *Expert Review of Obstetrics & Gynecology [Internet].*, 2012, 7(6), [605-13 pp.].

[118] Apostolidis, A; Dasgupta, P; Denys, P; Elneil, S; Fowler, CJ; Giannantoni, A; et al. *Recommendations on the use of botulinum toxin in the treatment of lower urinary tract disorders and pelvic floor dysfunctions: a European consensus report. European urology.*, 2009, 55(1), 100-19.

[119] Pr Botox® product monograph: Allergan Inc., 2014 [2016/01/10]. Available from: http://www.allergan.ca/assets/pdf/ca_botox_pm.pdf.

[120] Hermieu, JF; Ballanger, P; Amarenco, G; Chartier-Kastler, E; Cosson, M; Costa, P; et al. [Guidelines for practical usage of botulinum toxin type A (BoNTA) for refractory idiopathic overactive bladder management]. *Progres en urologie: journal de l'Association francaise d'urologie et de la Societe francaise d'urologie.*, 2013, 23(17), 1457-63.

[121] Dave, S. A pilot trial comparing the effects of onabotulinumtoxina and standard oxybutynin therapy as first line treatment for the poorly compliant pediatric neurogenic bladder [Electronic Thesis and Dissertation Repository.]: The University of Western Ontario, 2012.

[122] Dykstra, DD; Sidi, AA. Treatment of detrusor-sphincter dyssynergia with botulinum A toxin: a double-blind study. *Archives of physical medicine and rehabilitation.*, 1990, 71(1), 24-6.

[123] DasGupta, R; Murphy, FL. Botulinum toxin in paediatric urology: a systematic literature review. *Pediatric surgery international.*, 2009, 25(1), 19-23.

[124] Game, X; Mouracade, P; Chartier-Kastler, E; Viehweger, E; Moog, R; Amarenco, G; et al. Botulinum toxin-A (Botox) intradetrusor injections in children with neurogenic detrusor overactivity/neurogenic overactive bladder: a systematic literature review. *Journal of pediatric urology.*, 2009, 5(3), 156-64.

[125] Hoebeke, P; De Caestecker, K; Vande Walle, J; Dehoorne, J; Raes, A; Verleyen, P; et al. The effect of botulinum-A toxin in incontinent children with therapy resistant overactive detrusor. *The Journal of urology.*, 2006, 176(1), 328-30, discussion 30-1.

[126] Khan, MK; VanderBrink, BA; DeFoor, WR; Minevich, E; Jackson, E; Noh, P; et al. Botulinum toxin injection in the pediatric population with medically refractory neuropathic bladder. *Journal of pediatric urology.*

[127] Riccabona, M; Koen, M; Schindler, M; Goedele, B; Pycha, A; Lusuardi, L; et al. Botulinum-A toxin injection into the detrusor: a safe alternative in the treatment of children with myelomeningocele with detrusor hyperreflexia. *The Journal of urology.*, 2004, 171(2 Pt 1), 845-8, discussion 8.

[128] Rohrsted, M; Nordsten, CB; Bagi, P. Onabotulinum toxin a (botox(R)) in the treatment of neurogenic bladder overactivity. *Nephro-urology monthly.*, 2012, 4(2), 437-42.

[129] Akbar, M; Abel, R; Seyler, TM; Bedke, J; Haferkamp, A; Gerner, HJ; et al. Repeated botulinum-A toxin injections in the treatment of myelodysplastic children and patients with spinal cord injuries with neurogenic bladder dysfunction. *BJU international.*, 2007,100(3), 639-45.

[130] Marte, A; Borrelli, M; Sabatino, MD; Balzo, BD; Prezioso, M; Pintozzi, L; et al. Effectiveness of botulinum-A toxin for the treatment of refractory overactive bladder in children. *European journal of pediatric surgery: official journal of Austrian Association of Pediatric Surgery [*et al*] = Zeitschrift fur Kinderchirurgie.*, 2010, 20(3), 153-7.

[131] Binder, WJ; Brin, MF; Blitzer, A; Pogoda, JM. Botulinum toxin type A (BOTOX) for treatment of migraine. *Disease-a-month:DM.*, 2002, 48(5), 323-35.

[132] Blackburn, SC; Jones, C; Bedoya, S; Steinbrecher, HA; Malone, PS; Griffin, SJ. Intravesical botulinum type-A toxin (Dysport(R)) in the treatment of idiopathic detrusor overactivity in children. *Journal of pediatric urology.*, 2013, 9(6 Pt A), 750-3.

[133] Greer, T; Abbott, J; Breytenbach, W; McGuane, D; Barker, A; Khosa, J; et al. Ten years of experience with intravesical and intrasphincteric onabotulinumtoxinA in children. *Journal of pediatric urology.*, 2015.

[134] Verleyen, P; Hoebeke, P; Raes, A; Van Laecke, E; Vande Walle, J. The use of botulinum toxin A in children with a non-neurogenic overactive bladder: a pilot study. BJU INTERNATIONAL BLACKWELL PUBLISHING LTD., 2004, p 69–69.

[135] Nitti, VW; Dmochowski, R; Herschorn, S; Sand, P; Thompson, C; Nardo, C; et al. OnabotulinumtoxinA for the treatment of patients with overactive bladder and urinary incontinence: results of a phase 3, randomized, placebo controlled trial. *The Journal of urology.*, 2013, 189(6), 2186-93.

[136] Orasanu, B; Mahajan, ST. The use of botulinum toxin for the treatment of overactive bladder syndrome. *Indian journal of urology:IJU:journal of the Urological Society of India.*, 2013, 29(1), 2-11.

[137] Hassouna, T; Gleason, JM; Lorenzo, AJ. Botulinum toxin A's expanding role in the management of pediatric lower urinary tract dysfunction. *Current urology reports.*, 2014, 15(8), 426.

[138] Dowson, C; Watkins, J; Khan, MS; Dasgupta, P; Sahai, A. Repeated botulinum toxin type A injections for refractory overactive bladder: medium-term outcomes, safety profile, and discontinuation rates. *European urology.*, 2012, 61(4), 834-9.

[139] Pascali, MP; Mosiello, G; Boldrini, R; Salsano, ML; Castelli, E; De Gennaro, M. Effects of botulinum toxin type a in the bladder wall of children with neurogenic bladder dysfunction: a comparison of histological features before and after injections. *The Journal of urology.*, 2011, 185(6 Suppl), 2552-7.

[140] Kajbafzadeh, AM; Nikfarjam, L; Mahboubi, AH; Dianat, S. Antibody formation following botulinum toxin type A (Dysport) injection in children with intractable bladder hyper-reflexia. *Urology.*, 2010, 76(1), 233-7.

[141] Schulte-Baukloh, H; Herholz, J; Bigalke, H; Miller, K; Knispel, HH. Results of a BoNT/A antibody study in children and adolescents after onabotulinumtoxin A (Botox(R)) detrusor injection. *Urologia internationalis.*, 2011, 87(4), 434-8.

[142] Laschke, S; Carl, S. Repeated botulinum toxin a injections in children with detrusor hyperreflexia: long term follow up. *The Journal of urology.*, 2009, 181(4), 311.

[143] McDowell, DT; Noone, D; Tareen, F; Waldron, M; Quinn, F. Urinary incontinence in children: botulinum toxin is a safe and effective treatment option. *Pediatric surgery international.*, 2012, 28(3), 315-20.

[144] Berger, D; Berger, K; Genton, N. Endovesical transurethral electrostimulation in the rehabilitation of neurogenic bladder in children. 4 Years clinical experience. *European urology.*, 1978, 4(1), 33-45.

[145] Kaplan, WE; Richards, I. Intravesical bladder stimulation in myelodysplasia. *The Journal of urology.*, 1988, 140(5 Pt 2), 1282-4.

[146] Boone, TB; Roehrborn, CG; Hurt, G. Transurethral intravesical electrotherapy for neurogenic bladder dysfunction in children with myelodysplasia: a prospective, randomized clinical trial. *The Journal of urology.*, 1992, 148(2 Pt 2), 550-4.

[147] Gladh, G; Mattsson, S; Lindstrom, S. Intravesical electrical stimulation in the treatment of micturition dysfunction in children. *Neurourology and urodynamics.*, 2003, 22(3), 233-42.

[148] Hagerty, JA; Richards, I; Kaplan, WE. Intravesical electrotherapy for neurogenic bladder dysfunction: a 22-year experience. *The Journal of urology.*, 2007, 178(4 Pt 2), 1680-3, discussion 3.

[149] Trsinar, B; Kraij, B. Maximal electrical stimulation in children with unstable bladder and nocturnal enuresis and/or daytime incontinence: a controlled study. *Neurourology and urodynamics.*, 1996, 15(2), 133-42.

[150] Kajbafzadeh, AM; Sharifi-Rad, L; Baradaran, N; Nejat, F. Effect of pelvic floor interferential electrostimulation on urodynamic parameters and incontinency of children with myelomeningocele and detrusor overactivity. *Urology.*, 2009, 74(2), 324-9.

[151] Lordelo, P; Teles, A; Veiga, ML; Correia, LC; Barroso, U. Jr. Transcutaneous electrical nerve stimulation in children with overactive bladder: a randomized clinical trial. *The Journal of urology.*, 2010, 184(2), 683-9.

[152] Hagstroem, S; Mahler, B; Madsen, B; Djurhuus, JC; Rittig, S. Transcutaneous electrical nerve stimulation for refractory daytime urinary urge incontinence. *The Journal of urology.*, 2009, 182(4 Suppl), 2072-8.

[153] Hoebeke, P; Van Laecke, E; Everaert, K; Renson, C; De Paepe, H; Raes, A; et al. Transcutaneous neuromodulation for the urge syndrome in children: a pilot study. *The Journal of urology.*, 2001, 166(6), 2416-9.

[154] Foster, C; McKenzie, J; Hepburn, K; Hutchinson, R; Garriboli, M; Clothier, J; et al. Which is the best TENS programme to use for idiopathic bladder overactivity in children? *26th European Society for Paediatric Urology Congress; Prague, Czech Republic*, 2015.

[155] Barroso, U; Jr. Lordelo, P; Lopes, AA; Andrade, J; Macedo, A; Jr. Ortiz, V. Nonpharmacological treatment of lower urinary tract dysfunction using biofeedback and transcutaneous electrical stimulation: a pilot study. *BJU international.*, 2006, 98(1), 166-71.

[156] Bower, WF; Moore, KH; Adams, RD. A pilot study of the home application of transcutaneous neuromodulation in children with urgency or urge incontinence. *The Journal of urology.*, 2001, 166(6), 2420-2.

[157] Malm-Buatsi, E; Nepple, KG; Boyt, MA; Austin, JC; Cooper, CS. Efficacy of transcutaneous electrical nerve stimulation in children with overactive bladder refractory to pharmacotherapy. *Urology.*, 2007, 70(5), 980-3.

[158] Tugtepe, H; Thomas, DT; Ergun, R; Kalyoncu, A; Kaynak, A; Kastarli, C; et al. The effectiveness of transcutaneous electrical neural stimulation therapy in patients with urinary incontinence resistant to initial medical treatment or biofeedback. *Journal of pediatric urology.*, 2015, 11(3), 137 e1-5.

[159] Sillen, U; Arwidsson, C; Doroszkiewicz, M; Antonsson, H; Jansson, I; Stalklint, M; et al. Effects of transcutaneous neuromodulation (TENS) on overactive bladder symptoms in children: a randomized controlled trial. *Journal of pediatric urology.*, 2014, 10(6), 1100-5.

[160] Quintiliano, F; Veiga, ML; Moraes, M; Cunha, C; de Oliveira, LF; Lordelo, P; et al. Transcutaneous parasacral electrical stimulation vs oxybutynin for the treatment of overactive bladder in children: a randomized clinical trial. *The Journal of urology.*, 2015, 193(5 Suppl), 1749-53.

[161] Hutchinson, R; Garriboli, M; Clothier, J; Wright, A. Is parasacral neuromodulation using TENS a cost-effective first-line treatment for bladder overactivity in children? *26th European Society for Paediatric Urology Congress; Prague, Czech Republic*, 2015.

[162] Barroso, U; Jr. Sampaio, C; Hoffman, A; Nascimento, A; Bastos Netto, JM; Veiga, ML. Predictors of parasacral transcutaneous neurostimulation (TENS) failure in children with overactive bladder. *26th European Society for Paediatric Urology Congress; Prague, Czech Republic*, 2015.

[163] Capitanucci, ML; Camanni, D; Demelas, F; Mosiello, G; Zaccara, A; De Gennaro, M. Long-term efficacy of percutaneous tibial nerve stimulation for different types of lower

urinary tract dysfunction in children. *The Journal of urology*., 2009, 182(4 Suppl), 2056-61.

[164] De Gennaro, M; Capitanucci, ML; Mastracci, P; Silveri, M; Gatti, C; Mosiello, G. Percutaneous tibial nerve neuromodulation is well tolerated in children and effective for treating refractory vesical dysfunction. *The Journal of urology*., 2004, 171(5), 1911-3.

[165] Hoebeke, P; Renson, C; Petillon, L; Vande Walle, J; De Paepe, H. Percutaneous electrical nerve stimulation in children with therapy resistant nonneuropathic bladder sphincter dysfunction: a pilot study. *The Journal of urology*., 2002, 168(6), 2605-7, discussion 7-8.

[166] Patidar, N; Mittal, V; Kumar, M; Sureka, SK; Arora, S; Ansari, MS. Transcutaneous posterior tibial nerve stimulation in pediatric overactive bladder: A preliminary report. *Journal of pediatric urology*., 2015, 11(6), 351 e1-6.

[167] Boudaoud, N; Binet, A; Line, A; Chaouadi, D; Jolly, C; Fiquet, CF; et al. Management of refractory overactive bladder in children by transcutaneous posterior tibial nerve stimulation: A controlled study. *Journal of pediatric urology*., 2015, 11(3), 138 e1-10.

[168] Humphreys, MR; Vandersteen, DR; Slezak, JM; Hollatz, P; Smith, CA; Smith, JE; et al. Preliminary results of sacral neuromodulation in 23 children. *The Journal of urology*., 2006, 176(5), 2227-31.

[169] Groen, LA; Hoebeke, P; Loret, N; Van Praet, C; Van Laecke, E; Ann, R; et al. Sacral neuromodulation with an implantable pulse generator in children with lower urinary tract symptoms: 15-year experience. *The Journal of urology*., 2012, 188(4), 1313-7.

[170] Schober, MS; Sulkowski, JP; Lu, PL; Minneci, PC; Deans, KJ; Teich, S; et al. Sacral Nerve Stimulation for Pediatric Lower Urinary Tract Dysfunction: Development of a Standardized Pathway with Objective Urodynamic Outcomes. *The Journal of urology*., 2015, 194(6), 1721-7.

[171] Schober, MS; Alpert, SA. Subjective and objective outcomes of sacral neurmodulation in children with refractory lower urinary tract dysfunction and attention deficit hyperactivity disorder. *26th European Society for Paediatric Urology Congress; Prague, Czech Republic*, 2015.

Biographical Sketch

Name: Dr Stéphane Bolduc, MD, FRCSC, FAAP

Affiliation: CHU de Québec – Université Laval

Education: Medicine and Urology residency at Université Laval, Québec city, Canada 1990-2000

Fellowship in Pediatric Urology, The Hospital for Sick Children, Toronto, Canada 2000-2002

Address: 2705 Boul Laurier (R-1742), Québec, Québec, Canada, G1V 4G2

Email: Stephane.bolduc@fmed.ulaval.ca

Professional Appointments: Assistant Professor, Department of Surgery, Director of Regenerative Medicine of the CHU de Québec Research Center. Head of Pediatric Urology

Publications Last 3 Years (29):

1. Blais, A-S., Nadeau, G., Moore K., Genois, L., Bolduc, S. Prospective Pilot Study of Mirabegron in Pediatric Patients with Overactive Bladder Accepted Eur Urol Jan 2016.
2. Morin, F., Blais, A-S., Nadeau, G., Moore K., Genois, L., Bolduc, S. Dual Therapy for Refractory Overactive Bladder in Children: A Prospective Open-Label Study. Submitted Eur Urol, Jan 2016.
3. Fortin, A. Morin V., Ramsay, S. Gervais, P., Bolduc, S., Compliance to antimuscarinics in children with overactive bladder. Submitted Child and Pediatric Health, Jan 2016.
4. Blais, A-S., Bergeron, M., Nadeau, G., Ramsay, S., Bolduc, S. Persistance and Patterns of Anticholinergic Therapy in Pediatric. Accepted CUAJ Jan 2016.
5. Bureau, M., Pelletier, J., Rousseau, A., Bernard, G., Chabaud, S., Bolduc, S. Demonstration of the Direct Impact of Ketamine on Urothelium Using a Tissue Engineered Bladder Model. CUAJ Sept 2015, Volume 9, Number 9-10, pages 613-17.
6. Chabaud, S., Baratange, C. Boiroux, B., Rousseau, A., Bouhout, S., Bolduc, S. Urothelial cell expansion and urothelium maturation are improved by exposition to hypoxia. JTERM sept 2015, en révision.
7. Orabi H, Rousseau A, Laterreur, V. and Bolduc S Optimization of The current self-assembled urinary bladder model: Organ-specific Stroma and Smooth muscle inclusion. CUAJ Sept 2015, Volume 9, Number 9-10, pages 599-607.
8. Chabaud S, Marcoux TL, Rousseau A, Bouhout S, Morissette A, Bernard G, Deschênes Rompré MP, Bolduc S. Lysophosphatidic acid, but not L-arginine, enhances collagen deposition and matrix thickening in engineered tissue. Journal of Tissue Engineering and Regenerative Medicine, 2015 Nov; 9(11):E65-75.
9. Rousseau A, Bernard G, Marceau Fortier G, Gauvin R, Bouhout S, Fradette J, Bolduc S; Adipose-Derived Stem Cells for the Reconstruction of a Vesical Equivalent. Journal of Tissue Engineering and Regenerative Medicine, 2015 Nov; 9(11):E135-43.
10. Bouhout S. Tremblay J., Bolduc S. Maintenance of bladder urothelia integrity and successful urothelialization of various tissue-engineered mesenchymes in vitro. In Vitro Cellular & Developmental Biology – Animal, 2015 Oct;51(9):922-31. PMID: 26091628.
11. Blais, A-S., Morin F., Moore K., Bolduc, S. Efficacy of Dextranomer Hyaluronic Acid and Polyacrylamide Hydrogel in Endoscopic Treatment of Vesicoureteral Reflux: A Comparative Study. CUAJ June 2015, Volume 9, Number 5-6, pages 202-6.
12. Bouhout S., Bolduc S Novel observations in normal bladder urothelial cells differentiation: Naimi's structure and migration. Scientific Reports (Nature), en revision.
13. Bouhout S., Bolduc S A novel and faster method to obtain a differentiated three-dimensional tissue-engineered bladder J of Urology, Sept 2015, 194 (3), 834-41.
14. Bouhout S., Chabaud S., Bolduc S Development of a spherical tissue-engineered bladder for clinical applications. Nov 2015 Biofabrication, en revision.

15. Bouhout S., Janvier R., Tremblay T., Bolduc S Organ-specific matrix self-assembled by bladder mesenchymal cells improves the normal urothelial differentiation in vitro. World Journal of Urology: Epub May 2015.
16. Gibot L., Chabaud S., Bouhout S., Bolduc S., Auger FA., Moulin VJ. Anticancer properties of chitosan on human melanoma are cell line dependant Int J Biol Macromol. 2015 Jan;72:370-9.
17. Chabaud S, Rousseau A, Marcoux TL, Bolduc S Inexpensive production of near-native engineered tissues Journal of Tissue Engineering and Regenerative Medicine, Epub May 2015.
18. Moore K, Bolduc S; Prospective Randomized Study of Endoscopic Injection for Paediatric VUR: Macroplastique vs. Deflux J of Urology, Dec 2014, Volume 192 (6), 1794-1800.
19. Nadeau G., Schröder A., Moore K., Genois L., Lamontagne P., Hamel M., Pellerin E and Bolduc S. Long-Term Use of Solifenacin in Pediatric Patients with Overactive Bladder: Extension of a Prospective Open-Label Study CUAJ Mars 2014, Vol 8 (3-4), 118-23.
20. Orabi H, Goulet C, Rousseau A, Fradette J, and Bolduc S Adipose Derived Stem Cells for Treatment of Lower Genitourinary Dysfunction Stem Cell Research and Therapy, Invited review, Volume 4 (4), March 2014.
21. Nadeau G, Schröder A, Moore K, Genois L, Lamontagne P, Hamel M, Pellerin E and Bolduc S. Double Anticholinergic Therapy for Refractory Neurogenic and Non-Neurogenic Detrusor Overactivty in Children: Long-Term Results of a Prospective Open-Label Study CUAJ May 2014, Vol 8 (5), 175-80.
22. Orabi H, Bouhout S, Morissette A, Rousseau A, Chabaud S and Bolduc S Tissue Engineering of Urinary Bladder and Urethra: Advances from Bench to Patients The Scientific World Journal, Dec 2013, Review, 13 pages.
23. Morissette A, Imbeault A, Cattan V, Bernard G, Taillon G, Chabaud S and Bolduc S Strategies to Reconstruct a Functional Urethral Substitute by Self-Assembly Method Procedia Engineering 59(2013) 193-200.
24. Bergeron M, Bolduc S, Moore K Intrascrotal Extratesticular Schwannoma: a First Pediatric Case CUAJ Mars 2014, Vol 8 (3-4), E279-81.
25. Cloutier J, Blais AS, Moore K, Bolduc S; A prospective study using a new bulking agent for the treatment of pediatric vesicoureteral reflux: Polyacrylamide Hydrogel J. of Urology 2013 Sept; 190(3): 1034-7.
26. Deschênes Rompré, M-P; Nadeau, G.; Moore, K.; Ajjaouj, Y.; Braga, L.; Bolduc, S. Learning Curve for TIP Urethroplasty: a Single Surgeon Experience CUAJ Dec 2013, Vol 7 Number 12, 789-94.
27. Imbeault A, Bernard G, Rousseau A, Morissette A, Bouhout S, Chabaud S, Bolduc S; An endothelialized urothelial cell-seeded tubular graft for urethral replacement CUAJ 2013 Jan; 7(1): E4-9.
28. Boucher A, Cloutier J, Bolduc S; Is an initial endoscopic treatment for all ureteroceles appropriate? Journal of Pediatric Urology, 9 (2013), pp. 339-343.
29. Cloutier J, Haidar N, Rompré M.P, Grimard M, Bolduc S. Study Comparing the Applicability of Dorsal Lumbotomy in Older Children. Can Urol Assoc J. 2012 Dec; 6(6): 435-39.

Book Chapters, last 3 years (9):

1. Ramsay, S. Blais, AS., Nadeau, G., Moore, K., Bolduc, S. Chapter title: Overactive Bladder in the Pediatric Population.
   Book title: *Overactive Bladder (OAB): Prevalence, Risk Factors and Management* Editor: Eric Chung, Novapublishers 2016, Invitation.
2. Chabaud S. Saba I., Jakubowska W., Bolduc S. Chapter title: New and improved tissue engineering techniques: production of exogenous material-free stroma by the self-assembly technique for urologic applications. Book title: Extracellular Matrix», ISBN 978-953-51-4747-3. Editor: By In-Tech 2016, Invitation.
3. Ingrid Saba, Hazem Orabi, Stéphane Bolduc. Title of the chapter: Stem Cell Therapy and Tissue Engineering In Genitourinary Disorders.
   Book title: Advances in Stem Cell Therapy Editor: Prof Dr Nagwa El-Badri Publisher: Springer 2015.
4. Michelle Bergeron, Anne-Sophie Blais, S Bolduc, K Moore Pyelonephritis: Risk Factors, Clinical Outcomes and Potential Complications.
   Chapitre: Vesicoureteral reflux: Diagnosis and Treatment.
   Éditeurs: Rasheed A. Balogun, Emaad M. Abdel-Rahman, and Seki A. Balogun, Novapublishers 2014.
5. Bouhout S, Jadson Moreira Pereira, Franck Simon, Stéphane Chabaud, Stéphane Bolduc, Massimo Conti, Alex Therien, Eric Rousseau, Véronique Moulin, Jean-Pierre Lavoie, Michel Rouleau and Francine Goulet.
   Production of tissue-engineered human 3D bronchi *in vitro*. Regenerative Medicine and Tissue Engineering (ISBN 978-953-51-4114-3) Éditeur: Daniel Eberly, Sous presse Déc 2014.
6. Anne-Sophie Blais, S Bolduc, K Moore Vesicoureteral Reflux: Causes, Prevalence and Treatment Approaches Ureters: Anatomy, Physiology and Disorders.
   Chapitre: Endoscopic treatment of Vesicoureteral Reflux.
   Editeurs: Richard A. Santucci and Mang Chen, Novapublishers 2014.
7. Orabi, H., R Goulet, C., Fradette, J., Bolduc, S. Adipose-Derived Stem Cells: Are They The Optimal Cell Source For Urinary Tract Regeneration? Regenerative Medicine and Tissue Engineering (ISBN 978-953-51-4114-3).
   Éditeur: Daniel Eberly, Sous presse Déc 2014.
8. Bouhout Sara, Rousseau Alexandre, Chabaud Stéphane, Morissette Amélie, Bolduc Stéphane Potential of different tissue engineering strategies in bladder reconstruction. Editeur: Daniel Eberly, By In-Tech 2013, Invitation.
9. Bouhout S., Rousseau A., Bouchard F., Morissette A. Chabaud S., Bolduc Stéphane From bench to patients: advances in genitourinary regenerative medicine. Handbook of Genitourinary Medicine: new research, by Dr Rashmi R Singh, Nova Publication. 2013, Invitation.

In: Overactive Bladder (OAB)
Editor: Elvira Larson
ISBN: 978-1-63485-033-9

Chapter 4

CURRENT UPDATES ON OVERACTIVE BLADDER MANAGEMENT

Kirin K. Syed, DO, and Angelo E. Gousse, MD
Bladder Health and Reconstructive Urology Institute,
Miramar FL, US

ABSTRACT

The manuscript will provide the reader with a better understanding of the diagnosis and available treatment options for refractory non-neurogenic overactive bladder (OAB).

Non-neurogenic OAB is a symptom complex, which is defined by the International Continence Society (ICS) standardization committee as urgency, with or without urgency incontinence, usually with frequency and nocturia, in the absence of proven infection or other obvious pathology. It is diagnosed by patient symptomatology and does not rely on urodynamic findings and characteristics.

Previously published literature has estimated that approximately 16.5% of American adults have OAB and up to 37% of OAB patients have concomitant urinary incontinence (OAB-wet). In fact, OAB is one the most common urologic disorders, accounting for more than 2 million physician office visits in the United States (2007).

To date, there is a paucity of validated instruments to define urinary urgency and therefore there is no consensus on an appropriate definition of "refractory" OAB. The diagnosis is based on clinical judgment and management is often at the discretion of the clinician due to a lack of standardized and established clinical care pathways to guide the clinician and the patient.

The current established approaches for refractory OAB has been on third line options as outlined by the most recent American Urologic Association and Society of Urodynamics, Female pelvic medicine and Urogenital reconstruction (AUA/SUFU) guidelines.

Of these options, the pharmacologic use of onabotulinumtoxinA (Botox®) has the strongest rating of "standard" (strength of evidence grade B) and was recently approved by the FDA in 2013 for use in patients with OAB who did not adequately respond to oral medications. Other third line options include neuromodulation with posterior tibial nerve stimulation and sacral nerve modulation. These modalities received a rating of "recommended" (strength of evidence grade C) and will be discussed in greater detail in this manuscript.

INTRODUCTION

Non-neurogenic overactive bladder (OAB) syndrome is a chronic bothersome, debilitating condition that can have a significant impact on health-related quality of life (HRQL) and can be associated with considerable social and financial burden. Previously known as "idiopathic" OAB, it is a non-life threatening symptom complex. Previous studies have reported the negative impact of OAB on patients including less work productivity, higher rates of depressive symptoms less sexual satisfaction, erectile dysfunction and lower levels of overall health [1, 2].

Non-neurogenic OAB is a symptom complex, which is defined by the International Continence Society (ICS) standardization committee as urgency, with or without urgency incontinence, usually with frequency and nocturia, in the absence of proven infection or other obvious pathology [4]. It is important to note that urgency is the cornerstone component of OAB. Urgency with at least one other symptom is essential to diagnose OAB [13]. It is diagnosed by patient symptomatology and does not rely on urodynamic findings and characteristics. The most common symptomatic components of OAB include urgency, frequency, nocturia and urgency incontinence.

OAB is a costly disorder and total national cost, including community and institutional costs, was estimated at $65.9 billion in 2007 ($49.1 billion direct medical, $2.3 billion direct nonmedical, and $14.6 billion indirect) and total national costs are expected to increase to $82.6 billion by 2020, an increase of 25.3% [3]. In 2007, OAB was one the most common urologic disorders, accounting for more than 2 million physician office visits in the United States [4].

Urodynamically, OAB is characterized by the presence of involuntary bladder contractions (detrusor overactivity) that occur during bladder filling despite the patient's attempt to suppress them. Specifically, non- neurogenic detrusor overactivity (DO) refers to involuntary detrusor contractions noted in neurologically intact patients while neurogenic detrusor overactivity refers to those with an associated neurological disorder. DO may be spontaneous or provoked and may be demonstrated independent of sensation. DO in of itself is strictly a urodynamic finding and therefore distinct from OAB symptoms. Furthermore patients with OAB symptoms do not always demonstrate DO during urodynamic evaluation. OAB that is accompanied with urge incontinence is commonly referred to as OAB-wet whereas OAB without urge incontinence as OAB-dry.

NOMENCLATURE AND TERMINOLOGY

In addressing OAB it is essential to review the common set of definitions and terminology specific to OAB as standardized by the ICS. In 2002 [6] and then revised in 2010 [4], the International Continence Society (ICS) derived specific terminology and definitions to standardize terminology. (Note: nomenclature utilized in this manuscript is in accordance with the most up to date, 2010 ICS terminology).

Symptoms of OAB occur during the filling/storage phase of micturition and are commonly referred to as storage lower urinary tract symptoms (LUTS). Some of the most common symptoms are listed below.

- *Urgency* is a sudden compelling desire to void that is difficult to defer. It has been shown to be the strongest predictor of bother associated with OAB with the most impact on patients [7]. The compelling desire to void is associated with the fear of urinary leakage. Patients often fear that if they do not void, they will have an episode of incontinence. Urgency is also a symptom associated with other syndromes such as bladder pain syndrome (BPS). The key difference in urgency associated with OAB and BPS is the anxiety associated with deferment of voiding. While OAB patients fear urinary incontinence, BPS patients fear the pain and discomfort that is associated with bladder distension during filling and therefore often report dissipation of pain with voiding.
- *Nocturia* is the complaint of interruption of sleep one or more times due to the need to micturate. Each void is preceded and followed by sleep. It is important to differentiate nocturia from nocturnal polyuria and sleep disorders including sleep apnea, which have different pathophysiological etiologies.
- *Daytime urinary frequency* is a subjective perception by the patient that he/she voids too often by day. Healthy adults generally void every 3 to 4 hours with a normal fluid intake (approximately 64 ounces of fluid daily). There is no established number of voids to adequately define daytime frequency. Previously published clinical trials used a threshold of >8 void per day.
- *Urinary incontinence* (UI) is the involuntary loss of urine and *urgency urinary incontinence* (UUI) is involuntary loss of urine associated with urgency.

Prevalence

Determination of prevalence has proved to be challenging due several factors including subjective assessment of symptoms, data acquisition methods, variations in epidemiological studies and criteria utilized to define OAB. Since standardization of ICS terminology, several studies have attempted to determine the prevalence of OAB and lower urinary tract symptoms (LUTS).

The National Overactive BLadder Evaluation (NOBLE) study [7] estimated that approximately 16.5% of American adults have OAB and up to 37% of OAB patients have concomitant urinary incontinence (UI). Additionally "OAB dry" was noted to be more prevalent in men while "OAB wet" had a higher prevalence in women.

The EPIC study [8], based on the 2002 ICS definitions, reported an overall prevalence of OAB of 11.8% in 5 countries (Canada and four European countries) with nocturia being the most prevalent lower urinary tract symptom.

The EpiLUTs study [9] also based on the 2002 ICS definitions, reported storage symptoms associated with OAB were more prevalent in women than men with urgency and nocturia being the most prevalent in a general population study of USA, UK and Sweden. Data collected from the US indicated that 27% of men and 43% of women have OAB symptoms at least "sometimes" and 16% of men and 33% of women have OAB symptoms at least "often."

OAB has been shown to be a progressive chronic disorder [10] associated with aging and with symptoms of OAB dry preceding and progressing to OAB wet.

Risk Factors

The etiology and risk factors for OAB are not clearly established. However multiple studies have reported several factors that have been associated with OAB and urinary incontinence including age, gender, ethnicity, race, dietary and lifestyle factors, parity and medical and metabolic comorbidities such as diabetes, obesity and constipation [10, 11, 12].

Micturition Cycle

In addressing OAB it is essential to review the normal micturition cycle and establish a common set of definitions and nomenclature specific to OAB.

The lower urinary tract comprises of the bladder, the bladder neck, prostate (in men), urethra, urethral meatus and two urethral sphincters, the internal (smooth muscle) sphincter at the bladder neck and proximal urethra and the external (striated muscle) sphincter of the membranous urethra. These interrelated structures function together in a series of coordinated events that ensure bladder filling, urine storage without leakage and periodic volitional expulsion of urine to completion, all at low pressure. This coordinated effort is the micturition cycle and regulated primarily by the rostral brainstem where the pontine micturition center (a.k.a Barrington's nucleus) resides. Any dysfunction in the lower urinary tract can lead to a disruption of normal voiding.

The micturition cycle is usually divided into two separate and discrete phases which are under neuronal control [13].

1. Bladder filling/urine storage and
2. Bladder emptying/voiding.

The symptoms of the various dysfunctions in voiding are based upon deregulation of these two phases. Overall, bladder overactivity results in frequent urination, often before the bladder has reached full capacity.

The micturition cycle is a complex neuronal circuit system with several interconnecting pathways between the central and peripheral nervous systems. Attempts to describe this complicated neurophysiological system have been made by Wein, De Groat, Steers, Bradley's "loop system," Blaivas, Holstege and Griffiths [14]. Opinions regarding control of micturition mechanisms, reflex arcs and supraspinal connections vary and are at times contradictory. However, some key principles are generally agreed upon and are described below.

Inhibition of the voiding reflex is mediated by the sympathetic nervous system. This is required during the storage phase and is mainly facilitated by the sympathetic nervous system. During storage, the hypogastric nerve releases noradrenaline, which activates β-adrenergic inhibitory receptors in the detrusor muscle resulting in relaxation of the bladder. Concurrently, both smooth and striated urethral sphincters are activated to prevent involuntary bladder emptying and leakage. This is referred to as the "guarding reflex" [15].

Bladder filling and urine storage is a passive process with a gradual increase of volume under low pressure. This is referred to as bladder "compliance" and requires a closed bladder outlet to prevent leakage of urine and absence of DO. The sensation to void once the bladder has reached capacity is triggered by an intact neural pathway.

Voiding involves coordinated contractions of the detrusor muscles, increasing bladder pressure that is less than 40cm H2O to prevent upper tract damage, relaxation of the smooth and striated sphincters and subsequent active expulsion of urine without anatomic obstruction. Efferent nerves and interstitial cells trigger bladder contractility.

Activation of the voiding reflex commences the emptying phase and requires inhibition of storage reflexes. This is primarily mediated by cholinergic factors released by the parasympathetic Pelvic nerve and act as the major excitatory mechanism in the human bladder. Acetylcholine binds to bladder muscarinic receptors, mainly M2 and M3, and result in detrusor contraction [15].

The striated muscles of the external urethral sphincter are under somatic cholinergic control via motor nerves that arise in S2–S4 motor neurons in Onuf's nucleus and reach the periphery through the Pudendal nerve [15].

In regards to sensation, afferent input to the spinal cord from the bladder and urethra occur via the pelvic nerve and dorsal root ganglia whereas afferent input from the striated sphincteric muscle and pelvic floor occur via the pudendal nerve.

A.

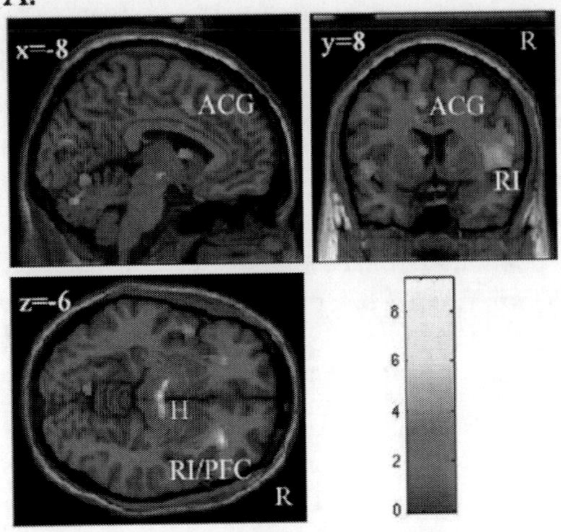

Figure 1. (continued).

B.

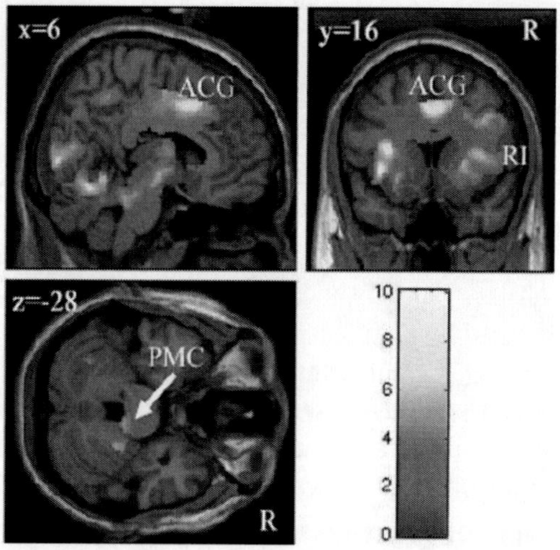

Griffiths D, Tadic SD, Schaefer W, Resnick NM. Cerebral control of the bladder in normal and urge-incontinent women. *NeuroImage*. 2007;37(1):1-7.

Figure 1. A. Responses to bladder infusion in normal controls at large bladder volumes. B. Responses to bladder infusion in subjects with urge incontinence at large bladder volumes B. Insular response is RI = right insula; ACG = anterior cingulate gyrus; H = hypothalamus; RI/. PFC = right anterior insula and/or lateral prefrontal cortex. R = right side. Color bar shows scale of student's t values.

The afferent components consist of myelinated (Aδ) and unmyelinated (C) axons. The Aδ -fibers convey information of bladder filling during the storage phase. They respond to passive distension. The C-fibers act on vanilloid receptors and respond to noxious stimuli such as chemical irritation. They are otherwise insensitive to bladder distension [15]. Vanilloid receptors have been associated with detrusor overactivity and increased expression of the TRPV1 receptor has been found in OAB patients [69].

The increasingly important role of the urothelium and the suburothelial layers of the bladder in signal transduction and the afferent input via the release of cytokines and other mediators has been shown in recent new data. Better understanding these sensory pathways is becoming more relevant as theoretically perceived hypersentivitiy associated with OAB maybe the product of increased sensory activity [12].

Due to lack of anatomic abnormality, OAB is considered a functional rather than anatomical or structural disorder. OAB has been likened to other functional disorders such as irritable bowel syndrome and both are associated with abnormal perception or interpretation of physiologic events by the brain. This is supported by a recent study that compared Functional Magnetic Resonance Imaging (fMRI) in women and with and without OAB. Increased brain activation associated with increased urinary urgency was noted in the Insula and Anterior Cingulate Gyrus (ACG) in the Limbic Cortex in patients with OAB compared to those without OAB. Results of this study are congruous with a similar study performed on patient with neurogenic DO [16, 17] (Figure 1).

MANAGEMENT

Non-neurogenic OAB is a syndrome complex without a perfect treatment and often may be challenging to manage. While there are various first, second and third line options to choose from, it is perhaps management of patient expectation that is paramount and a necessary first step prior to embarking on a treatment plan.

While OAB can have significant impact on QoL, it usually does not affect survival. The risks and benefits of therapy should be clearly and concisely discussed and reviewed with the patient. Potential benefits of treatment should be carefully weighed against possible adverse side effects. In addition, patients should be made aware that given OAB is non-life threatening, "no treatment" is an acceptable option. No treatment may be preferred in certain special patient population such as the old, frail and very elderly or those with dementia or other cognitive defects [15, 20].

If treatment is pursued, then it is essential to convey to the patient that the goal of treatment is to improve symptoms and therefore improve quality of life however 100% resolution of symptoms or "cure" can be an unrealistic goal and may not occur. The ideal regimen is often determined by a "trial and error" approach to ensure the patient obtains the most effect and benefit from the chosen therapy. This may require trials of multiple therapeutic options and dose adjustments with close follow up before adequate symptom control is achieved. Patient should also be made aware that treatment is generally life-long and benefits are reversible. Non- compliance or discontinuation of therapy will likely result in return to baseline bothersome symptoms.

Treatment should be initiated when the patient desires and treatment regimens are individualized and based upon the patient's unique and specific response (or lack thereof) to treatment options. Furthermore, therapy and treatment options should be approached in a step-wise fashion starting with first line options as determined by the AUA/SUFU Guidelines published in 2012 and amended in 2014 [19, 20]. The following discussion is in accordance with these guidelines.

FIRST LINE THERAPY: LIFESTYLE MODIFICATION AND BEHAVIOR THERAPIES

Treatment for OAB is broadly subdivided into two classifications: non-pharmacological and pharmacological.

Non- pharmacological, non-invasive, cost effective treatment options with limited side effects include lifestyle changes, dietary modification and behavioral therapies. Lifestyle changes pertain to fluid management, weight loss and smoking cessation while behavior therapies focus on bladder training, maneuvers to control bladder behavior and pelvic floor muscle training. These are the recommended standard first line therapies for OAB. These therapeutic options require active participation of the patient, family/care givers with support, encouragement and frequent follow up with the clinician. Additionally any and all components may be utilized simultaneously and must be tailored to the patient's unique and individual requirements.

Highlighted in the AUA/SUFU Guidelines [19, 20] are several previously published literature reviews of randomized trials comparing the effectiveness of various behavioral therapeutic options and medications. The results indicated that behavioral treatment was generally either equivalent or superior to medications in terms of reducing episodes of incontinence episodes and improving voiding parameters such as frequency and nocturia as well as improving QoL [19, 20].

Lifestyle and Dietary Modifications

- Fluid management: while water is the preferred fluid for OAB patients, the volume consumed per 24 hours should be monitored. The recommended fluid intake is reduction in fluid of 25% [15, 20] or 30mL/kg/day [21].
- Bladder irritants: there are several agents commonly consumed that are known bladder irritants. These include alcohol, carbonated beverages caffeine, spicy and acidic foods. Therefore intake of these should be moderated to limit exacerbation of OAB symptoms
    - Caffeine is known stimulant of detrusor muscle contraction and therefore intake should be limited to <400 mg/day.
- Weight loss: Obesity has a tremendous socioeconomic imprint and is a major contributor to multiple medical comorbidities in today's medical climate. Several well-organized epidemiological studies have identified obesity as a strong independent risk factor for urinary incontinence in women [22]. Consequently, several studies have shown that weight loss has been associated with a reduction in episodes of urinary incontinence [23, 24] and therefore must be discussed with the patient during OAB counseling.
- Nocturia: factors that can effect or worsen nocturia include evening fluid consumption, timing of medications and peripheral edema. To counter these, patients should be recommended to cease fluid intake 2 hours prior to bedtime and encouraged to consume the majority of their daily fluid intake in the morning and afternoon. In addition, timing of diuretic medications should be attenuated so that they are taken during daytime waking hours instead of bedtime. Finally patients suffering from peripheral edema are encouraged to elevate lower extremities to stimulate reabsorption of third spaced fluid and stimulate natural diuresis [26].
- Tobacco cessation: smoking has been shown to increase the risk of urinary incontinence. Nicotine is a known bladder irritant. Additionally, coughing due to smoking can increase risk of stress incontinence as well as urgency and urge incontinence.
- Bowel function: constipation has been associated dysfunction detrusor function and urinary incontinence [21]. Patients are encouraged to keep bowel function regulated with use of dietary fiber well-balanced meals and fluid intake.

Behavioral Therapy

This non-pharmacological treatment option consists of two components: one which tailors voiding habits and the other that concentrates on bladder training.

- Modifying voiding habits can be achieved via scheduled (timed) voiding, double voiding to ensure complete bladder emptying which facilitates in increasing time between voids, delayed voiding and monitoring voiding patterns with a bladder diary.
- Bladder training focuses on pelvic floor muscle training and rehabilitation to re-establish and improve control over the bladder and to suppress and resist urgency.
    - Pelvic floor rehabilitation includes performing exercises devised by Arnold Kegel to strength the muscles of the pelvic floor. This results in modification of the pelvic floor reflex, which can help temper detrusor contractions and urinary urgency. These Kegel exercises must be performed regularly and requires patience as symptomatic improvement may takes several weeks to months. Therefore this therapy should be offered to highly motivated patients with mild to moderate OAB symptoms.
    - Urge suppression strategies include performing "quick flicks" which are short successive contractions of the pelvic floor. Such contractions have been shown to have a reflexive inhibitory effect on detrusor overactivity. Additional techniques include avoiding the bathroom during an urge episode and delaying voiding until the urge has passed as well. Other tactics such as relaxation techniques with deep breathing are also recommended.

Behavioral therapy may be combined with pharmacological treatment to optimize symptom control. Timing of starting dual modality treatment is based on discretion of the clinician and patient feedback.

SECOND LINE THERAPY: PHARMACOLOGIC TREATMENT

Pharmacological management with anti- muscarinics (AM) or β3-adrenoceptor agonists (BA) are recommended second line treatment options.

The choice of which agent to start therapy with relies on the clinician and is based on the clinician's judgment of the patient's overall urological status, potential contraindications and cost analysis. A therapeutic trial of a minimum of 4 weeks and generally lasting 6-8 weeks, is typically instituted for the chosen agent. After the trial period, symptoms are re-evaluated before the chosen agent is deemed a success or failure.

Of note, current guidelines lack algorithms and evidence- based recommendations on length of treatment utilizing second line pharmacological agents and number of medications to attempt prior to moving forward with third line therapies.

If the medication does not adequately improve the patient's urinary symptoms, or the patient incurs unacceptable, bothersome side effects (SE) then the patient may benefit from dose modification or a different agent based on the clinician's assessment.

Medications should be started at the lowest available dose and titrated gradually. If symptom improvement is noted along with adverse side effects, then it is recommended to manage the SE prior to abandoning the therapy. This is of great importance to increase tolerability of the medication and ensure patient compliance.

Management may include increasing fiber intake, eating well balanced meals and exercising to counter constipation while oral lubricants, chewing sugar-free gum or eating sugar-free candy and using non-alcohol based mouthwashes may curb dry mouth symptoms.

Finally, extended release and long acting formulations are preferred over immediate release and they have been shown to have a more favorable adverse effect profile [15, 20, 70]. Additionally, transdermal preparations such as oxybutynin patch (Oxy-TDS, Oxytrol®) and oxybutynin topical gel (Oxy-TDS, Gelnique®) have shown similar efficacy as the oral drug with reduced systemic side effects due to bypass of first metabolism [27]. An additional advantage is less frequent dosing of transdermal agents.

Antimuscarinics

There are 5 known subtypes of the muscarinic receptor- M1, M2, M3, M4 and M5. The most abundant and predominate receptor is M2, however M3 mediates smooth muscle contraction, including bladder detrusor muscle.

Anticholinergic agents act to inhibit primarily M3 receptors thereby inhibiting the effects of acetylcholine on nicotinic or muscarinic receptors in the peripheral and central nervous system (CNS).

This results in suppression of detrusor contractions and decreases episodes and severity of urgency while increasing bladder capacity and time between voids [22]. They have been shown to decrease urinary urge incontinence, and frequency of urgency symptoms but have not shown to have a significant clinical impact on nocturia.

Randomized controlled trials have demonstrated comparable efficacy for several agents including (in alphabetical order): darifenacin, fesoterodine, oxybutynin (also available as transdermal patch and gel), solifenacin, tolterodine and trospium. These agents vary in pharmacological and chemical formulation but have all been shown to improve bladder capacity, modulate and decrease involuntary detrusor contractions, urgency, and frequency.

These agents have been endorsed by AUA/SUFU guidelines [19, 20] as acceptable second line agents and have been granted a grade A recommendation by the International Continence Society (ICS) [21].

Other agents including hyoscyamine sulfate (Levsin) and hyoscine hydrobromide (Scopolamine) are infrequently used and are not FDA approved for use in OAB. There are no reported head-to-head comparisons of these agents to another drug for OAB. Scopolamine was shown to be superior to placebo in women with OAB, however there are no placebo-controlled trials for Levsin [18].

Muscarinic receptors are ubiquitous and found in vital organs such as brain, salivary glands, gastrointestional system and eyes. Due to cross reactivity, adverse side effects range from dry eyes, blurred vision, dry mouth, constipation and impaired cognitive function. The adverse side effect profile varies with each agent and the degree of bother varies with individual patients. They are contraindicated in patients with narrow angle glaucoma, gastroparesis or those taking potassium supplements or oral potassium chloride as AMs can potentially decrease bowel motility thereby causing increase in absorption and hyperkalemic states.

The rate of urinary retention associated with these agents is relatively low and incidence of retention has been reported to be <5% [27]. Care must be taken when prescribing these agents to patients with incomplete bladder emptying and are contradicted in patients with urinary retention.

In addition, caution should be taken when prescribing AM to patients taking other agents with anti-cholinergic properties such as tricyclic antidepressants, medications for Alzheimer's disease, Parkinson's and other extra-pyramidal diseases as well as acetylcholinesterase inhibitors and select anti-emetics.

Previous studies have shown low long-term compliance and tolerability rate for anticholinergic therapy with almost 50% of patients failing to refill their initial prescription and only 8-29% continuing their prescribed therapy for 1 year. In addition compliance and adherence to medical regimen was noted to be higher for extended release than immediate release agents [29-34].

β3-Adrenoceptor Agonists (BA)

Mirabegron is the first in this class of medications that was FDA approved to treat OAB in 2012. It has shown similar efficacy to the anti-muscarinic class with lower rates of dry mouth and constipation.

There are 3 subtypes of β adrenoreceptors (AR), β1, β2 and β3. Of the 3, it is the β3-AR that has shown to be predominately expressed in human detrusor muscle. Mirabegron acts as an agonist with a high, almost exclusive selectivity for the β3-AR.

When stimulated, the β3-AR promotes detrusor relaxation during the storage cycle of micturition and has shown to increase cystometric capacity [35. The proposed pathway involves activation of adenyl cyclase, G proteins and increased levels of cyclic adenosine monophosphate which contribute to urine storage [35, 36]. Other hypothesized effects of β3-AR agonist include alteration in sensation by inhibition of efferent and afferent detrusor pathways via release of nitric oxide. Previous studies in rats demonstrated that β3-AR agonist can reduce bladder non-voiding micro-contractions that may have a role in sensory urgency. In addition, Mirabegron was shown to inhibit micro-contractions and Aδ fibers at low doses in rat urothelium and additionally inhibited C-fibers at higher doses, an effect that was not seen with Oxybutynin [35].

The efficacy and safety of Mirabegron has been previously demonstrated in randomized controlled trials [36-40]. Other β3-AR agonists currently in development and undergoing clinical trials include Ritobegron and Solabegron [41].

Since Mirabegron's mechanism of action is unique, the side effect profile is unlike that of antimuscarinics. The most common drug-related side effects associated with Mirabegron include hypertension and headache. When compared to placebo, an approximately 1 mmHg or less in systolic/diastolic blood pressure was noted along with a mean difference of one beat per minute for pulse rate. These were comparable to the incidence with placebo and tolterodine. The incidence of other anticholingeric related side effects such as dry mouth were less than tolterodine and equivalent to placebo [27, 37- 40].

OTHER AGENTS

Phosphodiesterase Type 5 Inhibitors (PDE5I)

The PDE5Is class is a new addition to the treatment armamentarium for BPH-LUTS in male voiding dysfunction. Tadalafil (Cialis®) was approved by the FDA in 2011 for concomitant treatment of BPH and erectile dysfunction. Other PDE5I's such as Vardenafil (Staxyn®, Levitra®) and Sildenafil (Viagra®) were all studied for their effects in reducing LUTS; however, in the United States, only Tadalafil received approval for this indication.

PDE5 receptors have found to be expressed and biologically active at the bladder neck, prostatic urethra and prostate, with a predominance at the bladder neck [41, 43, 44].

The addition of PDE5-I to treatment regimens showed improvement in continence after radical prostatectomy as well as improvement in urodynamic parameters in men with spinal cord injury [44, 45, 46].

The pathophysiology of male LUTs is complex and poorly understood. Several etiologies have been proposed such as impaired nitric oxide/cyclic guanosine monophosphate (NO/cGMP) signaling pathway, pelvic ischemia, autonomic overactivity, increased RhoA/Rho-kinase pathway activation and increased bladder/prostate afferent activity [41, 43, 44].

The exact mechanism of action of PDE5Is on detrusor muscle is unknown, however it is believed that this agent plays some part in all of the above mentioned factors. Some proposed effects include increasing the signaling of the NO/cGMP pathway resulting in reduction of smooth muscle tone in the lower urinary tract. Additionally, up-regulation of the Rho-kinase pathway has been associated with outflow obstruction, diabetic cystopathy and non-neurogenic detrusor overactivity [41] and these effects could be counteracted by PDE5-Is [43]. PDE5-Is have also been shown to improve arterial blood flow thereby countering pelvic ischemia that may be secondary to pelvic artery insufficiency, caused by metabolic syndrome and artheroscleorsis of hypertension [41-46].

Common side effects of these agents include headache, back pain, dizziness and dyspepsia. They are contraindicated in patients who use nitrates, and should be used with caution in patients treated with alpha-blockers as the combination may lead to hypotension.

Tadalafil is contraindicated in patients with a history of non-arteritic anterior ischemic optic neuropathy.

Finally it is recommended that the patient's cardiac status be assessed prior to prescribing this medication.

Tricyclic Antidepressants

TCAs are potent inhibitors of muscarinic, α-adrenergic and histamine H1 receptors [28]. They also inhibit norepinephrine and serotonin reuptake at nerve terminals and facilitate urinary storage by decreasing detrusor contractility and increasing bladder outlet resistance. Imipramine also has a local anesthetic effect on bladder mucosa.

The most commonly used agents in OAB are imipramine (Tofranil) or amitriptyline (Elavil). These agents do not have FDA approval for use in OAB and therefore their use is considered "off label."

The side effect profile is similar to other antimuscarinics including dry mouth, constipation and drowsiness. These agents should be used with care as they have been associated with serious side effects including arrhythmia, QT prolongation and urinary retention [28].

Propiverine

This is a dual action drug. It has components of nonselective antimuscarinic activity and calcium channel−blocking effects. Proposed mechanism of action is similar to other antimuscarinics with the addition of cellular calcium influx inhibition. It results in decrease of muscle contractions and spasm. Efficacy of propiverine has been demonstrated to be comparable to that of solifenacin, tolterodine and oxybutynin. Combination therapy with alpha-blockers in men with LUTs from BPH showed similar or superior efficacy than with alpha-blocker alone. The adverse event profile is similar to those associated with other antimuscarinic agents with dry mouth being the most frequently reported. No negative effects on cardiac function have been reported such as changes in QTc interval or arrhythmias [28, 47].

Desmopressin

Desmopressin (DDAVP) is a synthetic form of vasopressin- the antidiuretic hormone. It has primary use in the treatment of diabetes insipidous but has also been used for short- term treatment of nocturia and nocturnal enuresis in both children and adults. The intranasal formulation is no longer recommended due to reported side effects of severe hyponatremia and seizures. Other significant adverse events (particularly in the elderly) include fluid retention, hyponatremia, and worsening of underlying cardiac failure which make this agent a challenge to use [28].

Third Line Therapy

The current established third line options include neuromodulation and chemodenervation as outlined by the most recent American Urologic Association and Society of Urodynamics, Female pelvic medicine and Urogenital reconstruction (AUA/SUFU) guidelines [19, 20].

These options are offered to patients with refractory OAB symptoms despite treatment with antimuscarinics, have failed behavioral and/or pharmacologic therapy, were unable to tolerate or are not candidates for second line therapies.

Neuromodulation includes posterior tibial nerve stimulation and sacral nerve modulation. These modalities received a rating of "recommended" (strength of evidence grade C).

Chemodenervation is accomplished by pharmacologic use of onabotulinumtoxinA (Botox®). This modality was approved by the FDA in 2013 for use in patients with non-neurogenic OAB who did not adequately respond to oral medications. This therapeutic agent was recently upgraded and received the stronger rating of "standard" (strength of evidence grade B) by the amended 2014 AUA/SUFU guidelines [19].

Neuromodulation

This modality includes percutaneous posterior tibial nerve stimulation (PTNS) and sacral neuromodulation (SNS).

PTNS

Urgent PC® (Cogentix, Minnetonka, MN) is a minimally invasive neuromodulation system that delivers retrograde stimulation to the sacral nerve plexus through percutaneous electrical stimulation of the posterior tibial nerve via a 34-gauge needle. It results in central and peripheral suppression of efferent nerve activity thereby modulating detrusor activity. The patient is typically treated in an office setting once per week for 30 minutes for a period of 12 weeks. Periodic reevaluation of symptoms assists in determining success of treatment.

Multi institute randomized controlled trials and sham studies have demonstrated that compared to placebo, PTNS significantly improved symptoms of OAB and voiding parameters [41] and had comparable improvement in symptoms when compared with tolterodine ER 2-4 mg daily [49].

Of all the third line options, it has been found to be the most cost effective alternative [50] and longer follow-up studies have shown durability of treatment effects with on-going maintenance therapy at tapering intervals [51].

This type of therapy requires active participation by motivated patients who are willing to come to office weekly for 12 weeks, are willing to accept maintenance therapy and willing to accept low "cure/dry" rates.

Contraindications include: patients who are pregnant or planning to become pregnant while using therapy, patients with pacemakers or implantable defibrillators, patients prone to excessive bleeding and patients with nerve damage that could impact either percutaneous tibial nerve or pelvic floor function.

This type of therapy may not be ideal for special patient populations such as those with peripheral nerve injury, severe peripheral edema, morbid obesity and amputees.

SNS

Sacral neuromodulation directly stimulates the sacral plexus via the S3 nerve root. The Interstim ™ neuromodulator (Medtronic, Minneapolis, MN) is a peripherally implanted stimulator that utilizes electrical impulses to alter or modulate the S3 peripheral nerve. While the exact mechanism of action is not completely understood, effects on the lower urinary tract and pelvic nervous system are thought to occur via activation of somatic afferent nerves that alter bladder sensory pathways and inhibit reflex bladder hyperactivity [21].

The Interstim™ neuromodulator received FDA approval in 1997 for use in urinary urge incontinence. In 1999 it was approved for use of urinary urgency, frequency and non-obstructive urinary retention. Most recently it was approved for use in fecal incontinence in 2011.

Placement of the device is a minimally invasive procedure that has been described previously [52] and is typically staged. The patient initially undergoes a trial period with a tined permanent lead inserted into the S3 sacral foramen connected to an external stimulator (stage 1). This is usually done in an outpatient surgical setting. A variation can be performed in- office under local anesthesia at which time a thin wire (temporary lead) is placed into the S3 foramen instead of the permanent tined lead. This is referred to as peripheral nerve evaluation (PNE) and maybe performed with or without the use of fluoroscopy. Placement of the lead or PNE wire is confirmed by sensory and motor responses as confirmed by the patient. Correct lead placement will result in motor responses such as bellowing of the perineum and plantar flexion of the ipsilateral great toe. Sensory responses include patient report of pulling sensation of rectum with extension of sensation into vagina or labia (women) or scrotum (men).

A malpositioned lead may cause stimulation of S2 as evidenced by ipsilateral leg/hip rotation and plantar flexion of the foot while S4 stimulation will result in perineal bellowing without lower extremity motor response.

The trial period then extends for 7-14 days based on clinician preference during which time the patient's symptoms are monitored and evaluated closely. A 50% or more improvement in baseline symptoms is considered a success at which time the permanent lead (if PNE performed) and stimulator battery (implantable pulse generator or IPG) is placed under sedation in the operating room. If an unacceptable response is noted, then the lead or wire can be removed easily and atraumatically.

Success rate and efficacy of the Interstim ™ System has been demonstrated by one prospective, multicenter post-approval study that reported OAB therapeutic success rate of 85% at 12 months and statistically significant improvement in parameters of urinary incontinence and frequency. In addition 80% of the study patients reported improvement of their baseline voiding pattern at 12 months [53].

Similar results were reported by Moon et al. [54] who reported significant improvement in multiple voiding parameters at 12 months post-implant including episodes of daily urgency, urgency incontinence, severity of urgency episodes, daytime and night time micturition.

Adverse events of device placement have been reviewed extensively. Some of the most common AE's include lead migration, implant or lead site pain/infection, unexpected and undesirable change in stimulation/electric shock [19, 20, 52, 53].

Special considerations include patient selection and pre-procedural counseling. The initial trial period (PNE or stage 1) requires significant restricted activity including refraining from showering and bathing which may be bothersome to some patients. In addition patients should also be counseled on need for periodic battery replacements and therefore long-term treatment compliance is necessary.

This therapeutic option also requires cognitively intact patients who are capable of adjusting and optimizing their device settings.

Additional considerations: the equipment is costly and support from the local representative of the Medtronic company is necessary to ensure optimal patient care. Finally, MRI studies are contraindicated in patients with implanted Interstim™ device.

Chemodenervation

Chemodenervation is accomplished by pharmacologic use of intradetrusor onabotulinumtoxinA, a purified neurotoxin from *Clostridium botulinum*. It stems from the Latin word botulus, which means "sausage" as it was associated with "sausage poisoning" in the 18th century and lead to the term botulinum that was coined in Germany in 1870.

Today it has found many uses in the medical field from cosmetics to neurological disorders such cervical dystonia, blepharospasms, chronic migraine and upper limb spasticity. The first reported use of botulinum toxin in the lower urinary tract was in 1987, when it was injected into the external sphincter muscle to treat detrusor-external sphincter dyssynergia [62, 63].

This modality was approved by the FDA in 2011 for intra detrusor injection for neurogenic OAB. It was subsequently approved for urgency incontinence and non-neurogenic OAB in 2013. It was approved for use in patients with OAB who did not adequately respond to oral medications. This therapeutic agent was recently upgraded and received the stronger rating of "standard" (strength of evidence grade B) by the amended 2014 AUA/SUFU guidelines [19].

OnabotulinumtoxinA inhibits vesicle mediated neurotransmission by cleaving the SNARE protein SNAP-25, preventing docking and fusion of vesicles with the nerve terminal. This inhibits acetylcholine release from efferent nerves thereby causing relaxation of the detrusor muscle resulting in reversible muscle relaxation and weakness for several months.

There are seven serotypes of botulinum toxin (A–G). Botulinum toxin type A is the most commonly utilized in the lower urinary tract. Two formulations have been studied extensively, those manufactured as onabotulinumtoxinA (Botox®, Allergan, Inc., Irvine, CA, USA) and abobotulinumtoxinA (Dysport®, Ipsen Biopharm Ltd, Slough, UK) [62, 65]. Each formulation has its own specific dosing and these are not interchangeable. Our discussion focuses on Botox® (Allergan, Inc., Irvine, CA, USA) which is currently in use in the United States whereas Dysport® is available in Europe.

While various techniques for injection have been described [57, 58, 65] principle concepts include the following:

- Maximum cumulative dose should not exceed 360 U in a 3-month interval in adults. Therefore if patient is receiving Botox injection for other medical disorders such a

migraines, care must be coordinated between clinicians. In addition it is recommended that all Botox injections be performed within the same week.

- Prophylactic antibiotics for cystoscopy with manipula-tion are recommended by American Urological Association guidelines for all patients [66].
- Using a flexible or rigid cystoscope, injection needle is inserted approximately 2 mm into the detrusor in a trigone sparing manner.
- Injections are spaced approximately 1 cm apart and evenly distributed.
- The dose of Botox® varies with diagnosis. For non-neurogenic OAB 100 units are injected while neurogenic patients received 200 units.

Many clinicians are modifying their current injection technique to incorporate the trigone. Recent new published literature has demonstrated that including the trigone results in superior continence rates with improved incontinence noted in both neurogenic and non-neurogenic patients, although less effect was noted on urodynamic parameters in these studies [59-62].

A Phase 3, placebo controlled trial reported that when compared to placebo, intradetrusor Botox® significantly decreased the daily frequency of urinary incontinence and was associated with higher rates of complete continence [55]. In addition, long term follow up studies of idiopathic OAB show persistent durability with consistent reductions in urinary incontinence and improvement in urinary parameters with repeat injections [56].

Special considerations include patient selection and pre-procedural counseling. Patients must be counseled on risk of developing urinary retention, UTIs and must be informed that this is not a "permanent" solution and requires re-treatment every 3-6 months or as needed for return of baseline bothersome urinary symptoms.

Common adverse events include urinary tract infection and urinary retention with elevated PVRs.

Urinary retention requiring clean intermittent catheterization (CIC) was defined in many studies as an inability to void or a residual above 150–200mL causing urinary symptoms. A urinary retention rate of 6-7% has been shown in clinical trials [67]. Therefore pre-procedure counseling is imperative and patients should be counseled on technique of self-catheterization as well as educated on recognizing signs and symptoms of urinary retention which include inability to void, worsening incontinence, urgency and or frequency indicating overflow incontinence.

Increased risk of urinary tract infections are presumed to be secondary to increased PVRs in addition to the known risk of UTI with endoscopic procedures. Studies previously reported a 21% rate of UTIs in patients receiving 100 U and 33.3%–41.0% in those receiving higher doses [65].

In addition, this therapeutic option requires motivated patients that are willing and able to return for frequent re-evaluation and PVR checks and willing and able to return for re-treatment every 3-6 months as needed.

Contraindications to intradetrusor Botox® include active UTI, history of urinary retention, elevated PVR or bladder neck obstruction, patients who are unwilling or incapable of performing CIC and hypersensitivity to any component of botulinum toxin.

OTHER AGENTS

Capsaicin

This is a neurotoxin derived from red peppers of the genus Capsicum. It has been found to have a toxic effect on C-fiber afferent nerves by first stimulating then desensitizing unmyelinated C-fibers in high concentrations causing a reduction in bladder sensory input.

In previously reported studies, capsaicin has been shown to decrease neurogenic OAB related symptoms, improve urodynamic parameters and increase bladder capacity. Adverse effects of intravesical Capsaicin instillation include pain, discomfort, itch and urgency [68, 69].

While transient success has been reported in neurogenic OAB patients, use of this agent is still experimental and currently not FDA approved for use in OAB.

Resiniferatoxin

Research into capsaicin lead to the discovery of an alternate TRPV-1 binding agent, resiniferatoxin (RTX). This agent was found to be significantly more potent (up to 1000 times) than Capsacin. Invariably, RTX was shown to have a greater improvement in clinical outcomes and urodynamic parameters in neurogenic OAB when compared to capsaicin and without it's bothersome side effects.

When bound to TRPV-1 on C-fibers, RTX causes a significant influx of calcium resulting in release of neuropeptides and generation of action potentials. It is theorized that this effect causes a reduction in bladder sensory input and modulation of reflex detrusor contractions.

Commercial availability has been challenging due to lack of stable intravesical formulations and difficulties in determining therapeutic concentrations [68, 69].

This agent remains experimental and currently not approved by the FDA for use in OAB.

	Advantages	Disadvantages
PTNS	• Minimally invasive • Does not require anesthesia • Cost effective	• Requires multiple treatments • Requires active patient participation • Re-treatment often necessary
SNS	• Global management of pelvic floor • May address fecal and urinary incontinence • Treatment ½ life is approximately 5 years • No risk of urinary retention	• Requires minor surgical procedure • Staged procedure • Activity restriction with stage 1 • Unable to obtain MRI • Requires cognitively intact patients • Requires battery changes
Botox®	• Minimally Invasive • Does not require anesthesia	• Re-treatment often necessary • Risk of UTI and urinary retention

LAST RESORT OPTIONS

When all else fails, last resort options include augmentation cystoplasty, urinary diversion or bladder emptying with urethral or suprapubic catheters. These options are classified as expert opinions in the AUA/SUFU guidelines [19, 20] and are reserved for rare cases of severe, refractory, complicated OAB. The majority of reconstructive literature focuses on effects of augmentation cystoplasty and diversion on neurogenic patients and little is known regarding the impact of these procedures on non-neurogenic OAB patients and, particularly, on their quality of life.

REFERENCES

[1] Coyne KS, Sexton CC, Irwin DE, et al. The impact of overactive bladder, incontinence and other lower urinary tract symptoms on quality of life, work productivity, sexuality and emotional wellbeing in men and women: results from the EPIC study. *BJU Int.* 2008;101:1388-1395.

[2] Coyne KS, Sexton CC, Thompson CL, et al. Impact of overactive bladder on work productivity. *Urology.* 2012;80:97–103.

[3] Ganz ML, Smalarz AM, Krupski TL, et al. Economic costs of overactive bladder in the United States. *Urology.* 2010;75:526-532.

[4] Haylen BT, de Ridder D, Freeman RM et al: An International Urogynecological Association (IUGA)/International Continence Society (ICS) joint report on the terminology for female pelvic floor dysfunction. *Neurourol Urodyn* 2010; 29:4.

[5] Litwin MS, Saigal CS, editors. Urologic Diseases in America. US Department of Health and Human Services, Public Health Service, National Institutes of Health, National Institute of Diabetes and Digestive and Kidney Diseases. Washington, DC: US Government Printing Office, 2012; NIH Publication No. 12-7865.

[6] Abrams P, Cardozo L, Fall M, et al. The standardisation of terminology of lower urinary tract function. Report from the standardisation subcommittee of the International Continence Society. *Neurourol Urodyn* 2002; 21:167–78.

[7] Stewart WF, Van Rooyan JB, Cundiff GW, et al. Prevalence and burden of overactive bladder in the United States. *World J Urol.* 2003;20:327-336.

[8] Irwin DE, Milsom I, Hunskaar S, et al. Population-based survey of urinary incontinence, overactive bladder, and other lower urinary tract symptoms in five countries: results of the EPIC study. *Eur Urol* 2006;50:1306–15.

[9] Coyne KS, Sexton CC, Thompson CL, et al. The prevalence of lower urinary tract symptoms (LUTS) in the USA, the UK and Sweden: results from the Epidemiology of LUTS (EpiLUTS) study. *BJU Int* 2009;104:352–60.

[10] Irwin DE, Milsom I, Chancellor MB, et al: Dynamic progression of overactive bladder and urinary incontinence symptoms: a systematic review. *Eur Urol* 2010; 58: pp. 532-543.

[11] Milsom I, Kaplan SA, Coyne KS, et al: Effect of bothersome overactive bladder symptoms on health-related quality of life, anxiety, depression, and treatment seeking in the United States: results from EpiLUTS. *Urology* 2012; 80: pp. 90-96.

[12] Wein et al. Overactive Bladder. *Campbell-Walsh Urology 11th edition*. Philadelphia PA: Elsevier Saunders; 2016, 1796-1806.

[13] Wein et al. Pathophysiology and Classification of Lower Urinary Tract Dysfunction. *Campbell-Walsh Urology 11th edition*. Philadelphia PA: Elsevier Saunders; 2016, 1685-1696.

[14] Kinder, M. V, Bastiaanssen, E. H. C, Janknegt, R. A and Marani, E (1995). Neuronal circuitry of the lower urinary tract; central and peripheral neuronal control of the micturition cycle. *Anat. Embryol.*192, 195–209.

[15] Fowler CJ, Griffiths D, de Groat WC. The neural control of micturition. *Nature reviews Neuroscience*. 2008; 9(6):453-466.

[16] Komesu YM, Ketai LH, Mayer AR, Teshiba TM, Rogers RG. Functional MRI of the Brain in Women with Overactive Bladder: Brain Activation During Urinary Urgency. *Female pelvic medicine & reconstructive surgery*. 2011; 17(1):50-54.

[17] Griffiths D, Tadic SD, Schaefer W, Resnick NM. Cerebral control of the bladder in normal and urge-incontinent women. *NeuroImage*. 2007;37(1):1-7.

[18] McDonagh MS, Selover D, Santa J, et al. Drug Class Review: Agents for Overactive Bladder: Final Report Update 4 [Internet]. Portland (OR): Oregon Health & Science University; 2009 Mar. Results and Discussion. Available from: http://www.ncbi.nlm.nih.gov/books/NBK47181/.

[19] Diagnosis and Treatment of Overactive Bladder (Non-neurogenic) in Adults: AUA/SUFU Guideline. http://www.auanet.org/content/media/ OAB_guideline.pdf.

[20] Gormley EA, Lightner DJ, Burgio KL, Chai TC, Clemens JQ, Culkin DJ, et al. Diagnosis and treatment of overactive bladder (non-neurogenic) in adults: AUA/SUFU guideline. *J Urol*. 2012;188:2455–63.

[21] Wein AJ, Chapple C. Management of Overactive Bladder. *Overactive Bladder in Clinical Practice*. London: Springer; 2012, 75-82.

[22] Abrams P, Cardozo L, Khoury S, Wein A. Pharmacological Treatment of Urinary Incontinence. In: Abrams P, Cardozo L, Khoury S, Wein A, ed. *Incontinence*. Plymouth, UK: Plymbridge Distributors; 2002:479-513.

[23] Subak LL, Richter HE, Hunskaar S. Obesity and Urinary Incontinence: Epidemiology and Clinical Research Update. *J Urol*. 2009;182(6 Suppl):S2-S7.

[24] Subak LL, Wing R, West DS, et al.; PRIDE Investigators. Weight loss to treat urinary incontinence in overweight and obese women. *N Engl J Med* 2009; 360(5):481-490.

[25] Fantl JA, Wyman JF, McClish DK et al: Efficacy of bladder training in older women with urinary incontinence. *JAMA* 1991; 265: 609.

[26] Newman DK, Wein AJ (2009). Managing and Treating Urinary Incontinence, 2nd edn. Baltimore, MD: Health Professions Press.

[27] Hesch K. Agents for treatment of overactive bladder: a therapeutic class review. *Proc (Bayl Univ Med Cent)* 2011;20(3):307–14.

[28] Jayarajan J, Radomski SB. Pharmacotherapy of overactive bladder in adults: a review of efficacy, tolerability, and quality of life. *Res Rep Urol*. 2014;6:1–16.

[29] D'Souza AO, Smith MJ, Miller LA, Doyle J, Ariely R. Persistence, adherence, and switch rates among extended-release and immediate-release overactive bladder medications in a regional managed care plan. *J Manag Care Pharm*. 2008;14(3):291-301.

[30] Gopal M, Haynes K, Bellamy SL, Arya LA. Discontinuation rates of anticholinergic medications used for the treatment of lower urinary tract symptoms. *Obstet Gynecol.* 2008;112:1311-1318.

[31] Chancellor MB, Migliaccio-Walle K, Bramley TJ, et al. Long-term patterns of use and treatment failure with anticholinergic agents for overactive bladder. *Clin Ther.* 2013;35(11):1744-1751.

[32] Yu YF, Nichol MB, Yu AP, Ahn J. Persistence and adherence of medications for chronic overactive bladder/urinary incontinence in the California Medicaid program. *Value Health*. 2005;8(4):495-505.

[33] Shaya FT, Blume S, Gu A, Zyczynski T, Jumadilova Z. Persistence with overactive bladder pharmacotherapy in a Medicaid population. *Am J Manag Care.* 2005;11(4 Suppl):S121-S29.

[34] Varadharajan S, Jumadilova Z, Girase P, Ollendorf DA. Economic impact of extended-release tolterodine versus immediate- and extended-release oxybutynin among commercially insured persons with overactive bladder. *Am J Manag Care*. 2005;11(4 Suppl):S140-S49.

[35] Aizawa N, Homma Y, Igawa Y. Effects of mirabegron, a novel b3- adrenoceptor agonist, on primary bladder afferent activity and bladder microcontractions in rats compared with the effects of oxybutynin. *Eur Urol* 2012;62:1165–73.

[36] Novara G, Cornu JN. Mirabegron as a new class of oral drug for overactive bladder syndrome: many positive perspectives, some concerns. *Eur Urol*. 2013;63:306–308.

[37] Khullar V, Amarenco G, Angulo JC, et al. Efficacy and tolerability of mirabegron, a b3-adrenoceptor agonist, in patients with overactive bladder: results from a randomized European–Australian phase 3 trial. *Eur Urol* 2013;63:283–95.

[38] Chapple CR, Kaplan SA, Mitcheson D, et al. Randomized, double-blind, active-controlled phase 3 study to assess 12-month safety and efficacy of mirabegron, a b3 adrenoceptor agonist, in overactive bladder. *Eur Urol* 2013;63:296–305.

[39] Nitti VW, Auerbach S, Martin N, Calhoun A, Lee M, Herschorn S. Results of a randomized phase III trial of mirabegron in patients with overactive bladder. *J Urol.* 2013;189(4):1388–1395.

[40] Herschorn S, Barkin J, Castro-Diaz D, et al. A phase III, randomized, double-blind, parallel-group, placebo-controlled, multicentre study to assess the efficacy and safety of the β3 adrenoceptor agonist, mirabegron, in patients with symptoms of overactive bladder. *Urology.* 2013;82(2):313–320.

[41] Andersson K-E. Drug therapy of overactive bladder - What is coming next? *Korean Journal of Urology*. 2015;56(10):673-679.

[42] Liu L, Zheng S, Han P, Wei Q. Phosphodiesterase-5 inhibitors for lower urinary tract symptoms secondary to benign prostatic hyperplasia: a systematic review and meta-analysis. *Urology.* 2011;77(1):123-129.

[43] Gacci M, Corona G, Salvi M, Vignozzi L, McVary KT, Kaplan SA, et al. A systematic review and meta-analysis on the use of phosphodiesterase 5 inhibitors alone or in combination with α- blockers for lower urinary tract symptoms due to benign prostatic hyperplasia. *Eur Urol*. 2012;61:994–1003.

[44] Gacci M, Sebastianelli A, Salvi M, et al. PDE5-Is for the Treatment of Concomitant ED and LUTS/BPH. *Current Bladder Dysfunction Reports.* 2013;8(2):150-159.

[45] Gacci M, Del Popolo G, Macchiarella A, Celso M, Vittori G, Lapini A, et al. Vardenafil improves urodynamic parameters in men with spinal cord injury: results from a single dose, pilot study. *J Urol.* 2007;178:2040–3.

[46] Gacci M, Ierardi A, Rose AD, Tazzioli S, Scapaticci E, Filippi S, et al. Vardenafil can improve continence recovery after bilateral nerve sparing prostatectomy: results of a randomized, double blind, placebo-controlled pilot study. *J Sex Med.* 2010;7:234–43.

[47] McKeage K (2013). Propiverine: a review of its use in the treatment of adults and children with overactive bladder associated with idiopathic or neurogenic detrusor overactivity, and in men with lower urinary tract symptoms. *Clin Drug Investig* 33: 71–91.

[48] Peters KM, Carrico DJ, Perez-Marrero RA et al: Randomized trial of percutaneous tibial nerve stimulation versus Sham efficacy in the treatment of overactive bladder syndrome: results from the SUmiT trial. *J Urol* 2010.

[49] PetersKM, MacDiarmid SA, Wooldridge LS et al: Randomized trial of percutaneous tibial nerve stimulation versus extended-release tolterodine: Results from the overactive bladder innovative therapy trial. *J. Urol* 2009; 182: 1055.

[50] Staskin, D.R., Peters, K.M., MacDiarmid, S. et al, Percutaneous tibial nerve stimulation: a clinically cost effective addition to the overactive bladder algorithm of care. *Curr Urol Rep.* 2012;13:327.

[51] MacDiarmid SA, Peters KM, Shobeiri SA et al: Long-term durability of percutaneous tibial nerve stimulation for the treatment of overactive blad- der. *J Urol* 2010; 183: 234.

[52] Spinelli M, Sievert KD. Latest technologic and surgical developments in using InterStim Therapy for sacral neuromodulation: Impact on treatment success and safety. *European Urology* 2008;54:1287–96.

[53] Noblett K, Siegel S, Mangel J, et al. Results of a prospective, multicenter study evaluating quality of life, safety, and efficacy of sacral neuromodulation at twelve months in subjects with symptoms of overactive bladder. *Neurourol Urodyn.* 2014 doi: 10.1002/nau.22707. [Epub ahead of print].

[54] Moon, K. H.;Han, J. Y.;Kim, J. H.;Lee, H. N.;Lee, K. S.;Lee, J. G.;Oh, S. J.;Yoon, H. N.;Choo, M. S. Prospective Trial of Sacral Neuromodulation for Refractory Overactive Bladder Syndrome in Korean Patients. LUTS: Lower Urinary Tract Symptoms. 2013; [Epub ahead of print].

[55] Nitti VW, Dmochowski R, Herschorn S, Sand P, Thompson C, Nardo C, et al. OnabotulinumtoxinA for the treatment of patients with overactive bladder and urinary incontinence: results of a phase 3, randomized, placebo controlled trial. *J Urol.* 2013;189:2186–93.

[56] Chartier-Kastler E, Nitti V, De Ridder D, Sussman D, Sand P, Sievert K, Chapple C, Charmaine J, Magyar A, Radomski S. Durable improvements in urinary incontinence and positive treatment response in patients with idiopathic overactive bladder syndrome following long-term onabotulinumtoxinA treatment: Final results of 3.5-year study. *Prog Urol.* 2015 Nov;25(13):739.

[57] Shenot PJ, MarkJR. Intradetrusor onabotulinumtoxinA injection: how I do it. *Can J Urol* 2013;20(1):6649-6655.

[58] BOTOX® Clinical Data Overview https://www.botoxforincontinence.com/assets/pdf/Clinical_Data_Overview.pdf.

[59] Manecksha RP, Cullen IM, Ahmad S, McNeill G, Flynn R, McDermott TE, et al. Prospective randomised controlled trial comparing trigone-sparing versus trigone-including intradetrusor injection of abobotulinumtoxinA for refractory idiopathic detrusor overactivity. *Eur Urol.* 2012;61:928–35.
[60] Schulte-Baukloh H, Schobert J, Stolze T, Sturzebecher B, Weiss C, Knispel HH. Efficacy of botulinum-A toxin bladder injections for the treatment of neurogenic detrusor overactivity in multiple sclerosis patients: an objective and subjective analysis. *Neurourol Urodyn* 2006;25:110–5.
[61] Abdel-Meguid TA. Botulinum toxin-A injections into neurogenic overactive bladder—to include or exclude the trigone? A prospec- tive, randomized, controlled trial. *J Urol* 2010;184:2423–8.
[62] Sidi AA, Dykstra DD. Botulinum A toxin selective paralysis of the urethral rhabdosphincter: Pilot study of a new treatment for detrusor sphincter dyssynergia [abstract] *J Urol*. 1987;137(4 pt 2).
[63] Nitti VW. Botulinum Toxin for the Treatment of Idiopathic and Neurogenic Overactive Bladder: State of the Art. *Reviews in Urology*. 2006;8(4):198-208.
[64] Chapple CR. Which preparation of botulinum toxin a should be used, where should it be injected, and how should its efficacy be assessed? *Eur Urol*. 2012;61(5):936–937.
[65] Cox L, Cameron AP. OnabotulinumtoxinA for the treatment of overactive bladder. *Res Rep Urol*. 2014;6:79–89.
[66] Wolf JS Jr, Bennett CJ, Dmochowski RR, Hollenbeck BK, Pearle MS, Schaeffer AJ; Urologic Surgery Antimicrobial Prophylaxis Best Practice Policy Panel. Best practice policy statement on urologic surgery antimicrobial prophylaxis. *J Urol*. 2008;179(4):1379–1390.
[67] Liao C-H, Kuo H-C. Practical Aspects of Botulinum Toxin-A Treatment in Patients With Overactive Bladder Syndrome. *International Neurourology Journal*. 2015;19(4):213-219.
[68] Kennelly MJ, DeVoe WB. Overactive Bladder: Pharmacologic Treatments in the Neurogenic Population. *Reviews in Urology*. 2008;10(3):182-191.
[69] Kuo, H. Novel treatment of overactive bladder and detrusor overactivity with intravesical resiniferatoxin. Incont. *Pelvic Floor Dysfunction* 2 (2008): 17-20.
[70] Sussman D. O, Syed K. K. Diagnosing and Treating BPH-LUTS. AOA Health Watch-January 2015. https://www.docmeonline.com/Activity/ 3360070/Detail.aspx.

THE AUTHORS' BIOGRAPHIES

Dr. Angelo E. Gousse, M.D

One of the very few fellowship-trained reconstructive and neuro-urologists in Florida, Dr. Gousse is the Director of Bladder Health Program of South Florida, South Broward Hospital Districts. He is the Director of Female Pelvic Medicine and Reconstructive Urology at the Memorial Hospital Miramar. He is a former tenured Professor of Urology at the University of Miami Miller School of Medicine, Department of Urology, Vice-Chairman of the University of Miami Hospital and Clinics Urology service, where he was also the Urology Residency

Program Director and Fellowship Director for Female Urology, Urodynamics, and Reconstructive Surgery for more than ten years. He was also the Director of the Urodynamics Laboratory at the VA Medical Center where he also supervised the Neuro-Urologic care of the spinal cord injured patients. After graduating as the valedictorian of the City University of New York (York College) with a perfect GPA in his major, Dr. Gousse received his medical degree with highest honors from the Yale University School of Medicine. He completed his residency at the Baylor College of Medicine in Houston Texas and a postdoctoral fellowship in Urodynamics, female urology and pelvic floor reconstruction at the University of California, Los Angeles. Certified by the American Board of Urology, he has performed more than onethousand complex reconstructive procedures. He is one of a handful of urologists performing urethroplasty in the state of Florida and was the first to perform Sacral Nerve Modulation (InterstimTM) and intra-detrusor injection of Botox for urinary problems in South Florida. Dr. Gousse's research interests have focused on overactive bladder neuropharmacology, reconstruction, neurogenic urinary incontinence, as well as functional recovery from spinal cord injury. An international leader in voiding dysfunction, he pioneered the optimal dosage of neurotoxins (Botox®) to manage bladder dysfunction. His investigator-initiated research projects in Botox chemodernervation in human subjects led to the first FDA urologic indication of Botox in the United States. Dr. Gousse has also participated and co-authored in clinical trials which led to the FDA approval of the first Beta-3 drug to treat overactive bladder, Merebegron (marketed as Myrbetriq). He also collaborated on extramural NIH grants with Dr Vinata Lokeshwar to investigate urinary markers for interstitial cystitis. Dr. Gousse has authored or co-authored more than 60 peer-reviewed scientific publications and numerous textbook chapters, journal articles and abstracts. He participates as a guest professor in the United States and abroad on various aspects of reconstructive urology and voiding dysfunction, and he regularly lectures as an expert in the field of urology. He has been a panelist at the American Urologic Association (AUA) yearly meeting on numerous occasions. He is appointed to the board for the Society of Urodynamics, Female Pelvic Medicine & Urogenital Reconstruction (SUFU). He is the Chairperson for the AUA – SUFU meeting (2014). A former Genito-Urinary Reconstructive Surgeons (GURS) board member he led a group of reconstructive surgeons to train urologists in third world countries. In addition, Dr. Gousse served on the American Urology Association Female Urology Core Curriculum Committee and as the Section Editor of the Female Urology section in the journal Current Urology Reports. He is a reviewer for the Journal of Urology, Neuro-Urology and Urodynamics, Urology. A radio and TV personality in the Haitian community, Dr. Gousse is a regular guest on Island TV. He is the founder of the Radio Show " Urologic Consultation in Creole" dedicated to educate the Creole speaking population of South Florida and the Bahamas about urologic diseases. He recently developed a popular weekly Television Show "Urology Health" dedicated to the usage of visual aids in order to educate the general public on urologic problems. Listed in Best Doctors in America 2005-2013, Best Doctors US News and World Report 2011-2012, America's Top Urologists by the prestigious Consumer's Research Council of America 2008, Strathmore's Who's Who since 2001, the Miller University of Miami Medical School's Urology Teacher of the Year Award on numerous occasions, the Pfizer Scholars in Urology Award, the Cullen Research Award from the Scott Department of Urology, Baylor College of Medicine, and the Dr. Jonas Salk Scholar Award for his work on E.coli microbial genetics, Dr. Gousse remains a dedicated teacher, mentor, a researcher and community servant. He is co-founder and president of the Haitian American

Leadership Organization (HALO), a charitable organization established to further community outreach in underserved areas to benefit the less fortunate.

Dr. Kirin. K. Syed, D.O

Dr. Syed is originally from the New England area. She received a B.A. in microbiology from Ohio Wesleyan University and earned her medical degree from the University of Medicine and Dentistry of New Jersey-School of Osteopathic Medicine. She went on to complete her internship and residency in urological surgery at UMDNJ (now Rowan University) in Southern New Jersey. Her past research has been conducted at University of Massachusetts, Ohio Wesleyan University, Massachusetts General Hospital/Harvard Medical School, Rutgers University/Robert Wood Johnson University Hospital and Rowan University- School of Osteopathic Medicine. Her research efforts have been presented at national conferences, published in posters, abstracts, and journals. Dr. Syed is an active member in the Society of Urodynamics, Female Pelvic Medicine & Urogenital Reconstruction, American College of Osteopathic Surgeons, American Urological Association (AUA), Society of Women in Urology and American Osteopathic Association (AOA). She is currently completing a clinical fellowship in voiding dysfunction, female urology and urologic reconstruction at the Bladder Health and Reconstructive Urology Institute in Miami, Florida. Her clinical interests include refractory overactive bladder, pelvic organ prolapse, male and female stress incontinence, urethral stricture disease, urinary fistulae, neurourology, and general urology such as kidney stones, hematuria, and voiding dysfunction. Dr. Syed is devoted to serving the community as well as national and international public service. She has previously volunteered with AmeriCorps Volunteers In Service To America, the American Red Cross, underserved community outreach programs in southern New Jersey and a service- learning program in Quito, Ecuador through Child Family Health International- a global health, nongovernmental organization. She enjoys teaching and working with residents and medical students and received distinction as one of the 2015 National Guardian of the Profession by the AOA. She was also a member of the winning team at the 2013 MidAtlantic Section of AUA Regional Resident Jeopardy Bowl and a semifinalist at the 2014 AUA Annual Resident Jeopardy Bowl.

In: Overactive Bladder (OAB)
Editor: Elvira Larson

ISBN: 978-1-63485-033-9

Chapter 5

INVESTIGATIONAL AND PROMISING NOVEL THERAPEUTICS FOR THE OVERACTIVE BLADDER AND URGENCY URINARY INCONTINENCE

Emilio Sacco*[*], *MD, PhD, and Riccardo Bientinesi, MD
Urology Department, "Agostino Gemelli" Academic Hospital,
Catholic University of Sacred Heart, Rome, Italy

ABSTRACT

The increasing prevalence of overactive bladder (OAB) and the relevant limitations of current treatments urge the need for novel therapeutic approaches. To date, antimuscarinics dominate the first-line pharmacological treatment of OAB, together with β3-adrenergic agents, however side-effects and limited efficacy significantly affect patients compliance with these drugs. The growing knowledge of OAB pathophysiology fuelled a huge amount of basic and clinical research in this field of pharmacotherapy aiming to overcome these limitations. Several exiting hypothesis-driven pharmacological approaches for the future treatment of OAB have been suggested in the last few years and are shown in this chapter.

In particular, the exploratory agents alternative to available medications for OAB and that may ultimately prove to be therapeutically useful in the future management of OAB patients based on preclinical and early clinical data are presented. Many alternative pharmacological strategies have been discovered or are under investigation in disease-oriented studies. Several potential therapeutics are known for years but still find obstacles to pass the clinical stages of development, while other completely novel compounds, targeting new pharmacological targets, have been recently discovered and show a potential to translate into clinical therapeutic agents for idiopathic and neurogenic OAB syndrome.

[*] E-mail: emilio.sacco@gmail.com.

Introduction

Overactive bladder (OAB) is a complex of symptoms defined by urgency with or without urge urinary incontinence (UUI), usually associated with increased urinary frequency and nocturia [1]. It represents a very bothersome and debilitating chronic condition with a severe negative influence on the patient's quality of life [2]. OAB is highly prevalent in Western countries, its incidence increases with age, and is associated with very high socioeconomic burden due to the aging population, the OAB-associated comorbidities and the increased risk of hospitalization [3]. OAB is a heterogeneous disease with a multifactorial and still incompletely known pathophysiology; in fact, pathophysiology is largely unknown, although multiple causes have been proposed, such as a primary detrusor dysfunction, observed as detrusor overactivity (DO) during urodynamic studies, an overactivity of the afferent arm of the micturition reflex, a primary dysfunction of higher central nervous system (CNS) inhibitory centers [4]. The treatment is aimed at relieving symptoms improving quality of life (QOL), without interfering with the voiding bladder function. A multimodal approach is often required including behavioral therapy, functional electrical stimulation, clean intermittent catheterization, and pharmacological treatment. Pharmacological treatment has been based for years on antimuscarinic agents, but recently other two pharmacological principles have been approved for OAB by the United States Food and Drug Administration (FDA): the first β3-adrenergic agent, mirabegron (Myrbetriq®, Astellas, approved in June 2012), and the botulinum neurotoxin (Botox®, Allergan, approved in January 2013) [5, 6]. Although antimuscarinics represent the mainstay of pharmacological treatment [7], lack of both efficacy and bladder selectivity, leading to bothersome systemic adverse effects (AEs), considerably limits the long-term persistence with these drugs. Mirabegron, as alternative oral drug, only partly overcomes the limitations of antimuscarinics [8]. Consequently, there is a persistent need for new drugs with different mechanisms of action. A huge amount of preclinical studies is ongoing exploring the therapeutic potential of many novel compounds some of which already advanced to the clinical phases of development [9, 10].

Manipulation of Central Micturition Circuitry

Central Control of the Lower Urinary Tract Function

The lower urinary tract (LUT) consists of two major components, including the bladder and urethra. The bladder has abundant muscarinic M2 and M3 receptors and adrenergic beta 3 receptors, and is innervated by cholinergic (parasympathetic) and noradrenergic (sympathetic) fibres for contraction and relaxation, respectively [11]. The urethra presents many adrenergic alpha 1 A/D receptors and nicotinic receptors, and it is innervated by noradrenergic (sympathetic contraction) and cholinergic (somatic contraction) fibers. The LUT performs two opposite functions involving the storage and emptying of urine, both of which require an intact neuraxis that involves almost all parts of the nervous system [12]. Normal urinary storage is dependent on the spinal (sacral, bladder-inhibitory) autonomic reflex. The storage reflex is thought to be tonically facilitated by the brain, particularly the pontine storage centre [1, 13, 14].

The pontine storage centre is located ventrolateral to the pontine micturition centre (PMC). In addition to the pontine storage centre, the storage function is facilitated by the hypothalamus, cerebellum, basal ganglia, and frontal cortex. These areas have been shown to be activated during urinary storage using functional neuroimaging in humans [15]. Normal micturition is dependent on the brainstem (spino-bulbo-spinal, bladder-facilitatory) autonomic reflex and involves the midbrain periaqueductal grey matter (PAG) and the PMC. The PAG is thought to be central in regulating micturition and has a range of inputs from higher structures. The PMC is located in and adjacent to the locus coeruleus. The PMC is thought to project spinal descending fibres containing glutamate as a facilitatory neurotransmitter to activate the sacral bladder preganglionic nucleus. The PMC also projects fibres to sacral interneurons containing gamma-amino-butyric acid (GABA) and glycine as inhibitory neurotransmitters to suppresses the sacral urethral motor nucleus (the Onuf's nucleus) The voiding function is initiated and facilitated by higher brain structures, for example, the hypothalamus and prefrontal cortex, which overlap in the storage-facilitating area [16-18].

DO is a major cause of OAB and urinary incontinence [4]. In lesions above the brainstem, the micturition reflex arc is intact, and DO is considered to be an exaggerated micturition reflex.

The exaggeration of the micturition reflex may be due to more than simply the decreased inhibition of the brain, including further facilitation by glutamatergic and D2 dopaminergic mechanisms [19].

Central Acting Drugs

GABA-Ergics

Compounds with agonist activity on γ-aminobutyric acid (GABA) receptors in the CNS exploit the inhibitory effect of this neurotransmitter on micturition reflex [20]. Baclofen, the orthosteric agonist of the GABA-B receptor, is used in the treatment of neurological spasticity, particularly in the lower limb. Baclofen is pumped directly into the subarachnoid space by means of a programmable pump *via* a catheter system.

Also, as shown in several studies, baclofen dose-dependently inhibited bladder contractions and decreased micturition pressure in female rats showing DO as a result of spinal cord injury [21]. Importantly, baclofen has been shown to alleviate the symptoms of OAB in patients with idiopathic DO [22], neurogenic voiding disturbances [23] and non-neurogenic dysfunctional voiding [24]. Clinical studies based on urodynamic evaluations showed that the continuous intrathecal baclofen pump infusion is effective in the management of patients with medically-refractory neurogenic DO (NDO) and decreased bladder compliance [25]. Baclofen has gained approval for treatment of NDO in SCI patients, but the narrow therapeutic window and the tolerability profile (short half-life and long list of side effects) limited its clinical use. ADX71441, a novel, selective and orally bioavailable agonist of GABAB-receptor, in a recent study showed efficacy in two models of OAB in mice and guinea pigs with a good pharmacokinetic/pharmacodynamic relationship. Thus, ADX71441 could be considered as viable approach for the treatment of various forms of OAB in humans [26].

Anticonvulsants

Inhibition of the GABA transporters (GAT), that are thought to provide a GABA inactivation mechanism in the CNS, has been explored as a possible pharmacological principle aimed to treat DO. Tiagabine is an anticonvulsants that selectively inhibits GABA re-uptake increasing endogenous GABA concentrations.

In a study of 2002 by Pherson and Andersson, it has been shown that given intravenous or intrathecal in rats, Tiagabine decreases micturition pressure, decreases voided volume and improves storage phase parameters suggesting a potential utility for OAB treatment [27].

Gabapentin is an antiepileptic drug currently used for neuropathic pain and other conditions, that is free from antimuscarinic adverse effects; it is structurally related to the neurotransmitter GABA (gamma-aminobutyric acid) but it does not interact with GABA receptors, it is not converted metabolically into GABA or a GABA agonist, and it is not an inhibitor of GABA uptake or degradations. Gabapentin was approved by the FDA in 2000 for pediatric use [28].

Its mechanism of action is not fully clear although it appears to have inhibitory activity on afferent C-fibers likely by binding to a-2-delta subunit of voltage-dependent calcium channel [29]. The drug has also first been explored for the treatment of OAB in a study in which is reported that gabapentin improved both symptoms and urodynamic parameters in NDO patients [30]. Kim et al. [31] in 2004 reported that the drug was well tolerated and improved symptoms in 14 out of 31 antimuscarinics-refractory OAB patients.

In a recent study gabapentin used as an add-on therapy has shown good clinical effects in 16 out of 30 children with antimuscarinics-refractory OAB [32]. Phase II trials are ongoing comparing gabapentin with solifenacin in OAB patients [33] and evaluating the efficacy and tolerability of a combination of low doses of gabapentin and oxybutynin [34].

Pregabalin (Lyrica®, Pfizer) is an antiepileptic and analgesic medication that is similar to gabapentin in its mechanism of action, with the difference that pregabalin can be administered at considerably lower doses than gabapentin because of its higher bioavailability, more rapid adsorption, and greater potency [35]; it is mainly used for neuropathic pain and fibromyalgia. In a study by Marencak et al. [36], Pregabalin alone or with tolterodine ER showed efficacy and safety compared with tolterodine alone in subjects with idiopatic OAB.

A phase II trial is ongoing in patients with idiopathic OAB comparing pregabalin with tolterodine and their combination [37]. Furthermore, preclinical data showed significant improvement on the urodynamic parameters of an animal model of NDO providing a rationale for future proof-of-concept clinical trial on NDO patients [38].

Antidepressants

Inhibitory effects on micturition are known side-effects of drugs with inhibitory action on the monoamine reuptake, including tricyclic antidepressants. Furthermore, depression is more common in patients with OAB and a shared deficiency of monoamine (serotonin and noradrenaline) behind both depression and OAB has been suggested [39].

Imipramine, a tricyclic antidepressants, improves storage LUTS and DO at the cost of not negligible side-effects. Antidepressants selective serotonin reuptake inhibitors, such as escitalopram, are under evaluation for efficacy in OAB patients [40].

Duloxetine is a combined selective serotonin-norepinephrine reuptake inhibitor (SNRI) mainly used as antidepressive; however, its use in stress urinary incontinence has been recently analyzed in a metanalysis [41] and has also demonstrated significant efficacy compared to placebo in relieving urinary symptoms in women with OAB [41]. Duloxetine action on stress urinary incontinence seems to be linked to the inhibition of NE reuptake and 5-HT in the presynaptic space of the sacral Onuf's nucleus neurons. The effect of duloxetine in the lower urinary tract has been evaluated in an anesthetized cat model where a solution of acetic acid was infused in the bladder, mimicking human OAB [42]. In a recent pilot, single blinded study aimed to exstablish the efficacy and tolerability of duloxetine in the treatment of OAB in patients affected by Multiple Sclerosis, a statistically significant improvement in bladder disorder, as measured by OAB-Q, has been observed after treatment compared with both basal levels and placebo [43]. However, the side-effects of this compound significantly limit patient's compliance.

Desipramine is an active metabolite of imipramine. It is distinguished by the presence of only one n-methyl group on its side chain [44]. It has been shown in several studies to have less central nervous system (CNS) side effects than other tricyclic antidepressants agents including imipramine and amitriptyline. In a recent study, 43 patients (53% male and 47% female) were treated with desipramine for antimuscarinic refractory OAB. The study demonstrated that desipramine could be an useful potential treatment for patients with OAB refractory to first-line antimuscarinic therapy, possibly providing an alternative treatment modality with a mechanistically minimized risk of CNS side-effects compared to other tricyclic antidepressants [45].

Based on animal experiments showing that besipirdine, a SNRI that interacts also with a1 (agonist) and a2 (antagonist) receptors, significantly and dose-dependently improves storage function and external urethral sphincter activity, a human proof-of-concept study has been initiated by UroGene in patients with storage LUTS [46].

Serotoninergics

Increasing evidence indicates that serotonin [5-hydroxytryptamine (5-HT)] is involved in a complex way in the control of micturition at central and peripheral sites, with both inhibitory and facilitatory effects [47-50], although the serotonergic pathway generally enhances urine storage by facilitating the vesical sympathetic reflex pathway and inhibiting the parasympathetic voiding pathway. The 5-HT1A receptor agonist 8-OH-DPAT, as investigated in alpha-chloralose anesthetized or conscious chronic spinal cord injured (SCI) cats [50], significantly increased the bladder volume threshold for eliciting a large amplitude micturition contraction, but only slightly reduced the amplitude of the contractions. The inhibitory effect of 8-OHDPAT appeared mediated by an action on interneuronal pathways in the spinal cord or on the C-fibers afferent limb. Positive effects of this compound on voiding function have also been reported in a rat model of incomplete cauda equina injuries. 8-OH-DPAT also improved voiding efficiency and maximum intravesical pressure, and enhanced the external urethral sphincter tonic and bursting activity in a rat model of incomplete cauda equina/conus medullaris injury [51]. 5-HT2 and 5-HT3 receptors mediate excitatory effects on sympathetic and somatic reflexes to increase outlet resistance, and preclinical studies have shown that 5-HT2C and 5-HT3 receptors play an inhibitory role on micturition reflex suggesting that agonists at this site may have potential as candidate drugs for OAB [49].

Accordingly, in a pilot human study [52], a symptomatic benefit with sarpogrelate has been reported in patients with diabetes and refractory OAB. Selective antagonists of 5-HT4 and 5-HT1A receptors such as SB207266 (piboserod) and WAY100635, respectively, potently inhibited the micturition reflex in animal models and human detrusor [53, 54]. WAY100635 combined with duloxetine synergistically enhanced inhibition of DO in a cat model, indicating a potential novel treatment for OAB if duloxetine is combined with a 5-HT1A receptor antagonist agent [55, 56].

Antiserotoninergics

Serotonin is well known to have an increased peripheral excitatory function in disorders known to be associated with DO, such as bladder outlet obstruction (BOO) and diabetes mellitus [57]. The 5-HT2A receptor plays a facilitatory action on micturition reflex, as demonstrated in rats, and its overexpression has been observed in BOO rat bladder [58]. Accordingly, as observed in a study by Kodama et. al. in diabetic rat bladder, Sarpogrelate (a 5-HT2A selective antagonist) counteracted the increased contractile response to 5-HT in a dose-dependent manner [59]. As before, Takimoto et al. [60] reported a symptomatic benefit in patients with diabetes and refractory OAB treated with sarpogrelate.

5-HT4 and 5-HT1A receptors are also involved in micturition control and their selective antagonists such as Piboserod and WAY100635, respectively, potently inhibited the micturition reflex in animal models and human detrusor [47, 61]. However, disappointing results have been reported with a potent and selective antiserotoninergic in a proof-of-concept trial for the treatment of OAB patients [62].

Antipurinergics

The physiopathology of the "mucosal bladder network" (the functional unit consisting of the urothelium, interstitial cells and afferent nerves) has not yet completely understood and several pharmacological approaches have been driven to better define it. This theory postulates that stimulation of receptors and channels on urothelial cells can release mediators that target bladder nerves and other cell types; urothelial cells can also be targets for neurotransmitters released from nerves or other cell types. Urothelial cells can be activated by either autocrine (i.e., autoregulation) or paracrine (release from nearby nerves or other cells) mechanisms [63].

An interesting approach for the future treatment of OAB could be represented by purinergic receptors antagonists [64]. Many studies suggest that the adenosine 5'-triphosphate (ATP) and purinergic ionotropic (P2X) receptors are involved in pathogenesis of DO [65-67]. Purinergic transmission has in fact been found on both afferent and efferent signalling pathways within the lower urinary tract and appears to be abnormally enhanced with aging [68] and DO[69]. In particular, it has been seen that P2X3 receptors on sensory nerve terminals are involved in voiding dysfunctions of conscious chronic SCI rats, improving bladder function, raising the possibility that P2X3 receptor antagonists might be useful for the treatment of NDO [70]. An increase in P2X3 receptor expression was also observed in human bladder affected by DO [71]. P2X receptor-selective antagonists have been also tested as potential

therapeutics for pain management, on the basis of studies showing the role of purinergic receptors in mediating nociceptive neurotransmission [72]. A novel recently developed P2X3/P2X2/3 receptor antagonists, RO3 compound (Roche Palo Alto) and the AF-742

(Afferent Pharmaceuticals), seem to possess attributes that offer the potential for optimization into candidate drug molecules not only for inflammatory and painful bladder conditions but also for OAB. These compounds are ongoing a phase II trial for bladder pain syndrome [73]. Moreover, P2X3 antisense oligonucleotides and RNA interference-mediated treatment appear to be promising for neuropathic pain management and might open up new avenues for OAB therapeutic strategies [74].

Antineuropeptidergics

In the last years there has been a growing appreciation for the role of neuropeptidergic receptors in the pathophysiology of OAB. Studies using C fibers neurotoxins suggest that tachykinins, such as substance P (SP) and neurokinin A (NKA), may play a role as sensory transmitters in the micturition reflex. SP and NKA are neuropeptides with the highest affinity for NK1 and NK2 receptors, respectively. NK-receptors have been demonstrated to be widely expressed in various CNS regions involved in micturition control [75]; in particular, it has been seen that spinal and supraspinal NK1 and NK2 receptors may modulate the micturition reflex [76-77].

Tachykinins are also released from urothelial/suburothelial capsaicin-sensitive afferents and are able to stimulate muscle tone and bladder contractions (NKA > NKB > SP), and to influence vascular tone and permeability ("neurogenic inflammation") [78, 79].

Mixed clinical results have been reported on some compounds in this class. However, although the clinical evidence is still limited, NK-1 antagonists have attracted the interest of several companies and proof-of-concept studies are ongoing evaluating other compounds in this pharmacological class.

Aprepitant (Merck Sharp and Dohme Corp.) is a NK-1 receptor antagonist used for treatment of chemotherapy-induced nausea and vomiting; as shown in a well designed pilot randomized controlled trial (RCT), this drug significantly improved symptoms of OAB in 125 postmenopausal women with a history of urgency incontinence or mixed incontinence (urge urinary incontinence predominant) compared with placebo [80]. Aprepitant was generally well-tolerated and the incidence of side effects, including dry mouth, was low.

Serlopitant (MK0594, Merck Sharp and Dohme Corp.) has been evaluated in a RCT compared with tolterodine and, although it significantly decreased the primary endpoint of daily micturitions, no advantages in efficacy have been found [81]. Netupitant (by Helsinn Healthcare) is another potent and selective NK1 receptor antagonist, but has failed to demonstrate superiority over placebo in a phase II trial [82].

Opioids

μ-Opioid Receptor Agonists

μ-opioid receptor (MOR) agonists own a good analgesic efficacy and excellent tolerability. Tramadol, a weak MOR-agonist, is an effective and safe analgesic, but its metabolites have a stronger MOR-agonist effect and also have an inhibitory action on the noradrenaline and 5-HT reuptake; thus their effects are bound to indirectly activating serotonergic and α2-adrenergic receptors [83]. Promising clinical results in OAB patients were published on tramadol by Safarinejad et al. in 2006 [84], but the study contained statistical errors and therefore was retracted. Tramadol has been seen to increase the bladder capacity and compliance and to delay filling-sensations, without ill effect on voiding (also in patients affected by BOO), as shown in a study by Singh et al. in 15 subjects [85]. Tramadol-like compounds with less incidence of nausea might play a potential role in the treatment of patients suffering from NDO and the development of novel MOR-agonists is ongoing. KN203 (KeyNeurotek Pharma) is the first compound of this class to be developed against OAB, and the results of a proof-of-concept study are expected to clarify its role in this clinical setting [86].

δ-Receptor Agonists

A growing volume of information supports a role for the δ-receptor in the regulation of bladder activity [87]. In contrast to μ-agonists, δ-receptor agonists have a lower toxicity and no addiction; their most crucial safety aspect is the incidence of seizure-like convulsions in rodents. MCP-202 is a compound in this class and in the development pipeline of Mt Cook Pharma for the treatment of OAB. A novel nonpeptide, orally bioavailable δ-receptor agonist (DPI-221) with satisfactory safety profile and high potency in extending micturition interval in mice has been recently developed [88].

Targeting the Afferent Signalling Pathway

TRP-Antagonists

The transient receptor potential (TRP) channel superfamily represents another potential target for OAB treatment. The TRP has been demonstrated to be involved in nociception and mechano-sensory transduction in various organ systems. Studies of the lower urinary tract have indicated that several TRP channels, including TRPV1, TRPV2, TRPV4, TRPM8 and TRPA1, are expressed in the bladder and may act as sensors of stretch and/or chemical irritation, as well as in storage bladder function and DO, offering the possibility to target bladder dysfunctions at the level of sensory signal initiation (Figure 1) [89, 90].

The capsaicin-sensitive ion channel, TRPV1 (Transient receptor potential vanilloids 1) is the principal transduction channel for nociception; it has been linked with normal bladder function in addition to the generation of urgency sensation [91]. An increase in TRPV1 expression has been reported in bladder urothelium and suburothelial nerve fibers from patients with sensory urgency and idiopathic detrusor overactivity [92]. TRPV1 is also found in myelinated Aδ-fibres and sensory unmyelinated C-fibres located in the pelvic nerve afferents and in a sub/intraurothelial plexus [93]. C-fibres are normally silent but can become active and to convey signal to the spinal cord in pathological situation such as OAB, NDO and SCI, resulting in the bothersome sensation of urinary urgency [94].

Capsaicin is a well known natural TRPV1 agonists and several trials showed that, given intravesically, it could determinate a sustained activation of the TRPV1 receptor resulting in a desensitization of C-fibers with beneficial effects in patients with neurogenic or idiopathic DO; on the other side, capsaicin presents many side-effects [95, 96].

Potent orally-available small-molecule TRPV1 antagonists are undergoing clinical trials for chronic pain, but the lack of bladder-selectivity and potential effects on thermoregulation seems to be a serious hindrance for the clinical development [97, 98]. XEN-D0501 (Provesica Ltd.), a highly potent oral TRPV1 antagonist, has been seen to improve storage bladder function and reduce the strength of capsaicin-induced bladder contractions in animal models; a phase I study reported a good tolerability and safety [99] and an international phase II trial is currently evaluating XEN-D0501 for efficacy in OAB. JTS-653 (Japan Tobacco), MCP-101 (Mt. Cook Pharma) and SAF312 (Novartis Pharmaceuticals) [100], are other compounds in this drug class under investigation for the treatment of NDO.

Recent preclinical observations have shown that TRPA1 [101, 102] and TRPV4 [103, 104], other TRP channels expressed in the lower urinary tract, could have a critical role in bladder storage function and overactivity. Selective antagonists for these ion channels are already available making the superfamily of TRP channels a very interesting class of potential targets for drugs aimed to treat LUTS/OAB/DO.

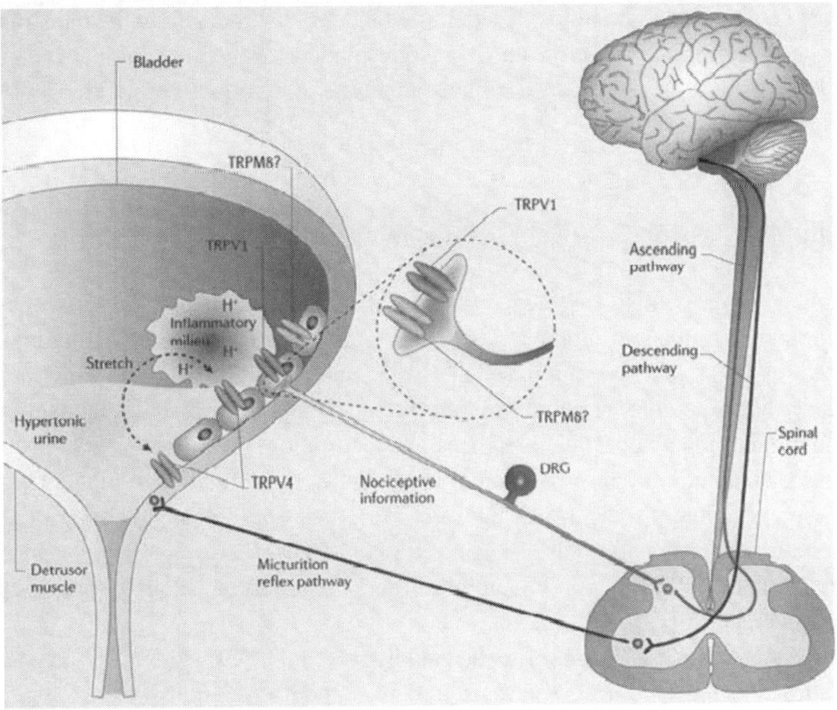

With permission of Nature Publishing Group.

Figure 1. Roles of TRP channels in bladder functions [179].

However, so far the potential of any of the channel antagonists developed for nonbladder indications has not been explored clinically in lower urinary tract (LUT) dysfunction, and the adverse effect of hyperthermia of the first generation TRPV1 antagonists has delayed development. Nevertheless, TRP channels still may be most exciting targets for future LUT drugs. LUT dysfunctions may not have been given the highest priority in TRP drugs development, but research carried out for non-bladder diseases may be possible to apply also to LUT disorders.

In conclusion, there seem to be several links between activation of different members of the TRP superfamily and OAB, and further exploration of the involvement of these channels in LUT function and dysfunctions may be rewarding.

The micturition reflex is mediated by transient receptor potential cation channel subfamily V, member 1 (TRPV1)-positive nerves and probably — albeit to a lesser degree — also by TRP cation channel subfamily M, member 8 (TRPM8)-positive nerves. These same neurons convey nociceptive information (for example, bladder pain that is secondary to cystitis) to the central nervous system. TRPV4 is a key player in bladder function because it is present in both the urothelium and the detrusor muscle, and it is activated by stretch (bladder distension) and hypo-osmolar urine. The activator of TRPM8 in the bladder remains to be determined. The micturition reflex is under the control of a descending central nervous system pathway; when this pathway is disrupted (for example, as a result of spinal cord injury or multiple sclerosis), it becomes autonomous and partly driven by TRPV1. Collectively, these findings imply a therapeutic potential of TRPV1 antagonists (or TRPV1 desensitization) and/or TRPM8 agonists as therapies in painful bladder disorders (and in pain induced by benign prostatic hyperplasia) and in an overactive bladder. These findings also suggest that TRPV4 blockers could be useful in the management of an overactive bladder. DRG, dorsal root ganglion.

Cannabinoids

Cannabis Sativa (also known as "marijuana") contains approximately 60 pharmacologically active compounds ("cannabinoids"). Δ-9-Tetrahydrocannabinol (THC) was isolated in 1964 and the nonpsychoactive cannabidiol (CBD) in 1963; the ratio in botanical and pharmaceutical preparations determines therapeutic versus psychoactive effects, with the latter emerging when THC is higher in concentration.

The endocannabinoid system is widely distributed in the brain and spinal cord [105] and comprises the cannabinoid receptors (CB1 and CB2), their endogenous ("endocannabinoids") and exogenous ("exocannabinoids," such as plant-derived and synthetic cannabinoids) ligands, and related enzymes for biosynthesis and degradation, such as fatty acid amide hydrolase (FAAH) [106].

Clinical studies with the use of exocannabinoids on OAB symptoms are scarce and essentially restricted to multiple sclerosis patients, and the results have so far not been convincing. However, amplification of the activity of endocannabinoids by FAAH inhibitors may be an attractive approach [107].

Recently, a human G-protein coupled receptor called GPR55 was claimed to be a novel cannabinoid receptor [108]. These receptors have been showed to be located in animal and human urinary tract tissues (detrusor, bladder afferent nerves, and, particularly, urothelium) and are thought to be involved in regulation of bladder function and bladder inflammation [106, 108-111]. CB-agonists (intravesical, intrathecal and systemic administered) are reported to inhibit bladder afferent signalling as shown in animal models of bladder inflammation and to improve urodynamic parameters in naive and DO animals models [111-113].

Cannabis extracts and delta-9-tetrahydrocannabinol (THC) were found to reduce OAB symptoms in patients suffering from MS in open-label [114] and randomized trials [115].

Nabiximols (Sativex, GW Pharmaceuticals) is a specific extract of Cannabis approved as a botanical drug in the United Kingdom as a mouth spray for MS patients; he drug is a pharmaceutical product standardised in composition, formulation, and dose. Its principal active cannabinoid components are the cannabinoids THC) and CBD. In a RCT including patients suffering from NDO due to MSO, it failed to achieve primary endpoint (incontinence episodes); however significantly improved other OAB symptoms (e.g., voids per 24 h, nocturia, and bladder symptom severity) [116]. A systematic review in 2014 by the American Academy of Neurology found that nabiximols was 'probably effective' for spasticity, pain, and urinary dysfunction in MS patients [117].

Neurological side-effects of CB1-agonists, together with the unknown consequences of long-term use of such drugs, generated concern about their safety [118]. However, the intravesical administration of CB-agonists, the possible exploitation of CB2 (mainly peripheral) receptors and the inhibition of the FAAH by systemic, intravesical or intratecal-administered inhibitors may be alternative approaches to target the endocannabinoid system avoiding CNS side-effects [106, 110, 119, 120].

Modulation of Second Messengers

Specific modulation of intracellular second messenger pathways, shared by different but synergistic receptors, offers the possibility of a more complete and organ selective manipulation of tissue function, avoiding the inhibition/stimulation of a single receptor being bypassed by another acting on the same pathway.

PDE-Inhibitors

Phosphodiesterases (PDE) are enzymes that, degrading cyclic nucleotides (cAMP and cGMP), are able to reverse the cholinergic-induced contraction of human detrusor and to enhance cAMP/cGMP-mediated detrusor relaxation (Figure 2) [121]. The presence of PDE isoenzymes PDE1, PDE2, PDE3, PDE4 and PDE5 in the human detrusor was initially shown by Truss et al. [122]. They also demonstrated relaxant responses of human detrusor strip preparations contracted by the muscarinic agonist carbachol to papaverine (a nonspecific PDE inhibitor) and the PDE1 inhibitor vinpocetine. These effects were paralleled by an increase in cyclic AMP and cyclic GMP. Thus, based on these findings, they concluded that the PDE1 may be of significance in the control of the detrusor smooth muscle [123]. A randomized, double-blind, placebo-controlled study assessing the effects of vinpocetine in patients with urgency and urgency incontinence who had failed standard pharmacological therapy demonstrated that the PDE1 inhibitor was superior to placebo with regards to the outcome parameters of micturition frequency, bladder volume at first sensation, bladder volume at voiding desire, maximum detrusor pressure and voided volume [124].

The observation that patients treated for erectile dysfunction with PDE5 inhibitors had an improvement of their LUTS, has sparked a new interest in also using these drugs for treatment of LUTS and OAB. The mechanism behind the beneficial effect of the PDE5 inhibitors on LUTS/OAB and their site(s) of action are not still totally clear and several theories remain regarding the mechanism of action of PDE inhibitors. Studies have shown the involvement of the cAMP, cGMP, K^+-channel modulated pathways and the *l*-cysteine/H_2S pathway as possible pathways through which PDE5 inhibitors exert their effects on the bladder [125]. Animal models have also produced conflicting results as to the location of the bladder where the PDE5 inhibitors exert their effects, whether it is the muscle cells, nerve fibers, or interstitial cells. The drugs obviously do not interfere with the emptying ability of the bladder, and thus do not reduce the contractility of the detrusor muscle in response to parasympathetic (mainly cholinergic) activation. Like the β_3-AR agonists, the PDE5 inhibitors seem to act mainly during bladder filling. Sildenafil, a PDE5-Inhibitor, reversed the tonic cholinergic-induced contraction of human detrusor smooth muscle and produced relaxation *via* activation of cGMP- and cAMPdependent pathways, K+ channels and the hydrogen sulfide [H(2)S] signaling pathway [126]. Recently, the efficacy of the PDE5 inhibitor vardenafil was assessed in a randomized, double-blind, placebo-controlled trial in a cohort of 25 male patients with micturition disorders secondary to spinal cord injuries, all undergoing oxybutynin treatment; in this study, vardenafil decreased maximum detrusor pressure, improved cystometric capacity and increased volume at first sensation compared with placebo [127]. Different randomized controlled trials provided evidence about the efficacy and tolerability of PDE5-Is (sildenafil, tadalafil, vardenafil, and United Kingdom-369003) for the treatment of LUTS in male patients with or without erectile dysfunction, confirmed by meta-analyses [128, 129]. Tadalafil received the FDA approval in October 2011 for the treatment of males with LUTS secondary to BPH or concurrent LUTS and ED.

PDE-Is require further evaluations in order to better define their mechanism and site of action in LUT, their role and optimal dosage in different group of patients and in women, long-term safety and efficacy and cost-effectiveness. Stretch stimuli, or acetylcholine release, increase internal Ca^{2+} levels in NOS-expressing urothelial cells. NOS produces NO, which signals to detrusor smooth muscle cells. NO is thought to have a modulatory role in the lower urinary tract, including the relaxation of urethral smooth muscle, modulation of neurotransmitter release from efferent nerves, regulation of urothelial permeability, and modulation of afferent nerve activity. Moreover, a pathophysiological role of NO has been suggested because injury or chronic inflammation can upregulate the expression of inducible NOS. Guanylyl cyclases located in the cytoplasm or plasma membrane synthesize cGMP in response to NO or CNP, respectively. cAMP is synthesized by adenylyl cyclases, either associated with G protein-coupled receptors in the plasma membrane, or in the cytoplasm.

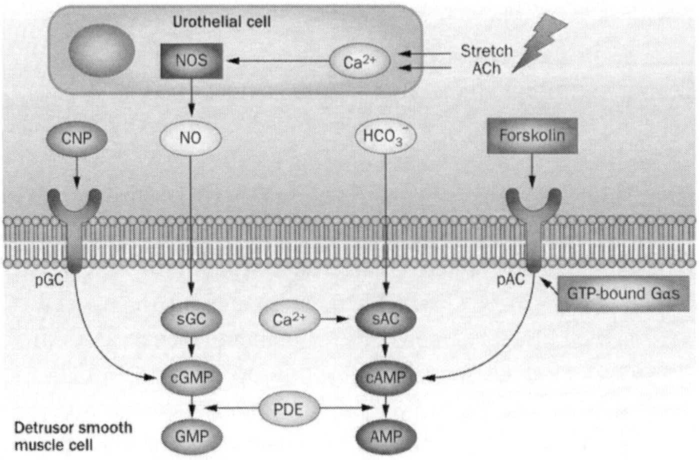

With permission of Nature Publishing Group.

Figure 2. Schematic diagram of the cyclic nucleotide signalling pathways [180].

Membrane-associated adenylyl cyclases are activated by GTP-bound $G_s\alpha$ and forskolin, whereas cytoplasmic adenylyl cyclases are regulated by HCO_3^- and Ca^{2+}, but insensitive to forskolin or activated $G_s\alpha$. cAMP and cGMP are hydrolysed to AMP and GMP, respectively, by phosphodiesterases (PDEs). Abbreviations: ACh, acetylcholine; CNP, C-like natriuretic peptide; NOS, nitric oxide synthase; pAC, particulate (plasma membrane) adenyl cyclase; PDE, phosphodiesterase; pGC, particulate (plasma membrane) guanylyl cyclase; sAC, soluble (cytoplasmic) adenyl cyclase; sGC, soluble guanylyl cyclase.

Nitric Oxid Donors

Nitric oxide (NO) is a potent biological messenger that promotes detrusor relaxation, likely *via* the elevation of intracellular cGMP. NO is thought to have a modulatory role in the LUT, including the relaxation of urethral smooth muscle, modulation of neurotransmitter release from efferent nerves, regulation of urothelial permeability, and modulation of afferent nerve activity. Moreover, a pathophysiological role of NO has been suggested because injury or chronic inflammation can upregulate the expression of inducible NOS.

HCT-1026 (nitroflurbiprofen, by NicOx SA) is a NO-releasing derivative of the nonsteroidal anti-inflammatory drugs (NSAID) flurbiprofen [130] and is thought to combine the analgesic and anti-inflammatory effects of flurbiprofen with the smooth muscle relaxant effect of the NO moiety. HCT1026 was shown to be more potent than flurbiprofen in inhibiting carbachol-induced bladder strip contractions in vitro. Phase I trials showed good safety and acceptability, potent prostaglandin inhibition and reduced gastric toxicity by means of gastroscopic evaluation [131, 132]. In a pilot phase IIa study in patients with neurogenic bladder, an improvement in urodynamic parameters and clinical symptoms was observed [132], providing a rationale for phase III trials.

Cox-Inhibitors

The role of prostaglandins (PGs) in the modulation of the bladder function has been suggested in several studies [133]. PGF2α, PGE1, and PGE2 are involved in inducing slow contractions in isolated animal and human detrusor and a role of PGs in the maintenance of detrusor tone and in the modulation of efferent and afferent neurotransmission has been suggested [134]. In patients affected by DO due to SCI [135] or BOO [136, 137] has been shown that the release of PGE2, which acts *via* mainly EP receptors, is elevated. Intravesical instillation of PGE2 has been also shown to induce DO, urgency and decreases bladder capacity in humans [138]. PGs are locally synthesized in human bladder by constitutive (COX-1) and inducible (COX-2) cyclooxygenase [133]. Several factors including stretch, nerve stimulation, injury, exposure to ATP and other inflammatory mediators may induce the synthesis of PGs [134]. COX-inhibitors such as NSAID seem to be able to increase bladder capacity and increase micturition interval without affecting voiding phase in rats, and favorable clinical effects have been reported in OAB patients treated with aspirin, indometacin, flurbiprofen, ketoprofen and loxoprofen [139, 140].

Cardozo et al. [139] performed a double-blind controlled study including 30 women with DO using the prostaglandin synthesis inhibitor flurbiprofen at a dosage of 50 mg three times daily. The drug was shown to have favourable effects, although it did not completely abolish DO. There was a high incidence of side effects (43%) including nausea, vomiting, headache and gastrointestinal symptoms. Other preclinical findings have also indicated COX-2-selective inhibitors as potential drugs in the treatment of OAB, also by intravesical instillation [141, 142]. NSAIDs might open a novel treatment opportunity for OAB although clinical evidence of efficacy of COX-inhibitors in OAB patients remains low and side-effects are important issues with these drugs [143].

ROCK Inhibitors

The Ras homologue family member A (RhoA) is a guanosine triphosphate hydrolase (GTPase) that, together with one of its downstream effectors, the type I and type II Rho-kinases, have a central role in the regulation of bladder smooth muscle from human and various animal species. Rho-kinase pathway modulates the level of phosphorylation of the myosin light chain, mainly through the inhibition of myosin phosphatase. Recent experimental data indicate that its role might be exacerbated in local and systemic pathological conditions which affect the bladder, as well as OAB [144-146]. It seems that Rho-kinase inhibitors, such as Y27632 and HA-1077 (fasudil), may turn out to be an effective group of drugs in pharmacotherapy of OAB, which will influence the storage phase of the micturition cycle, without interfering with the physiological voiding [147]. In a study on spontaneous hypertensive rats with OAB the role of RhoA/Rho-kinase pathway in DO was examined by evaluating the effect of Y-27632 on bladder function. Results showed that inhibition of Rho-kinase activity with Y-27632 produced a significant suppression of DO [148]. Identification of Rho-kinase isoforms that are bladder-tissue specific and their selective inhibitors may help to disassociate the unwanted hypotensive effects of this approach, making ROCK inhibitors begin a new pharmacological approach to treat OAB/DO.

Elocalcitol

Elocalcitol, which had been under development by BioXell SpA, is a synthetic derivative of vitamin D3 that regulates cell proliferation and apoptosis via its binding to the vitamin D receptor. Elocalcitol appears to modulate bladder contractility by decreasing calcium sensitization and increasing L-type mediated calcium entry [149]. In preclinical studies, elocalcitol inhibited the androgen-dependent and androgen-independent proliferation of benign prostatic hyperplasia (BPH) cells more potently than finasteride, a 5alpha-reductase inhibitor [150]. A proof-of-concept clinical study prompted a phase IIb RCT including 308 OAB women with encouraging results: although elocalcitol failed to meet the primary endpoint (change in bladder volume at the first involuntary detrusor contraction), it demonstrated a good efficacy on patients' symptoms perception and a favorable efficacy/tolerability profile [151]. Given the novel mechanism of action, efficacy profile and improved tolerability of elocalcitol over existing classes of drugs, the compound could have potentially added to the armamentarium in the expanding therapeutic markets of OAB, BPH, and male infertility. However, this possibility appears to have been negated by BioXell's recent decision to terminate all further development of elocalcitol.

GENE THERAPIES

The bladder is ideally suited for molecular medicine. Through gene therapy we can replace, supplement, or suppress a protein or cytokine to correct a disease process. Here we present potential targets for OAB gene therapy, as well as GABAergic therapy, ion channels selective drugs and liposome-delivered therapies.

GABAergic Therapy

As previously seen, glycine and GABA inhibitory mechanisms have been identified in rat spinal cord in local interneuronal inhibitory pathways, projecting directly in periganglia neurons [20]. Intratecal injection of $GABA_A$ and $GABA_B$ agonists increase bladder capacity and decrease voiding pressure in rats [152]. Increasing GABA in the spinal cord *via* viral-mediated gene delivery could be considered an alternative strategy in treating OAB symptoms. Recently, gene therapy using intravesical injection in SCI rats of HSV-GAD (replication-defective herpes simplex virus vectors encoding genes of glutamic acid decarboxylase, the GABA synthesis enzyme) significantly decreased the number and amplitude of non-voiding contractions compared with controls, without blunting micturition pressure likely *via* the inhibition of the afferent limb of the micturition reflex [153]. *GAD* gene therapy mainly inhibits DO mediated by C-fibers bladder afferent pathways via activation of $GABA_A$ receptors.

Thus, *GAD* gene therapy gives promise to become a novel therapy of urinary dysfunctions in SCI patients.

Potassium Channels Openers

One promising class of drugs that a number of pharmaceutical companies are considering for the treatment of OAB is potassium channel openers (KCOs).

Many types of potassium channels have been demonstrated in the detrusor smooth muscle [154]: (1) big, intermediate and small calcium-activated channels (BK or maxi-K, IK and SK, respectively); (2) voltage-dependent (KV) channels; (3) inward-rectifying ATP-dependent channels (KATP, also known as Kir6 channels, a subtype of the Kir channels family); and (4) two-poredomain (K2P) channels (also known as “leak potassium channels”).

Drugs such as cromakalim, pinacidil, and ZD6169, that open ATP-sensitive K^+ (K_{ATP}) channels and produce membrane hyperpolarization, are effective in suppressing spontaneous action potentials and isolated contractions of bladder smooth muscle. K_{ATP} channel openers are more effective in blocking spontaneous bladder contractions than neurally evoked ones, and therefore should be more active in suppressing involuntary bladder contractions during bladder filling without interfering with normal voiding. ZD6169, a K_{ATP} channel opener, orally administered reduces voiding frequency in rats and dogs without lowering blood pressure [155]. Intravesical administration in rats increases the bladder volume at which a micturition reflex is induced and also decreases the frequency and amplitude of spontaneous bladder contractions and reduces voiding pressure in both normal and outlet-obstructed animals [155, 156]. It has been suggested that the drug acts not only on bladder smooth muscle but also on capsaicin-sensitive bladder afferents to reduce afferent firing induced by bladder distention or chemical irritation of the mucosa [156].

The role of K_V channels in normal and pathological detrusor activity remains controversial and largely unexplored [157]. A reduction in potassium currents through K_V channels has been involved in the hyperexcitability of the afferent neurons [158]. A phase II trial on flupirtine, a K_{V7} channel opener, is ongoing (EudraCT Number:2006-004854-26) but another one (NCT00439192) has been terminated because the AE profile did not match expectations.

Although their role is still debated, interesting preclinical observations are also available on openers of SK channel [159, 160], combined SK/IK channel [161] and putative TREK-1 K2P channel [162]. Nevertheless, ongoing efforts are aimed at developing new classes of more potent and selective KCOs that may lead to the development of a bladder-selective clinical therapeutic agent.

Maxi-K

The most physiologically important, and consequently the most extensive investigated K^+ channel subtype, is the large conductance $Ca2^+$-activated K^+ (big potassium or BK) channel, also called *Maxi-K* or *slo1*. *Maxi-K* channels play a role in modulating contraction and relaxation responses in smooth muscle cells. Bladder injection of human *maxi-K* channel DNA blocked detrusor hyperactivity in partially urethral-obstructed female rats [163]. It is hypothesized that expression of *hSlo* in rat bladder functionally antagonizes the increased contractility normally observed in obstructed animals and thereby ameliorates bladder overactivity [163].

NGF Blokade

In the urinary tract, nerve growth factor (NGF) is produced by urothelium and smooth muscle [164]. It has been suggested that selective inhibitors of NGF may be a new way to treat OAB [165]. Clinical and experimental data corroborate this hypothesis: urinary NGF levels increased in patients with bladder outlet obstruction and OAB symptoms and decreased after successful treatment of OAB with oral antimuscarinics or intradetrusorial injection of Botulinum Toxin A [166-168]. NGF overexpression in the bladder and bladder afferent pathways has also been reported to be involved in the emergence of hyperexcitability in bladder C-fiber sensory pathways [169]; on the other side, intrathecal administration of NGF antibodies decreased NGF levels in bladder afferent pathways and normalized bladder/urethral function in SCI rats [170]. It has been demonstered by Jang et coll that intravesical instillation with COX-2 inhibitors can reduce cyclophosphamide-induced OAB by acting on NGF expression [171]. However, NGF inhibitors are not jet available as a current treatment for OAB and is still under investigation.

Intravesical liposome-delivered *antisense* NGF-suppressing therapy could be an attractive approach for OAB, avoiding the toxicity of systemic nonspecific blockade [172], although there is nonclinical evidence that the local instillation of antisense oligonucleotides against the NGF can suppress DO and the expression of NGF and chemokines [172]. The term *antisense* therapeutics emerged from seminal studies done 4 decades using a short synthetic oligonucleotide for sequence-specific gene silencing.

Empty liposomes itself can act as a topical healing agent and same has been demonstrated in treatment of dry eye [173]. Either empty or with entrapped drugs, liposomes have also been used in ophthalmology to ameliorate keratitis, corneal transplant rejection, uveitis, endophthalmitis, and proliferative vitreoretinopathy [174]. These reports encouraged investigation of empty liposomes as a therapeutic agent for bladder injury. Interaction of liposomes with cultured urothelium cells suggested that liposomes can be adsorbed and be endocytosed [175]. Previous studies showed that binding of large multilamellar liposomes to the bladder cells was stronger than of sonicated small size liposomes. Bladder reflex activity of female Sprague-Dawley rats before and after treatment was evaluated by continuous cystometry under urethane anaesthesia (1.0 g/kg). Intravesical liposomes were effective in doubling the intercontractile interval (ICI) compared with PPS, while acute instillation of DMSO failed to produce any protective effect in this animal model [176].

In 2008, Lee et al. [177] further improved this model of DO induced by intravesical infusion by combining it with systemic metabolic alteration through fructose feeding. Metabolic syndrome created by feeding of fructose to rats can lead to DO and urination frequency [177]. Cystometric bladder capacity of fructose fed rats can be further decreased by instillation of acidic ATP solution, which provokes reflex micturition via afferent noise. Evidence suggests that increased expression or release of neurotransmitters in the mucosal layer of the bladder can generate afferent noise via C-fiber pathway and result in DO [178]. Compared to infusion with normal saline, ATP solution decreased bladder capacity and increased phasic contractions.

REFERENCES

[1] Abrams P., Cardozo L., Fall M. et al. The standardisation of terminology of lower urinary tract function: report from the Standardisation Sub-committee of the International Continence Society (ICS). *Neurourol. Urodyn.,* 2002; 21(2):167–178.

[2] Kelleher C. J., Kreder K. J., Pleil A. M., Burgess S. M., Reese P. R. Longterm health-related quality of life of patients receiving extendedrelease tolterodine for overactive bladder. *Am. J. Manag. Care,* 2002; 8:S616-S630.

[3] Sacco E., Tienforti D., D'Addessi A., Pinto F., Racioppi M., Totaro A., D'Agostino D., Marangi F., Bassi P. Social, economic, and health utility considerations in the treatment of overactive bladder. *Open Access J. Urol.,* 2010; 2: 11-24.

[4] Sacco E. Physiopathology of overactive bladder syndrome. *Urologia,* 2012; 79: 24-35.

[5] Sacco E., Bientinesi R., Tienforti D., Racioppi M., Gulino G., D'Agostino D., Vittori M., Bassi P. Discovery history and clinical development of mirabegron for the treatment of overactive bladder and urinary incontinence. *Expert Opin. Drug Discov.,* 2014; 9:433-448.

[6] Duthie J. B., Vincent M., Herbison G. P., Wilson D. I., Wilson D. Botulinum toxin injections for adults with overactive bladder syndrome. *Cochrane Database Syst. Rev.,* 2011; (12): CD005493.

[7] Chapple C. R., Khullar V., Gabriel Z., Muston D., Bitoun C. E., Weinstein D. The effects of antimuscarinic treatments in overactive bladder: an update of a systematic review and metaanalysis. *Eur. Urol.,* 2008; 54(3):543–562.

[8] Sacco E., Bientinesi R. Mirabegron: a review of recent data and its prospects in the management of overactive bladder. *Ther. Adv. Urol.,* 2012; 4(6):315–324.

[9] Sacco E., Pinto F., Bassi P. Emerging pharmacological targets in overactive bladder therapy: experimental and clinical evidences. *Int. Urogynecol. J. Pelvic Floor Dysfunct.,* 2008; 19: 583-598.

[10] Sacco E., Bientinesi R. Innovative pharmacotherapies for women with overactive bladder: where are we now and what is in the pipeline? *Int. Urogynecol. J.,* 2015; 26: 629-640.

[11] de Groat W. C. Integrative control of the lower urinary tract: Preclinical perspective. *BJP,* 2006; 147:S25–40.

[12] akakibara R., Fowler C. J. Brain disease (Chapter 9). In: Seminars in Clinical Neurology (by World Federation of Neurology). Neurologic bladder, bowel, and sexual function. Edited by Fowler C. J., Boston: Elsevier; 2001:229–43.

[13] Blok B. F. The central control of micturition and continence: Implications for urology. *Br. J. Urol. Int.,* 1999; 83(Suppl. 2):1–6.

[14] Sakakibara R., Nakazawa K., Shiba K., et al. Firing patterns of micturition-related neurons in the pontine storage centre in cats. *Auton. Neurosci.,* 2002; 99:24–30.

[15] Kavia R. B. C., Dasgupta R., Fowler C. J. Functional imaging and the central control of the bladder. *J. Comp. Neurol.,* 2005; 493:27–32.

[16] Matsumoto G., Hisamitsu T., De Groat W. C. Role of glutamate and NMDA receptors in the descending limb of the spinobulbospinal micturition reflex pathway of the rat. *Neurosci. Lett.,* 1995; 183:58–61.

[17] Blok B. F., de Weerd H., Holstege G. The pontine micturition center projects to sacral cord GABA immunoreactive neurons in the cat. *Neurosci. Lett.,* 1997; 233:109–12.

[18] Fowler C. J. Integrated control of lower urinary tract: Clinical perspective. *BJP,* 2006; 147:S14–24.

[19] Yokoyama O., Yoshiyama M., Namiki M., et al. Changes in dopaminergic and glutamatergic excitatory mechanisms of micturition reflex after middle cerebral artery occlusion in conscious rats. *Exp. Neurol.,* 2002; 173:129–35.

[20] Miyazato M., Yoshimura N., Nishijima S., Sugaya K. Roles of Glycinergic and Gamma-aminobutyric-ergic Mechanisms in the Micturition Reflex in Rats. *Low Urin Tract Symptoms,* 2009; 1:S70-S73.

[21] Miyazato M., Sasatomi K., Hiragata S., Sugaya K., Chancellor M. B., de Groat W. C. et al. GABA-receptor activation in the lumbosacral spinal cord reduces detrusor overactivity in spinal cord injured rats. *J. Urol.,* 2008; 179: 1178–1183.

[22] Taylor C. M., Bates C. P. A double-blind crossover trial of baclofen-a new treatment for the unstable bladder syndrome. *Br. J. Urol.,* 1979; 51: 504–505.

[23] Haubensak K. A double-blind trial with the antispasticity drug Lioresal in 15 paraplegics with upper neuron lesions. *Urol. Int.,* 1977; 132: 198–201.

[24] Xu D., Qu C., Meng H., Ren J., Zhu Y., Min Z. et al. Dysfunctional voiding confirmed by transdermal perineal electromyography, and its effective treatment with baclofen in women with lower urinary tract symptoms: a randomized doubleblind placebo-controlled crossover trial. *BJU Int.,* 2007;100: 588–592.

[25] Steers W. D., Meythaler J. M., Haworth C., Herrell D., Park T. S. Effects of acute bolus and chronic continuous intrathecal baclofen on genitourinary dysfunction due to spinal cord pathology. *J. Urol.,* 1992; 148: 1849-1855.

[26] Kalinichev M., Palea S., Haddouk H., Royer-Urios I., Guilloteau V., Lluel P., Schneider M., Saporito M., Poli S. ADX71441, a novel, potent and selective positive allosteric modulator of the GABA(B) receptor, shows efficacy in rodent models of overactive bladder. *Br. J. Pharmacol.*, 2014 Feb.; 171(4):995-1006.

[27] Pehrson R., Andersson K. E. Effects of tiagabine, a gammaaminobutyric acid re-uptake inhibitor, on normal rat bladder function. *J. Urol.,* 2002; 167: 2241-2246.

[28] A. M. Chung, L. S. Eiland Use of second-generation antiepileptic drugs in the pediatric population. *Paediatr. Drugs*, 10 (4) (2008), pp. 217–254.

[29] Maneuf Y. P., Gonzalez M. I., Sutton K. S., Chung F. Z., Pinnock R. D., Lee K. Cellular and molecular action of the putative GABA-mimetic, gabapentin. *Cell Mol. Life Sci.,* 2003; 60: 742-750.

[30] A. Carbone, A. Tubaro, P. Morello, R. Parascani, C. Catalani, G. Palleschi The effect of gabapentin on neurogenic detrusor over activity, a pilot study. *Eur. Urol. Suppl.*, 2 (2003), pp. 141–155.

[31] Kim Y. T., Kwon D. D., Kim J., Kim D. K., Lee J. Y., Chancellor M. B. Gabapentin for overactive bladder and nocturia after anticholinergic failure. *Int. Braz. J. Urol.,* 2004; 30: 275-278.

[32] Ansari M. S., Bharti A., Kumar R., Ranjan P., Srivastava A., Kapoor R. Gabapentin: a novel drug as add-on therapy in cases of refractory overactive bladder in children. *J. Pediatr. Urol.,* 2013; 9: 17-22.

[33] St. Luke's Medical Center, Philippines. Efficacy and Safety of Gabapentin in Treating Overactive Bladder (OAB). In: ClinicalTrials.gov [Internet]. Bethesda (MD): National Library of Medicine (US). Available from: URL: https://clinicaltrials.gov/ct2/show/NCT01486706.

[34] DDP-200. DrugBank. Available from: URL: http://www.drugbank. ca/drugs/DB05919 Accession Number: DB05919.

[35] Wesche D., Bockbrader H. A pharmacokinetic comparison of pregabalin and gabapentin [abstract]. *J. Pain,* 2005; 6:S29.

[36] Marencak J., Cossons N. H., Darekar A., Mills I. W. Investigation of the clinical efficacy and safety of pregabalin alone or combined with tolterodine in female subjects with idiopathic overactive bladder. *Neurourol. Urodyn.*, 2011 Jan.; 30(1):75-82.

[37] Pfizer. Investigation of Tolterodine, Pregabalin and a Tolterodine - Pregabalin Combination for the Treatment of Overactive Bladder. In: ClinicalTrials.gov [Internet]. Bethesda (MD): National Library of Medicine (US). Available from: URL: http://clinicaltrials.gov/show/ NCT00746681 NLM Identifier: NCT00746681.

[38] Loutochin O., Al Afraa T., Campeau L., Mahfouz W., Elzayat E., Corcos J. Effect of the anticonvulsant medications pregabalin and lamotrigine on urodynamic parameters in an animal model of neurogenic detrusor overactivity. *Neurourol. Urodyn.,* 2012; 31:1197-1202.

[39] Kafri R., Kodesh A., Shames J., Golomb J., Melzer I. Depressive symptoms and treatment of women with urgency urinary incontinence. *Int. Urogynecol. J.,* 2013; 24: 1953-1959.

[40] Samsung Medical Center. Efficacy and Safety of Selective Serotonin Reuptake Inhibitor (SSRI) in Overactive Bladder Patients. In: ClinicalTrials.gov [Internet]. Bethesda (MD): National Library of Medicine (US). Available from: URL: http: //clinicaltrials.gov/show/ NCT00902421 NLM Identifier: NCT00902421.

[41] Mariappan P., Alhasso A., Ballantyne Z., et al. Duloxetine, a serotonine and noradrenaline reuptake inhibitor (SNRI), for the treatment of stress urinary incontinence: a systematic review. *Eur. Urol.,* 2007; 51(1): 67Y74.

[42] Steers W. D., Herschorn S., Kreder K. J., Moore K., Strohbehn K., Yalcin I., Bump R. C.; Duloxetine OAB Study Group. Duloxetine compared with placebo for treating women with symptoms of overactive bladder. *BJU Int.,* 2007; 100: 337-345. Thor K. B. Serotonin and norepinephrine involvement in efferent pathways to the urethral rhabdosphincter: implications for treating stress urinary incontinence. *Urology,* 2003; 62:3Y9.

[43] Di Rezze S. 1., Frasca V., Inghilleri M., Durastanti V., Cortese A., Giacomelli E., Millefiorini E. Duloxetine for the treatment of overactive bladder syndrome in multiple sclerosis: a pilot study. *Clin. Neuropharmacol.,* 2012; 35(5):231-4.

[44] Dimascio A., Heninger G., Klerman G. L.. Psychopharmacology of Imipramine and Desipramine: A Comparative Study of Their Effects in Normal Males. *Psychopharmacologia,* 1964; 5:361-71.

[45] Hillelsohn J. H., Rais-Bahrami S., Bagadiya N., Kashan M., Weiss G. H. Use of desipramine for the treatment of overactive bladder refractory to antimuscarinic therapy. *Urol. J.,* 2014. 4;10(4):1114-8.

[46] UROGENE. Besipirdine. Available from: URL: http: //urogene.free. fr/besipirdine.php.

[47] Yoshiyama M., Kakizaki H., de Groat W. C. Suppression of the micturition reflex in urethane-anesthetized rats by intra-cerebroventricular injection of WAY100635, a 5-HT(1A) receptor antagonist. *Brain Res.,* 2003; 980: 281-287.

[48] D'Agostino G., Condino A. M., Gallinari P., Franceschetti G. P., Tonini M. Characterization of prejunctional serotonin receptors modulating [3H]acetylcholine release in the human detrusor. *J. Pharmacol. Exp. Ther.,* 2006; 316: 129-135.

[49] Mbaki Y., Gardiner J., McMurray G., Ramage A. G. 5-HT 2A receptor activation of the external urethral sphincter and 5-HT 2C receptor inhibition of micturition: a study based on pharmacokinetics in the anaesthetized female rat. *Eur. J. Pharmacol.,* 2012; 682: 142-152.

[50] Tai C., Miscik C. L., Ungerer T. D., Roppolo J. R., de Groat W. C. Suppression of bladder reflex activity in chronic spinal cord injured cats by activation of serotonin 5-HT1A receptors. *Exp. Neurol.,* 2006; 199: 427-437.

[51] Chang H. H., Havton L. A. Serotonergic 5-HT(1A) receptor agonist (8-OH-DPAT) ameliorates impaired micturition reflexes in a chronic ventral root avulsion model of incomplete cauda equina/conus medullaris injury. *Exp. Neurol.,* 2013; 239: 210-217.

[52] Takimoto Y., Kodama M., Sugimoto S., Hamada T., Fuse T., Kawata N. et al. (1999) The effect of 5-HT2 antagonist for urinary frequency symptom on diabetes mellitus patients. *Nippon Hinyokika Gakkai Zasshi,* 90:731–740.

[53] Dardable B., Behr-Roussel D., Gorny D., Lebret T., Benoit G., Hieble J. P. et al. (2005) Piboserod (SB 207266), a selective 5-HT4 receptor antagonist, reduces serotonin potentiation of neurally-mediated contractile responses of human detrusor muscle. *World J. Urol.,* 23(2):147–151.

[54] Kakizaki H., Yoshiyama M., Koyanagi T., De Groat W. C. Effects of WAY100635, a selective 5-HT1A-receptor antagonist on the micturition-reflex pathway in the rat. *Am. J. Physiol. Regul. Integr. Comp. Physiol.,* 2001; 280:R1407–R1413.

[55] Schwen Z., Matsuta Y., Shen B., Wang J., Roppolo J. R., de Groat W. C., Tai C. (2013) Inhibition of bladder overactivity by duloxetine in combination with foot stimulation or WAY-100635 treatment in cats. *Am. J. Physiol. Renal Physiol.,* 305(12):F1663–F1668.

[56] Reese J., Xiao Z., Schwen Z., Matsuta Y., Shen B., Wang J., Roppolo J. R., de Groat W. C., Tai C. Effects of duloxetine and WAY100635 on pudendal inhibition of bladder overactivity in cats. *J. Pharmacol. Exp. Ther.,* 2014; 349(3):402–407.

[57] Kodama M., Takimoto Y. Influence of 5-hydroxytryptamine and the effect of a new serotonin receptor antagonist (sarpogrelate) on detrusor smooth muscle of streptozotocin-induced diabetes mellitus in the rat. *Int. J. Urol.,* 2000; 7: 231-235.

[58] Mbaki Y., Gardiner J., McMurray G., Ramage A. G. 5-HT 2A receptor activation of the external urethral sphincter and 5-HT 2C receptor inhibition of micturition: a study based on pharmacokinetics in the anaesthetized female rat. *Eur. J. Pharmacol.,* 2012; 682: 142-152.

[59] Kodama M., Takimoto Y. Influence of 5-hydroxytryptamine and the effect of a new serotonin receptor antagonist (sarpogrelate) on detrusor smooth muscle of streptozotocin-induced diabetes mellitus in the rat. *Int. J. Urol.,* 2000; 7: 231-235.

[60] Takimoto Y., Kodama M., Sugimoto S., Hamada T., Fuse T., Kawata N., Hirakata H., Hosokawa H. The effect of 5-HT 2 antagonist for urinary frequency symptom on diabetes mellitus patients. *Nihon Hinyokika Gakkai Zasshi,* 1999; 90: 731-740.

[61] Darblade B., Behr-Roussel D., Gorny D., Lebret T., Benoit G., Hieble J. P., Brooks D., Alexandre L., Giuliano F. Piboserod (SB 207266), a selective 5-HT4 receptor antagonist, reduces serotonin potentiation of neurally-mediated contractile responses of human detrusor muscle. *World J. Urol.,* 2005; 23: 147-151.

[62] Recordati S.p.A. Available from: URL: http://www.recordati.it/ ~/media/Files/R/Recordati-V2/investors/presentations/2005it/2005-09-22.pdf.

[63] Birder L. A., de Groat W. C. Mechanisms of disease: involvement of the urothelium in bladder dysfunction. *Nat. Clin. Pract. Urol.,* 2007; 4:46-54.

[64] Burnstock G. Therapeutic potential of purinergic signalling for diseases of the urinary tract. *BJU Int.,* 2011; 107: 192-204.

[65] Ruggieri M. R. Mechanisms of disease: role of purinergic signaling in the pathophysiology of bladder dysfunction. *Nat. Clin. Pract. Urol.,* 2006; 3: 206-215.

[66] Zhang H. P., Li C. L., Lu P., Zheng J. C., Yu L. L., Yang W. M., Xiong F., Zeng X. Y. The function of P2X3 receptor and NK1 receptor antagonists on cyclophosphamide-induced cystitis in rats. *World J. Urol.,* 2014; 32: 91-97.

[67] Uvin P., Boudes M., Menigoz A., Franken J., Pinto S., Gevaert T., Verplaetse R., Tytgat J., Vennekens R., Voets T., De Ridder D. Chronic administration of anticholinergics in rats induces a shift from muscarinic to purinergic transmission in the bladder wall. *Eur. Urol.,* 2013; 64: 502-510.

[68] Yoshida M., Homma Y., Inadome A., Yono M., Seshita H., Miyamoto Y., Murakami S., Kawabe K., Ueda S. Age-related changes in cholinergic and purinergic neurotransmission in human isolated bladder smooth muscles. *Exp. Gerontol.,* 2001; 36: 99-109.

[69] O'Reilly B. A., Kosaka A. H., Knight G. F., Chang T. K., Ford A. P., Rymer J. M., Popert R., Burnstock G., McMahon S. B. P2X receptors and their role in female idiopathic detrusor instability. *J. Urol.,* 2002; 167:157-164.

[70] Burnstock G. Therapeutic potential of purinergic signalling for diseases of the urinary tract. *BJU Int.,* 2011; 107: 192-204.

[71] Brady C. M., Apostolidis A., Yiangou Y., Baecker P. A., Ford A. P., Freeman A., Jacques T. S., Fowler C. J., Anand P. P2X3-immunoreactive nerve fibres in neurogenic detrusor overactivity and the effect of intravesical resiniferatoxin. *Eur. Urol.,* 2004; 46: 247-253.

[72] North R. A., Jarvis M. F. P2X receptors as drug targets. *Mol. Pharmacol.*, 2013; 83: 759-769.

[73] Kaan T. K. Y., Yip P. K., Grist J., Gever J. R., Cefalu J. S., Nunn P. A., Ford A. P., Zhong Y., McMahon S. B. Selective Blockade of Spinal P2X3 and P2X2/3 Receptors with a Novel and Selective Antagonist, AF-742, Reveals Central Endogenous Purinergic Regulation of Bladder Activity. Abstract 602 at 2010 Joint Annual Meeting of the International Continence Society and the International Urogynecological Association in Toronto, Canada. Available from: URL: http://www.ics.org/ Abstracts/Publish/105/000602.pdf.

[74] Hemmings-Mieszczak M., Dorn G., Natt F. J., Hall J., Wishart W. L. Independent combinatorial effect of antisense oligonucleotides and RNAi-mediated specific inhibition of the recombinant rat P2X3 receptor. *Nucleic Acids Res.,* 2003; 31: 2117-2126.

[75] Lecci A., Maggi C. A. Tachykinins as modulators of the micturition reflex in the central and peripheral nervous system. *Regul. Pept.,* 2001; 101: 1-18.

[76] Seki S., Erickson K. A., Seki M., Nishizawa O., Igawa Y., Ogawa T., de Groat W. C., Chancellor M. B., Yoshimura N. Elimination of rat spinal neurons expressing neurokinin 1 receptors reduces bladder overactivity and spinal c-fos expression induced by bladder irritation. *Am. J. Physiol. Renal Physiol.,* 2005; 288: F466-F473.

[77] Ishizuka O., Igawa Y., Nishizawa O., Andersson K. E. Role of supraspinal tachykinins for volume- and L-dopa-induced bladder activity in normal conscious rats. *Neurourol. Urodyn.,* 2000; 19:101-109.

[78] Andersson K. E., Wein A. J. Pharmacology of the lower urinary tract: basis for current and future treatments of urinary incontinence. *Pharmacol. Rev.,* 2004; 56: 581-631.

[79] Abdel-Gawad M., Dion S. B., Elhilali M. M. Evidence of a peripheral role of neurokinins in detrusor hyperreflexia: a further study of selective tachykinin antagonists in chronic spinal injured rats. *J. Urol.,* 2001; 165: 1739-1744.

[80] Green S. A., Alon A., Ianus J., McNaughton K. S., Tozzi C. A., Reiss T. F. Efficacy and safety of a neurokinin-1 receptor antagonist in postmenopausal women with overactive bladder with urge urinary incontinence. *J. Urol.,* 2006; 176: 2535-2540; discussion 2540.

[81] Frenkl T. L., Zhu H., Reiss T., Seltzer O., Rosenberg E., Green S. A multicenter, double-blind, randomized, placebo controlled trial of a neurokinin-1 receptor antagonist for overactive bladder. *J. Urol.,* 2010; 184: 616-622.

[82] Haab F., Braticevici B., Krivoborodov G., Palmas M., Zufferli Russo M., Pietra C. Efficacy and safety of repeated dosing of netupitant, a neurokinin-1 receptor antagonist, in treating overactive bladder. *Neurourol. Urodyn.,* 2014; 33: 335-340.

[83] Grond S., Sablotzki A. Clinical pharmacology of tramadol. *Clin. Pharmacokinet.*, 2004; 43: 879-923.

[84] Safarinejad M. R., Hosseini S. Y. Safety and efficacy of tramadol in the treatment of idiopathic detrusor overactivity: a double-blind, placebo-controlled, randomized study. *Br. J. Clin. Pharmacol.*, 2006; 61: 456-463.

[85] Singh S. K., Agarwal M. M., Batra Y. K., Kishore A. V., Mandal A. K. Effect of lumbar-epidural administration of tramadol on lower urinary tract function. *Neurourol. Urodyn.*, 2008; 27: 65-70.

[86] KeyNeurotek Pharma GmbH. Double-blind placebo-controlled proof of concept study with the μ-receptor agonist KN203 in patients with overactive bladder syndrome. Double-blind, randomized, parallel groups prospective phase II-a study for 8 weeks with two dosages of KN203 (20 and 40 mg b.i.d.) and placebo. National Competent Authority: Germany - BfArM. Available from: URL:http://www.clinicaltrialsregister.eu [EudraCT Number: 2009-013334-24] EudraCT Number: 2009-013334-24.

[87] Dray A., Nunan L., Wire W. Central delta-opioid receptor interactions and the inhibition of reflex urinary bladder contractions in the rat. *Br. J. Pharmacol.*, 1985; 85: 717-726.

[88] Holt J. D., Watson M. J., Chang J. P., O'Neill S. J., Wei K., Pendergast W., Gengo P. J., Chang K. J. DPI-221 [4-((alpha-s)-alpha-((2s,5r)-2,5-dimethyl-4-(3-fluorobenzyl)-1-piperazinyl)benzyl)-N,Ndiethylbenzamide]: a novel nonpeptide delta receptor agonist producing increased micturition interval in normal rats. *J. Pharmacol. Exp. Ther.*, 2005; 315: 601-608.

[89] Andersson K. E., Gratzke C., Hedlund P. The role of the transient receptor potential (TRP) superfamily of cation-selective channels in the management of the overactive bladder. *BJU Int.*, 2010; 106: 1114-1127.

[90] Streng T., Axelsson H. E., Hedlund P., et al. Distribution and function of the hydrogen sulfide-sensitive TRPA1 ion channel in rat urinary bladder. *Eur. Urol.*, 2008;53:391–9.

[91] Gunthorpe M. J., Szallasi A. Peripheral TRPV1 receptors as targets for drug development: new molecules and mechanisms. *Curr. Pharm. Design*, 2008;14:32–41.

[92] Liu H. T., Kuo H. C. Increased expression of transient receptor potential vanilloid subfamily 1 in the bladder predicts the response to intravesical instillations of resiniferatoxin in patients with refractory idiopathic detrusor overactivity. *BJU Int.*, 2007;100:1086–1090.

[93] Birder L. A., de Groat W. C. Mechanisms of disease: involvement of the urothelium in bladder dysfunction. *Nat. Clin. Pract. Urol.*, 2007; 4:46-54.

[94] de Groat W. C., Yoshimura N. Changes in afferent activity after spinal cord injury. *Neurourol. Urodyn.*, 2010; 29: 63-76.

[95] Wiart L., Joseph P. A., Petit H., Dosque J. P., de Sèze M., Brochet B., Deminière C., Ferrière J. M., Mazaux J. M., N'Guyen P., Barat M. The effects of capsaicin on the neurogenic hyperreflexic detrusor. A double blind placebo controlled study in patients with spinal cord disease. Preliminary results. *Spinal Cord*, 1998; 36: 95-99.

[96] de Sèze M., Gallien P., Denys P., Labat J. J., Serment G., Grise P., Salle J. Y., Blazejewski S., Hazane C., Moore N., Joseph P. A. Intravesical glucidic capsaicin versus glucidic solvent in neurogenic detrusor overactivity: a double blind controlled randomized study. *Neurourol. Urodyn.*, 2006; 25: 752-757.

[97] Santos-Silva A., Charrua A., Cruz C. D., Gharat L., Avelino A., Cruz F. Rat detrusor overactivity induced by chronic spinalization can be abolished by a transient receptor potential vanilloid 1 (TRPV1) antagonist. *Auton. Neurosci.,* 2012; 166: 35-38.

[98] Gavva N. R., Treanor J. J., Garami A., Fang L., Surapaneni S., Akrami A., Alvarez F., Bak A., Darling M., Gore A., Jang G. R., Kesslak J. P., Ni L., Norman M. H., Palluconi G., Rose M. J., Salfi M., Tan E., Romanovsky A. A., Banfield C., Davar G. Pharmacological blockade of the vanilloid receptor TRPV1 elicits marked hyperthermia in humans. *Pain,* 2008; 136: 202-210.

[99] Round P., Priestley A., Robinson J. An investigation of the safety and pharmacokinetics of the novel TRPV1 antagonist XEN-D0501 in healthy subjects. *Br. J. Clin. Pharmacol.,* 2011; 72: 921-931.

[100] Novartis Pharmaceuticals. Safety and Efficacy of SAF312 in Patients With Neurogenic Detrusor Overactivity Due to Spinal Cord Lesions. In: ClinicalTrials.gov [Internet]. Bethesda (MD):National Library of Medicine (US). Available from: URL: http: //clinicaltrials.gov/show/ NCT01598103 NLM Identifier: NCT01598103.

[101] Juszczak K., Ziomber A., Thor P. J. Effect of partial and complete blockade of vanilloid (TRPV1-6) and ankyrin (TRPA1) transient receptor potential ion channels on urinary bladder motor activity in an experimental hyperosmolar overactive bladder rat model. *J. Physiol. Pharmacol.,* 2011; 62: 321-326.

[102] Andrade E. L., Forner S., Bento A. F., Leite D. F., Dias M. A., Leal P. C., Koepp J., Calixto J. B. TRPA1 receptor modulation attenuates bladder overactivity induced by spinal cord injury. *Am. J. Physiol. Renal Physiol.,* 2011; 300: F1223-F1234.

[103] Mochizuki T., Sokabe T., Araki I., Fujishita K., Shibasaki K., Uchida K., Naruse K., Koizumi S., Takeda M., Tominaga M. The TRPV4 cation channel mediates stretch-evoked Ca2+ influx and ATP release in primary urothelial cell cultures. *J. Biol. Chem.,* 2009; 284:21257-21264.

[104] Aizawa N., Wyndaele J. J., Homma Y., Igawa Y. Effects of TRPV4 cation channel activation on the primary bladder afferent activities of the rat. *Neurourol. Urodyn.,* 2012; 31: 148-155.

[105] Joy J. E., Watson S. J., Bensen J. A. Jr., editors., eds. Institute of Medicine. Marijuana and Medicine: Assessing the Science Base. Washington, DC: National Academies Press; 1999.

[106] Hedlund P. Cannabinoids and the endocannabinoid system in lower urinary tract function and dysfunction. *Neurourol. Urodyn.,* 2014; 33: 46-53.

[107] Ruggieri M. R. Sr. Cannabinoids: potential targets for bladder dysfunction. *Handb. Exp. Pharmacol.,* 2011;(202):425-51.

[108] Zhao P., Abood M. E.. GPR55 and GPR35 and their relationship to cannabinoid and lysophospholipid receptors. *Life Sci.,* 2013; 92:453-457.

[109] Hayn M. H., Ballesteros I., de Miguel F., Coyle C. H., Tyagi S., Yoshimura N., Chancellor M. B., Tyagi P. Functional and immunohistochemical characterization of CB1 and CB2 receptors in rat bladder. *Urology,* 2008; 72: 1174-1178.

[110] Strittmatter F., Gandaglia G., Benigni F., Bettiga A., Rigatti P., Montorsi F, Gratzke C., Stief C., Colciago G., Hedlund P. Expression of fatty acid amide hydrolase (FAAH) in human, mouse, and rat urinary bladder and effects of FAAH inhibition on bladder function in awake rats. *Eur. Urol.,* 2012; 61: 98-106.

[111] Tyagi V., Philips B. J., Su R., Smaldone M. C., Erickson V. L., Chancellor M. B., Yoshimura N., Tyagi P. Differential expression of functional cannabinoid receptors in human bladder detrusor and urothelium. *J. Urol.,* 2009; 181: 1932-1938.

[112] Campeau L., Fullhase C., Russo A. Intrathecal cannabinoid agonist effects in cystometric evaluation of normal rats [abstract MP-09.06]. *Can. Urol. Assoc. J.,* 2012; 6: S65.

[113] Gratzke C., Streng T., Stief C. G., Downs T. R., Alroy I., Rosenbaum J. S., Andersson K. E., Hedlund P. Effects of cannabinor, a novel selective cannabinoid 2 receptor agonist, on bladder function in normal rats. *Eur. Urol.,* 2010; 57: 1093-1100.

[114] Brady C. M., DasGupta R., Dalton C., Wiseman O. J., Berkley K. J., Fowler C. J. An open-label pilot study of cannabis-based extracts for bladder dysfunction in advanced multiple sclerosis. *Mult. Scler.,* 2004; 10: 425-433.

[115] Freeman R. M., Adekanmi O., Waterfield M. R., Waterfield A. E., Wright D., Zajicek J. The effect of cannabis on urge incontinence in patients with multiple sclerosis: a multicentre, randomised placebocontrolled trial (CAMS-LUTS). *Int. Urogynecol. J. Pelvic Floor Dysfunct.,* 2006; 17: 636-641.

[116] Kavia R. B., De Ridder D., Constantinescu C. S., Stott C. G., Fowler C. J. Randomized controlled trial of Sativex to treat detrusor overactivity in multiple sclerosis. *Mult. Scler.,* 2010; 16: 1349-1359.

[117] Koppel B. S., Brust J. C. M., Fife T., Bronstein J., Youssof S., Gronseth G., Gloss D. Systematic review: efficacy and safety of medical marijuana in selected neurologic disorders: report of the Guideline Development Subcommittee of the American Academy of Neurology. *Neurology*, 2014; 82 (17): 1556–1563.

[118] Apostolidis A. Taming the cannabinoids: new potential in the pharmacologic control of lower urinary tract dysfunction. *Eur. Urol.,* 2012; 61: 107-109; discussion 109-111.

[119] Aizawa N., Hedlund P., Füllhase C., Ito H., Homma Y., Igawa Y. Inhibition of peripheral FAAH depresses activities of bladder mechanosensitive nerve fibers of the rat. *J. Urol.,* 2014; 192: 956-963.

[120] Walczak J. S., Price T. J., Cervero F. Cannabinoid CB1 receptors are expressed in the mouse urinary bladder and their activation modulates afferent bladder activity. *Neuroscience,* 2009; 159: 1154-1163.

[121] Rahnama'I M. S., Ückert S., Hohnen R., van Koeveringe G. A. The role of phosphodiesterases in bladder pathophysiology *Nat. Rev. Urol.,* 2013; 10(7):414-24.

[122] Truss M. C., Uckert S., Stief C. G., Kuczyk M., Jonas U. Cyclic nucleotide phosphodiesterase (PDE) isoenzymes in the human detrusor smooth muscle. I. Identification and characterization. *Urol. Res.*, 1996; 24(3), 123–128.

[123] Truss M. C., Uckert S., Stief C. G., Forssmann W. G., Jonas U. Cyclic nucleotide phosphodiesterase (PDE) isoenzymes in the human detrusor smooth muscle. II. Effect of various PDE inhibitors on smooth muscle tone and cyclic nucleotide levels *in vitro. Urol. Res.*, 1996; 24(3), 129–134.

[124] Truss M. C., Stief C. G., Uckert S. et al. Phosphodiesterase 1 inhibition in the treatment of lower urinary tract dysfunction: from bench to bedside. *World J. Urol.,* 2001; 19(5), 344–350.

[125] F. Fusco, Rd di Villa Bianca, E. Mitidieri, G. Cirino, R. Sorrentino, V. Mirone. Sildenafil effect on the human bladder involves the L-cysteine/hydrogen sulfide

pathway: a novel mechanism of action of phosphodiesterase type 5 inhibitors. *Eur. Urol.*, 2012;62.
[126] Oger S., Behr-Roussel D., Gorny D., Lebret T., Validire P., Cathelineau X., Alexandre L., Giuliano F. Signalling pathways involved in sildenafil-induced relaxation of human bladder dome smooth muscle. *Br. J. Pharmacol.,* 2010; 160: 1135-1143.
[127] Gacci M., Del Popolo G., Macchiarella A. et al. Vardenafil improves urodynamic parameters in men with spinal cord injury: results from a single dose, pilot study. *J. Urol.,* 2007; 178(5), 2040–2043.
[128] Liu L., Zheng S., Han P., Wei Q. Phosphodiesterase-5 inhibitors for lower urinary tract symptoms secondary to benign prostatic hyperplasia: a systematic review and meta-analysis. *Urology,* 2011; 77: 123-129.
[129] Gacci M., Corona G., Salvi M., Vignozzi L., McVary K. T., Kaplan S. A., Roehrborn C. G., Serni S., Mirone V., Carini M., Maggi M. A systematic review and meta-analysis on the use of phosphodiesterase 5 inhibitors alone or in combination with α-blockers for lower urinary tract symptoms due to benign prostatic hyperplasia. *Eur. Urol.,* 2012; 61: 994-1003.
[130] Scatena R. Nitroflurbiprofen (NicOx). *Curr. Opin. Investig. Drugs,* 2004; 5: 551-556.
[131] Donnelly M. T., Stack W. A., Courtauld E. M., Garlick N., Del Soldato P., Hawkey C. J. Nitric oxide donating flurbiprofen (HCT1026) causes less endoscopic damage in healthy volunteers than flurbiprofen. British Society of Gastroenterology - 1997.
[132] Costa P., Perrouin-Verbe B., Rouays-Mabit H., Turlan J. L. Effects of an new drug, HCT1026, in patients with neurogenic bladder overactivity. *Int. Urogyn. J.*, 2000; 11 Suppl. 1.
[133] Jeremy J. Y., Tsang V., Mikhailidis D. P., Rogers H., Morgan R. J., Dandona P. Eicosanoid synthesis by human urinary bladder mucosa: pathological implications. *Br. J. Urol.,* 1987; 59: 36-39.
[134] Khan M. A., Thompson C. S., Mumtaz F. H., Jeremy J. Y., Morgan R. J., Mikhailidis D. P. Role of prostaglandins in the urinary bladder: an update. *Prostaglandins Leukot. Essent. Fatty Acids,* 1998; 59:415-422.
[135] Masunaga K., Yoshida M., Inadome A., Iwashita H., Miyamae K., Ueda S. Prostaglandin E2 release from isolated bladder strips in rats with spinal cord injury. *Int. J. Urol.,* 2006; 13: 271-276.
[136] Schröder A., Newgreen D., Andersson K. E. Detrusor responses to prostaglandin E2 and bladder outlet obstruction in wild-type and Ep1 receptor knockout mice. *J. Urol.,* 2004; 172: 1166-1170.
[137] Lee T., Hedlund P., Newgreen D., Andersson K. E. Urodynamic effects of a novel EP(1) receptor antagonist in normal rats and rats with bladder outlet obstruction. *J. Urol.,* 2007; 177: 1562-1567.
[138] Schüssler B. Comparison of the mode of action of prostaglandin E2 (PGE2) and sulprostone, a PGE2-derivative, on the lower urinary tract in healthy women. A urodynamic study. *Urol. Res.,* 1990; 18:349-352.
[139] Cardozo L. D., Stanton S. L., Robinson H., Hole D. Evaluation of flurbiprofen in detrusor instability. *Br. Med. J.,* 1980; 280: 281-282.
[140] Cardozo L. D., Stanton S. L. A comparison between bromocriptine and indomethacin in the treatment of detrusor instability. *J. Urol.,* 1980; 123: 399-401.

[141] Angelico P., Guarneri L., Velasco C., Cova R., Leonardi A., Clarke D. E., Testa R. Effect of cyclooxygenase inhibitors on the micturition reflex in rats: correlation with inhibition of cyclooxygenase isozymes. *BJU Int.*, 2006; 97: 837-846.

[142] Jang J., Park E. Y., Seo S. I., Hwang T. K., Kim J. C. Effects of intravesical instillation of cyclooxygenase-2 inhibitor on the expression of inducible nitric oxide synthase and nerve growth factor in cyclophosphamide-induced overactive bladder. *BJU Int.*, 2006; 98: 435-439.

[143] Ratz P. H., Speich J. E., Klausner A. P. COX Inhibitors and Overactive Bladder: The Potential for Future Therapy. *Curr. Bladder Dysfunct. Rep.*, 2010; 5: 4-12.

[144] Teixeira C. E., Jin L., Priviero F. B., Ying Z., Webb R. C. Comparative pharmacological analysis of Rho-kinase inhibitors and identification of molecular components of Ca2+ sensitization in the rat lower urinary tract. *Biochem. Pharmacol.*, 2007; 74: 647-658.

[145] Marx J. O., Basha M. E., Mohanan S., Hypolite J. A., Chang S., Wein A. J., Zderic S. A., Laping N. J., Chacko S. Effects of Rho-kinase inhibition on myosin light chain phosphorylation and obstruction-induced detrusor overactivity. *Int. J. Urol.*, 2014; 21: 319-324.

[146] Kirschstein T., Protzel C., Porath K., Sellmann T., Köhling R., Hakenberg O. W. Age-dependent contribution of Rho kinase in carbachol-induced contraction of human detrusor smooth muscle in vitro. *Acta Pharmacol. Sin.*, 2014; 35: 74-81.

[147] Wróbel A, Adamiak A, Skorupski P, Rechberger T. Rho kinase--a new target for pharmacological treatment of an overactive bladder. *Ginekol. Pol.*, 2008; 79(5):364-9.

[148] Rajasekaran M., Wilkes N., Kuntz S., E. Albo M. Rho-kinase inhibition suppresses bladder hyperactivity in spontaneously hypertensive rats. *Neurourol. Urodyn.*, 2005; 24: 295-300.

[149] Morelli A., Squecco R., Failli P., Filippi S., Vignozzi L., Chavalmane A. K., Fibbi B., Mancina R., Luciani G., Gacci M., Colli E., Francini F., Adorini L., Maggi M. The vitamin D receptor agonist elocalcitol upregulates L-type calcium channel activity in human and rat bladder. *Am. J. Physiol. Cell Physiol.*, 2008; 294: C1206-C1214.

[150] Morelli A., Vignozzi L., Filippi S., Vannelli G. B., Ambrosini S., Mancina R., Crescioli C., Donati S., Fibbi B., Colli E., Adorini L., Maggi M. BXL-628, a vitamin D receptor agonist effective in benign prostatic hyperplasia treatment, prevents RhoA activation and inhibits RhoA/Rho kinase signaling in rat and human bladder. *Prostate,* 2007; 67: 234-247.

[151] Digesu G. A., Verdi E., Cardozo L., Olivieri L., Khullar V., Colli E. Phase IIb, multicenter, double-blind, randomized, placebocontrolled, parallel-group study to determine effects of elocalcitol in women with overactive bladder and idiopathic detrusor overactivity. *Urology,* 2012; 80: 48-54.

[152] Igawa Y., Mattiasson A., Andersson K. E.: Effects of GABA-receptor stimulation and blockade on micturition in normal rats and rats with bladder outlet obstruction. *J. Urol.*, 1993;150:537-542.

[153] Miyazato M., Sugaya K., Goins W. F., Wolfe D., Goss J. R., Chancellor M. B., de Groat W. C., Glorioso J. C., Yoshimura N. Herpes simplex virus vector-mediated gene delivery of glutamic acid decarboxylase reduces detrusor overactivity in spinal cord-injured rats. *Gene Ther.*, 2009; 16: 660-668.

[154] Petkov G. V. Role of potassium ion channels in detrusor smooth muscle function and dysfunction. *Nat. Rev. Urol.,* 2012; 9: 30-40.

[155] Hu S., Kim H. S. Modulation of ATP-sensitive and large-conductance Ca2+ activated K+ channels by Zeneca ZD6169 in guinea pig bladder smooth muscle cells. *J. Pharmacol. Exp. Ther.*, 1997;280:38–45.

[156] de Groat W. C. Basic neurophysiology and neuropharmacology. In: Abrams P., Khoury S., Wein A., editors. Incontinence. Plymouth, UK: Health Publications Limited; 1999. pp. 105–154.

[157] Thorneloe K. S., Nelson M. T. Properties and molecular basis of the mouse urinary bladder voltage-gated K+ current. *J. Physiol.,* 2003; 549: 65-74.

[158] Yoshimura N., Bennett N. E., Hayashi Y., Ogawa T., Nishizawa O., Chancellor M. B., de Groat W. C., Seki S. Bladder overactivity and hyperexcitability of bladder afferent neurons after intrathecal delivery of nerve growth factor in rats. *J. Neurosci.,* 2006; 26: 10847-10855.

[159] Parajuli S. P., Hristov K. L., Soder R. P., Kellett W. F., Petkov G. V. NS309 decreases rat detrusor smooth muscle membrane potential and phasic contractions by activating SK3 channels. *Br. J. Pharmacol.,* 2013; 168: 1611-1625.

[160] Soder R. P., Parajuli S. P., Hristov K. L., Rovner E. S., Petkov G. V. SK channel-selective opening by SKA-31 induces hyperpolarization and decreases contractility in human urinary bladder smooth muscle. *Am. J. Physiol. Regul. Integr. Comp. Physiol.,* 2013; 304:R155-R163.

[161] Nielsen J. S., Rode F., Rahbek M., Andersson K. E., Rønn L. C., Bouchelouche K., Nordling J., Bouchelouche P. Effect of the SK/IK channel modulator 4,5-dichloro-1,3-diethyl-1,3-dihydrobenzoimidazol-2-one (NS4591) on contractile force in rat, pig and human detrusor smooth muscle. *BJU Int.,* 2011; 108: 771-777.

[162] Tertyshnikova S., Knox R. J., Plym M. J., Thalody G., Griffin C., Neelands T., Harden D. G., Signor L., Weaver D., Myers R. A., Lodge N. J. BL-1249 [(5,6,7,8-tetrahydro-naphthalen-1-yl)-[2-(1H-tetrazol-5-yl)-phenyl]-amine]: a putative potassium channel opener with bladder-relaxant properties. *J. Pharmacol. Exp. Ther.,* 2005; 313:250-259.

[163] Christ G. J., Day N. S., Day M., et al. Bladder injection of "naked" hSlo/pcDNA3 ameliorates detrusor hyperactivity in obstructed rats in vivo. *Am. J. Physiol. Regulatory Integrative Comp. Physiol.*, 2001; 281: R100–R1709.

[164] Steers W. D., Kolbeck S., Creedon D., Tuttle J. B.: Nerve growth factor in the urinary bladder of the adult regulates neuronal form and function. *J. Clin. Invest.,* 1991;88:1709-1715.

[165] Steers W. D., Kolbeck S., Creedon D., Tuttle J. B. Nerve growth factor in the urinary bladder of the adult regulates neuronal form and function. *J. Clin. Invest.,* 1991; 88: 1709-1715.

[166] Liu H. T., Kuo H. C.: Urinary nerve growth factor level could be a potential biomarker for diagnosis of overactive bladder. *J. Urol.,* 2008; 179:2270-2274.

[167] Liu H. T., Chancellor M. B., Kuo H. C. Decrease of urinary nerve growth factor levels after antimuscarinic therapy in patients with overactive bladder. *BJU Int.,* 2009; 103: 1668-1672.

[168] Liu H. T., Chancellor M. B., Kuo H. C. Urinary nerve growth factor levels are elevated in patients with detrusor overactivity and decreased in responders to detrusor botulinum toxin-A injection. *Eur. Urol.,* 2009; 56: 700-706.

[169] Schnegelsberg B., Sun T. T., Cain G., Bhattacharya A., Nunn P. A., Ford A. P., Vizzard M. A., Cockayne D. A. Overexpression of NGF in mouse urothelium leads to neuronal hyperinnervation, pelvic sensitivity, and changes in urinary bladder function. *Am. J. Physiol. Regul. Integr. Comp. Physiol.,* 2010; 298: R534-R547.

[170] Seki S., Sasaki K., Fraser M. O., Igawa Y., Nishizawa O., Chancellor M. B., de Groat W. C., Yoshimura N. Immunoneutralization of nerve growth factor in lumbosacral spinal cord reduces bladder hyperreflexia in spinal cord injured rats. *J. Urol.,* 2002; 168: 2269-2274.

[171] Jang J., Park E. Y., Seo S. I., Hwang T. K., Kim J. C.: Effects of intravesical instillation of cyclooxygenase-2 inhibitor on the expression of in-ducible nitric oxide synthase and nerve growth factor in cyclophosphamide-induced overactive bladder. *BJU Int.,* 2006; 98:435-439.

[172] Kashyap M., Kawamorita N., Tyagi V., Sugino Y., Chancellor M., Yoshimura N., Tyagi P. Down-regulation of nerve growth factor expression in the bladder by antisense oligonucleotides as new treatment for overactive bladder. *J. Urol.,* 2013; 190: 757-764.

[173] Lee S., Dausch S., Maierhofer C. and Dausch D. A new therapy concept with a liposome eye spray for the treatment of the 'dry eye.' *Klinische Monatsblatter fur Augenheilkunde*, 2004. 221;10, 825–836.

[174] Ebrahim S., Peyman G. A., and Lee P. J. Applications of liposomes in ophthalmology. *Survey of Ophthalmology,* 2005;50:2, 167–182.

[175] Nirmal J., Tyagi P., Dang L. et al. Endocytosis uptake of liposomes in urothelium cells detected by transmission electron microscopy. *J. Urol.,* 2012; 187.

[176] Tyagi P., Hsieh V. C., Yoshimura N., Kaufman J., and Chancellor M. B. Instillation of liposomes vs dimethyl sulphoxide or pentosan polysulphate for reducing bladder hyperactivity. *BJU Int.,* 2009; 104;11. 1689–1692.

[177] Lee W. C., Chien C. T., Yu H. J., and Lee S. W. Bladder dysfunction in rats with metabolic syndrome induced by long-term fructose feeding. *J. Urol.*, 2008;179,6 pp. 2470–2476.

[178] Gillespie J. I., Van Koeveringe G. A., De Wachter S. G., and De Vente J. On the origins of the sensory output from the bladder: the concept of afferent noise. *BJU Int.*, 2009; 103, 10, pp. 1324–1333, 2009.

BIOGRAPHICAL SCKETCH

Name: **Emilio Sacco**

Affiliation: Urologic Clinic, Department of Surgical Sciences, "Agostino Gemelli" Hospital, Catholic University Medical School of Rome
Date of Birth: 12/11/1974

Education:
October 13, 1999: Degree in Medicine and Surgery with full honors, University of Padua, School of Medicine, Padua, Italy

June 26, 2000: Certified Specialization in Urology, University of Padua, School of Medicine, Padua, Italy
July, 10, 2009: Ph.D. in Urologic Andrology, School of Urology, Catholic University Medical School, Rome, Italy

Address: Clinica Urologica, Policlinico "Agostino Gemelli," Largo Gemelli 8, 00168, Roma, Italy

Research and Professional Experience:
From October 01, 2013 - up to now: Contract Professor of Urology, School of Obstetrics and Gynecology, Catholic University Medical School, Rome, Italy (current position).
From February 01, 2006 - up to now: Medical Doctor, Specialist in Urology (current position).
From February 01, 2006 - up to now: Lead Clinician for Infection Control, Incontinence and Lower Urinary Tract Dysfunctions, Urodynamics and Pelvic Floor Rehabilitation, Urologic Robot-assisted Surgery (current position).
From October 01, 2007 - up to now: Contract Professor at School of Specialization in Urology, Catholic University Medical School, Rome, Italy (current position).
From October 01, 2007 to July 30 2013: Contract Professor of Urology, School of Physiotherapy, Catholic University Medical School, Campobasso, Italy.
From 09/2004 to 08/2005: Research fellowship at Urology Clinic, Oncology Department, Addenbrooke's Hospital, University of Cambridge, UK.
Research activities in the field of general urology, uro-oncology, functional urology, urogynaecology, endourology. With more than 150 publications in these fields.

Professional Appointments: "Agostino Gemelli" Hospital, Largo Gemelli 8, Roma, Italy

Honors: 2004: International grant from Eugenio Litta Foundation, Geneva, Switzerland

Publications Last 3 Years:
50 national and international abstracts, 40 scientific articles

Name: Riccardo Bientinesi

Affiliation: Urology Department, "Agostino Gemelli" Academic Hospital, Catholic University of Sacred Heart, Rome (Italy).

Date of Birth: Jan 23, 1986

Education: Medicine and Surgery Degree

Address: L.go F. Vito, 1 - 00166 Rome (IT)

Research and Professional Experience:

CLINICAL: all fields of Urology, particularly oncologic urology.
RESEARCH: Basic and Clinical (urologic oncology, molecular medicine, immunotherapy, development of new drugs) Assistant Editor of "Urologia" Professional Appointments: none.

Publications Last 3 Years:
Ten national and international scientific articles.

In: Overactive Bladder (OAB)
Editor: Elvira Larson

ISBN: 978-1-63485-033-9

Chapter 6

OVERACTIVE BLADDER (OAB): IS THERE A PLACE FOR DRUGS TARGETING THE PURINERGIC CASCADE?

M. Silva-Ramos[1,2,3], I. Silva[1,2], F. Ferreirinha[1,2], M. Faria[1,2] and P. Correia-de-Sá[1,2*]

[1]Laboratório de Farmacologia e Neurobiologia,
[2]Center for Drug Discovery and Innovative Medicines (MedInUP), Instituto de Ciências Biomédicas de Abel Salazar (ICBAS),
Universidade do Porto
[3]Serviço de Urologia, Centro Hospitalar do Porto (CHP),
Porto, Portugal

ABSTRACT

It is widely accepted that purines, in particular ATP, are important regulators of urinary bladder functions in animals, as well as in humans. The nucleotide regulates both afferent and efferent signaling pathways. ATP (i) activates sensory nerves during bladder filling conveying both normal and abnormal sensations like urgency and pain, (ii) acts as a co-transmitter with acetylcholine (ACh) in the parasympathetic control of bladder contraction during voiding, and (iii) participates in the central control of bladder reflexes. Bladder ATP originates from both neuronal and non-neuronal sources, such as urothelial cells, interstitial cells, fibroblast-like cells and smooth muscle fibers. The mechanisms regulating the release of ATP in the urinary bladder are still a matter of debate, but may include vesicle exocytosis and translocation via pannexin-1 containing hemichannels among others.

The purinergic tone increases significantly with age and is responsible for up to 40% of nerve-evoked atropine-resistant bladder contractions in pathological conditions, including hypertrophic unstable bladder, overactive detrusor, neurogenic bladder and

* Address for correspondence: P. Correia-de-Sá, MD, PhD, Laboratório de Farmacologia e Neurobiologia – Center for Drug Discovery and Innovative Medicines (MedInUP), Instituto de Ciências Biomédicas de Abel Salazar (ICBAS) - Universidade do Porto (UP), Rua Jorge Viterbo Ferreira, 228, 4050-312 Porto, Portugal. Tel.: 351-22-0428212. *E-mail address*: farmacol@icbas.up.pt.

interstitial cystitis. Recent data from our group showed that the release of ATP from urothelial cells and cholinergic nerves increases several fold in patients with overactive bladder (OAB). The greater purinergic tone may be partially related to the impairment of ecto-NTPDase1/CD39 activity, thus limiting the extracellular breakdown of ATP.

Excess of extracellular ATP released from the urothelium in response to stretch and chemical irritants may contribute to hyperexcitation of suburothelial nerve afferents via homomeric P2X3 and/or heteromeric P2X2/P2X3 receptors. In OAB patients, the increase in ATP release by the mucosa is associated with an increase in the expression of P2X3 receptors on nerves fibres, thus potentiating the sensory input. Although there is scant pharmacological data characterizing the P2 receptor involved in ATP-mediated detrusor contractions, quantitative mRNA studies and experiments with P2X1 knockout mice suggest that the P2X1 receptor might have a significant role. Few attempts have been made so far to investigate the pathophysiological role of P2Y and P1 receptors in the context of bladder overactivity, *vis-a-vis* the deficient formation of ATP metabolites, respectively ADP and adenosine.

The mechanisms underlying OAB are largely unknown, but these are usually divided into urothelial, myogenic and neurogenic. It thus, appears that ATP plays a chief role in all of these. Therefore, one may anticipate benefits in the treatment of OAB using a combination of drugs targeting the purinergic cascade, including ATP release sites, ectonuleotidases, and purinoceptors.

INTRODUCTION

ATP is a molecule with a wide range of metabolic and signalling functions. It acts intracellularly as an energy source and also extracellularly as a signalling transducer in a variety of physiological and pathological processes. Extracellular ATP binds to plasma membrane P2 purinoceptors, which include 8 G protein-coupled metabotropic P2Y receptors ($P2Y_1$, $P2Y_2$, $P2Y_4$, $P2Y_6$, $P2Y_8$, $P2Y_{11}$, $P2Y_{12}$, and $P2Y_{13}$) and 7 ligand-gated ionotropic receptors, called P2X (P2X1-P2X7) (Alexander et al., 2013a, 2013b). Once released from cells, ATP and other nucleotides are metabolized by a variety of cell-surface ectonucleotidases. These enzymes control ATP inactivation and ADP, AMP and adenosine formation and, therefore, are important regulators of purinergic signals. The end product of ATP metabolism is adenosine (ADO) that acts through G protein-coupled P1 receptors (A_1, A_{2A}, A_{2B} and A_3) (Fredholm et al., 2011).

Evidence for the role of ATP in bladder physiology, comes right from the beginning of the purinergic hypothesis formulated by Geoffrey Burnstock in the seventies. Indeed non-adrenergic and non-cholinergic (NANC) neurotransmission were first studied in the gut and in the urinary bladder (Burnstock, 1972; Burnstock et al., 1972). Since then, the knowledge of purinergic signalling in the lower urinary tract has expanded considerably. Purines are important regulators of normal bladder function, but also changes in purinergic signalling are associated with bladder dysfunction, particularly the overactive bladder (OAB). Although OAB is symptomatically complex, often idiopathic, it can be originated from multiple aetiologies. Mounting evidences indicate that bladder outflow obstruction (BOO) and neurologic disorders are common causes of OAB and this is why much fundamental research on OAB comes from studying obstructed and neurogenic bladders.

PURINERGIC EFFERENT MECHANISMS

Pioneering evidences that non-cholinergic non-adrenergic (NANC) contractions are caused by ATP came from similarities between NANC and ATP-induced contractile activity and from the depression of NANC responses owed to tachyphylaxis produced by previous application of high ATP concentrations (Burnstock et al., 1972). In agreement with this, it was demonstrated that desensitization of P2 purinoceptors with the enzymatically stable ATP analogue, α,β-meATP, abolished nerve-induced NANC contractions of the urinary bladder (Brading & Williams, 1990). More direct evidences came later on by measuring the release of ATP during stimulation of NANC nerves using the luciferin-luciferase bioluminescence assay (Burnstock et al., 1978). *In vivo* experiments in rats demonstrated that electrical stimulation of the spinal cord triggered increases in intravesical pressure, which were antagonized by pre-treatment with α,β-meATP or pyridoxalphosphate-6-azophenyl-2',4'-disulphonic acid (PPADS, a non-selective P2 receptor antagonist) (Hegde et al., 1998). Furthermore, cystometry experiments using non-anaesthetized rats showed that intra-arterial administration of ATP or α,β-meATP close to the bladder produced a dose dependent increase in bladder pressure (Igawa et al., 1993). Despite all these evidences, the study of the pos-junctional effect of ATP in the detrusor has been hampered by its metabolism into other biologically-active nucleotides with opposing effects and by P2 purinoceptors desensitization. Notwithstanding this, it is generally accepted that ATP released from efferent nerves cause bladder contractions in rodents via the activation of α,β-meATP-sensitive ionotropic P2X receptors, both *in vitro* and *in vivo* (Lukacsko & Krell, 1982; Hegde et al., 1998).

A slightly different scenario is observed in humans, where normal bladder contractions are mediated predominantly through the activation of muscarinic cholinergic receptors located in the detrusor smooth muscle, with a very limited participation of ATP-sensitive P2 receptors (see Figure 1A). Human detrusor smooth muscle expresses muscarinic receptors of M_2 and M_3 subtypes, with the M_2 receptor (66%) exceeding the M_3 receptor (33%) in number, but the latter being more active to cause smooth muscle contraction and voiding command under normal circumstances. The role of the M_2 receptor is still a matter of debate, even though it may contribute to bladder contraction in certain disease conditions (e.g., denervated bladder, neurogenic bladder dysfunction). Atropine-resistant contractions have been reported in the normal human detrusor, but these do not substantially contribute to bladder emptying under physiological conditions in contrast to that occurring in small laboratory animals (Ruggieri, 2006). The atropine-resistant purinergic component of the human bladder contraction may increase up to 40% in pathological conditions, such as OAB secondary to prostatic obstruction, interstitial cystitis, neurogenic bladders and aged bladders (reviewed in Burnstock, 2014). It is also noteworthy that detrusor sensitivity to acetylcholine decrease significantly ($P < 0.05$) in bladders from patients with BOO due to benign prostatic hyperplasia (BPH) (Figure 1A). Under these circumstances, which resemble the normal function of the bladder in laboratory animals, atropine-resistant contractions are attributed to ATP and may be due to (i) increased ATP release from nerves, (ii) impaired catabolism of ATP, and/or (iii) higher sensitivity of the detrusor smooth muscle to the nucleotide.

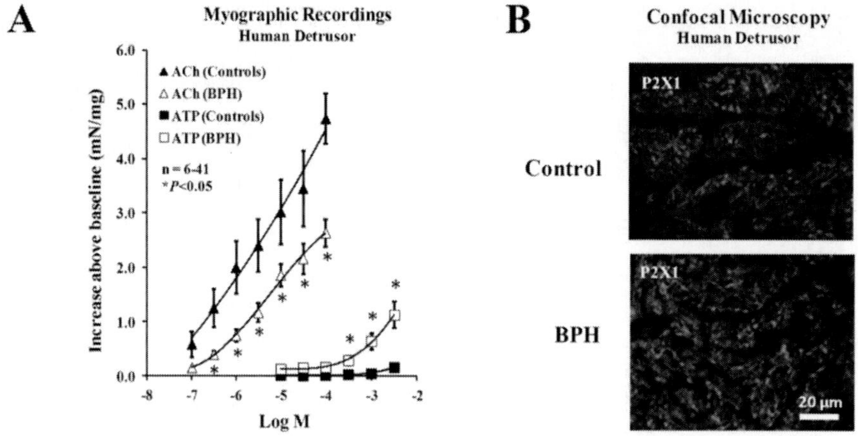

Figure 1. (A) Concentration-response curves of acetylcholine (ACh, 0.1-100 µM, triangles)- and ATP (0.01-3 mM, squares)-induced contractions of detrusor strips from cadaveric organ donors (Controls, filled symbols) and patients with BOO (BPH, open symbols). Bladder samples from BOO patients were obtained during transvesical prostatectomy. Each point represents mean ± SEM from a *n* number of individuals.*$P < 0.05$ (unpaired Student's t test with Welch's correction) represents significant differences from control samples. (B) Representative confocal micrographs showing the P2X1 receptor immunoreactivity (green fluorescence) in the detrusor of a cadaveric organ donor (Control) and a patient with BOO (due to BPH). Similar results were obtained in 4 additional experiments. Scale bar = 20 µm.

Evidence for the first hypothesis was lacking until very recently. Our group showed that ATP released from electrically-stimulated detrusor smooth muscle preparations from patients with BOO due to BPH was 2.5-fold higher than that obtained from control organ donors (Silva-Ramos et al., 2015a). We also proved that ATP hydrolysis and adenosine formation was significantly slower in the detrusor of obstructed patients that in the control population, a situation that has been attributed to downregulation of ecto-NTPDase1 and ecto-5'-nucleotidase enzymes which convert ATP directly into AMP and the latter into adenosine, respectively (Silva-Ramos et al., 2015a). Deficits in ATP catabolism have been previously demonstrated by others using a mixed population of patients with detrusor overactivity and/or bladder outlet obstruction (Harvey et al., 2002).

Concerning hypersensitivity of the detrusor smooth muscle to ATP, Figure 1A shows that ATP (0.01-3 mM) was virtually devoid of effect on detrusor contractions in control preparations, but it significantly ($P < 0.05$) increased the tone of the detrusor isolated from patients with BOO due to BPH; ATP (3 mM) increased the contractile tone of the detrusor from BOO patients up to 40% of the effect caused by 100 µM acetylcholine (ACh, Figure 1A). Although ATP evokes more potent contractions in isolated detrusor samples from overactive or obstructed bladders compared with that from normal bladders, its stable analogue, α,β-meATP, produces similar contractions in both groups (Harvey et al., 2002). Moreover, using isolated myocytes from normal and overactive detrusor, ATP evoked a similar increase in intracellular Ca^{2+} (Wu et al., 1999). While these observations are more consistent with the higher ATP bioavailability hypothesis due to downregulation of the nucleotide catabolism than with a different sensitivity of the detrusor to ATP in diseased samples (see above), one cannot easily discard the possibility that fast receptor desensitization induced by α,β-meATP might limit full detrusor contractions in overactive or obstructed bladders.

The recent availability of P2X receptor antagonists with subtype selectivity and of knockout mice allowed confirmation of the involvement of the P2X1 receptor in atropine-resistant contractions. In anesthetized rats the P2X1 receptor antagonist, RO116-6446, caused a significant attenuation of phasic isovolumetric contractions, without affecting volume and pressure thresholds (King et al., 2004). Moreover, ATP-induced contractions are completely absent in P2X1 receptor knockout mice (Vial & Evans, 2000). The P2X1 receptor has also been shown to be the dominant P2X receptor in the human detrusor using quantitative reverse transcription polymerase chain reaction (RT-PCR) (O'Reilly et al., 2001). Furthermore, immunohistochemistry studies showed that P2X1 receptor subunits are localized in the periphery of detrusor smooth muscle fibres (Elneil et al., 2001). Altogether these data strongly suggest that the dominant receptor mediating purinergic contractions in the detrusor smooth muscle is the P2X1 receptor. Despite this, evidences for the role of the P2X1 receptor in the pathophysiology of bladder syndromes are conflicting. Using RT-PCR, some authors reported no differences in P2X1 receptor transcripts among normal and obstructed bladder samples (Chua et al., 2007), while others showed increased amounts of these transcripts in obstructed samples (O'Reilly et al., 2001). Because RT-PCR results do not necessarily correlate with the presence of functional receptors on the plasma membrane, we evaluated the expression of the P2X1 receptor subtype in the human detrusor by immunofluorescence confocal microscopy. Figure 1B shows that patients with BOO due to BPH exhibit increased P2X1 immunoreactivity in detrusor smooth muscle fibres compared to control preparations. This result contributes to explain, at least partially, the increased purinergic tone of the detrusor from BOO patients.

P2Y receptors may also have a role in mediating detrusor response to ATP stimulation. At least in laboratory animals, pharmacological studies show that P2Y may be involved in relaxation of pre-contracted detrusor (McMurray et al., 1998). On the other hand P2Y agonists like ADP and ADPβS are capable of inducing detrusor smooth muscle contractions (Aronsson et al., 2010; McMurray et al., 1998; Palea et al., 1994; Suzuki & Kokubun, 1994; Yu et al., 2014). This effect was recently attributed to activation of the $P2Y_{12}$ receptor because it was blocked by the selective $P2Y_{12}$ receptor antagonist, PSB0739, but was unaffected by antagonists displaying affinity for other ADP-sensitive P2Y receptors, like $P2Y_1$ and $P2Y_{13}$ (Yu et al., 2014). However, the identified $P2Y_{12}$ receptor mediating ADP-induced bladder contractions has unique pharmacological properties because its effect on detrusor smooth muscle is temporally regulated by ectonucleotidases, both NTPDase1 and ecto-5'-nucleotidase, and by adenosine signalling. The crosstalk between $P2Y_{12}$ and adenosine receptors may be at the second messenger level since inhibition of the adenylate cyclase via $G_{\alpha i}$ provided by the $P2Y_{12}$ receptor activation may counteract the smooth muscle relaxation attributed to A_{2A}/A_{2B} receptors positively coupled to activation of this enzyme by $G_{\alpha s}$ proteins. The therapeutic significance of $P2Y_{12}$ in hemostasis and thrombosis has long been recognized due to the potent anti-thrombotic compounds, ticlopidine and clopidogrel, which selectively inhibit $P2Y_{12}$ receptors in platelets. Given the recent data implicating the expression and function of $P2Y_{12}$ receptors in the detrusor smooth muscle contraction, these receptors may open new therapeutic avenues for the use of thienopyridine compounds in human bladder disorders like lower urinary tract symptoms (LUTS).

Although $P2Y_1$ receptor transcripts have been found in cells from the detrusor, ADP-induced detrusor contractions were not inhibited by MRS2179. On the other hand, electrophysiological recordings in platelet-derived growth factor receptor-α-positive (PDGFRα$^+$) interstitial cells in the detrusor muscle showed that ATP elicited large amplitude outward currents and hyperpolarization mediated by small conductance Ca^{2+}-activated K^+ (SK) channels sensitive to apamin. The $P2Y_1$ receptor agonist, MRS2365, mimicked the effect of ATP, and a $P2Y_1$ antagonist, MRS2500, inhibited ATP-activated SK currents (Lee et al., 2014). Localization of purinergic inhibitory effects in PDGFRα$^+$ cells may provide the basis for a novel neural regulatory mechanism for the stabilization of bladder excitability during the filling phase. These authors observed that during extended neural stimulation of bladder muscles, the sustained component of contraction is significantly reduced by $P2Y_1$-mediated purinergic regulation. Thus, adenine nucleotides released from autonomic neurons may have dual, temporally-distinctive, actions in micturition: activation of detrusor contraction via P2X1-receptors in smooth muscle cells during voiding and stabilization of membrane potential and excitability during bladder filling through the activation of $P2Y_1$ receptors in PDGFRα$^+$ cells. The purinergic inhibitory input mediated by $P2Y_1$ receptors may potentiate detrusor relaxation during urine storage caused by activation of adrenergic β_3 receptors (Afeli et al., 2012; Brown et al., 2008). This synergism may be pathophysiologically relevant considering that discrete inhibitory neurons are extremely rare in the bladder (Lee et al., 2014).

In contrast to the compelling evidence for the extracellular signaling role of ATP and related adenine nucleotides, the hypothesis that uracil nucleotides exert autocrine/paracrine roles has only recently gained experimental support. UDP-sensitive $P2Y_6$ receptors have been involved in the generation of large spontaneous contractions and propagating waves of intracellular Ca^{2+} and membrane depolarization originating in suburothelial myofibroblasts and spreading to the detrusor smooth muscle in rats submitted to spinal cord transaction (Fry et al., 2012). Furthermore, using myographic recordings it has been demonstrated that UDP, acting on $P2Y_6$ receptors, interplays with P2X1 receptors in a synergistic manner to increase bladder smooth muscle tone (Yu et al., 2013). We confirmed that UDP increased the frequency and the amplitude of spontaneous detrusor contractions in the isolated rat bladder when the nucleotide was applied in high concentrations (300 μM) outside the bladder wall, but not when it was infused into the bladder lumen (Carneiro et al., 2014). However, increments of spontaneous bladder twitching caused by UDP (300 μM) were minimal (<10%) when compared to muscarinic and P2X1 receptors activation, respectively with oxotremorine (30 μM) and α,β-meATP (30 μM). A significant discrepancy was also observed between the lack of effect of intraluminal UDP in the isolated bladder and the increase in the voiding frequency when the nucleotide was infused into the bladder lumen in anaesthetized rats. Overall, our results indicate that direct activation of smooth muscle via co-expressed $P2Y_6$ and P2X1 receptors might represent a minor component of the urodynamic response to UDP that is mediated predominantly by the sequential activation of urothelial $P2Y_6$ receptors and ATP release resulting in stimulation of urothelial/sub-urothelial P2X3 receptors in the rat (Carneiro et al., 2014; Timoteo et al., 2014) and in humans (Silva et al., 2015).

Appearance of atropine-resistant P2 purinergic tone in patients with idiopathic detrusor overactivity has been related to decreased ecto-NTPDase activity (see above), but this may have also impact on endogenous adenosine formation and P1 receptors activation. In addition, to the well-characterized post-junctional effect of ATP, the nucleotide enhances parasympathetic motor drive through pre-synaptic P2X3 receptors (D'Agostino et al., 2012; King et al., 1997). On the other hand, the ATP metabolite adenosine partially relaxes pre-contracted urinary bladder detrusor strips in rodents (Acevedo et al., 1992; Brown et al., 1979; Burnstock et al., 1978; King et al., 1997; Nicholls et al., 1992), as well as in humans (Rubinstein et al., 1998). Besides direct actions of adenosine predominantly via A_{2A} and/or A_{2B} receptors located on detrusor smooth muscle fibers, the nucleoside may act indirectly by inhibiting nerve-evoked contractions. Recently, we provided evidence that adenosine-induced detrusor contractions require "unphysiological" millimolar concentrations of the nucleoside, which were 30-fold higher than those needed to reduce nerve-evoked ACh release from the human detrusor through the activation of A_1 receptors (Silva-Ramos, et al., 2015a; 2015b). Data from those studies suggest that reduced ATP hydrolysis leads to deficient adenosine formation and A_1 receptor-mediated inhibition resulting in cholinergic nerve hyperactivity in obstructed human bladders. Thus, we propose that pharmacological manipulation of A_1 receptors activity and/or endogenous adenosine levels (e.g., with inhibitors of adenosine deaminase and/or nucleoside uptake blockers) may be useful to control bladder overactivity (Silva-Ramos et al., 2015a), in parallel to the novel, potent and orally bioavailable P2X antagonists (Gever et al., 2010)

Purinergic Signaling during Bladder Filling

Most afferent nerves conveying sensitive information from the urinary bladder to the spinal cord originate in dorsal root ganglia (DRG). In the dorsal horn of the spinal cord, information received enters (1) via ascending nerve afferents, giving rise to conscious perception of bladder sensations, or (2) via interneurons, affecting motor pathways. At the bladder wall, C-fibre axons possess endings in the suburothelial layer and may also penetrate the urothelium (Birder et al., 2010). It is now accepted that the urothelium is more than a physical barrier and responds to mechanical and chemical stimuli transmitting the information to underlying nervous and muscular systems. Therefore, urothelium and suburothelial layers can be regarded as a functional transduction unit playing a pivotal role in generating afferent signals to bladder intrinsic relay circuits and to control centres in the central nervous system (CNS).

The urothelium is a transitional epithelium composed of three to five cell layers: a basal layer attached to the basement membrane, an apical layer with large umbrella cells and an intermediate layer. The suburothelium is composed of nerves, interstitial cells, blood vessels and connective tissue; it closely interacts with the urothelial layer above, the detrusor layer below and acts as a functional unit. The umbrella cell layer has the ability to incorporate additional membrane into the luminal surface as it is stretched, increasing the surface area during bladder filling. This is done by fusion and exocytosis of a subapical pool of discoidal/fusiform-shaped vesicles (Truschel et al., 2002). Upon voiding, the mucosa refolds, and the membrane added to the apical surface of the umbrella cells is thought to be recovered by endocytosis. Besides changes in membrane capacity, pressure-induced membrane traffic in apical urothelial cells can dramatically change drugs targeting to membrane-bound receptors and their coupling to downstream signalling cascades. This leads to dynamic modifications of urothelial signals in a moment-to-moment basis in order to accommodate urine storage and/or trigger bladder emptying. However, little is known about the events underlying these changes in both physiological and pathological conditions.

ATP was the first transmitter shown to be released directly by the urothelium (Ferguson et al., 1997). The release of the nucleotide can be triggered both by chemical stimuli and by stretching the uroepithelium during bladder filling. Non-neuronal release of ATP plays an important role as an autocrine and/or paracrine signalling molecule. Once in the suburothelial layer, ATP may act on vimentin-positive interstitial cells and on afferent nerve fibres conveying sensory information to the CNS through the activation of P2X2 and P2X3 receptors, respectively (Silva et al., 2015). Immunohistochemistry experiments have shown immunoreactivity against the P2X3 receptor on nerve fibres in the *lamina propria*, urothelium and detrusor muscle (Ford & Cockayne, 2011). Mice lacking P2X3 receptor exhibited reduced inflammatory pain, prolonged voiding intervals and higher voided volumes (Cockayne et al., 2000). Experiments using an *in vitro* bladder-pelvic nerve preparation, show that prolonged exposure to a desensitizing dose of α,β-meATP significantly reduces the activity of mechanosensitive pelvic nerve afferents in response to bladder distension (Namasivayam et al., 1999). Likewise, intravesical applications of ATP induce rapid excitation of bladder afferents, which was counteracted by PPADS and 2′,3′-*O*-(2,4,6-trinitrophenyl)-ATP (TNP-ATP) (Vlaskovska et al., 2001). Similarly, P2X3 knockout mice exhibited a diminished response to bladder distension and to instillation of P2X receptor agonists manifested by delayed bladder emptying and increased threshold of activation of sensory afferents when compared to wild-type mice (Vlaskovska et al., 2001). In keeping with functional and immunohistochemistry data from our group in the human bladder (Silva et al., 2015), a sensory role for the P2X2 receptor subtype has been revealed using P2X2 and P2X2/P2X3 knockout mice (Cockayne et al., 2005).

The mechanisms underlying ATP release from urothelial cells is a matter of debate in the literature (Sui et al., 2014). ATP can be released from both surfaces of isolated uroepithelium through multiple mechanisms, including vesicular excocytosis, conductance of ATP through ABC or nucleoside transporters or translocation across hemichannels containing either connexins or pannexins. ATP released from the uroepithelium or surrounding tissue may act as a trigger for discoidal/fusiform vesicle exocytosis and membrane recovery through signal at uroepithelial P2 receptors (Wang et al., 2005). Several studies using real-time PCR, Western blotting and immunocytochemistry techniques have demonstrated that the urothelium expresses almost all purinoceptor subtypes. These include all ionotropic P2X receptor subunits and metabotropic $P2Y_1$, $P2Y_2$, $P2Y_4$ and $P2Y_6$ receptors (Carneiro et al., 2014; Chopra et al., 2008; Elneil et al., 2001; Lee et al., 2000; Shabir et al., 2013; Vial & Evans, 2000). Cooperation between metabotropic $P2Y_6$ and ionotropic P2X3 and/or P2X2/3 receptor subunits contributes to promote ATP and ACh release from non-neuronal sources in healthy human urothelium, but the positive feedback mechanism operated by released ATP through fast desensitizing P2X3 and/or P2X2/3 receptors is impaired in obstructed patients, without much affecting the $P2Y_6$ mediated facilitation (Silva et al., 2015). Our group reported that activation of the $P2Y_6$ receptor increases the voiding frequency in anesthetized rats indirectly by releasing ATP from the urothelium via pannexin-1 hemichannels (Timóteo et al., 2014) and subsequent activation of P2X3 receptors on suburothelial nerve afferents. These results suggest that down-modulation of the release of signalling molecules, such as ATP and ACh, from the bladder uroepithelium with selective $P2Y_6$ receptor antagonists may constitute a novel strategy to control hyperactivity of sensory nerves and persistent storage symptoms in patients with BOO.

Once released from the urothelium, ATP is rapidly dephosphorylated by membrane-bound ectonucleotidases. The four members of the NTPDase family, as well as 5′-nucleotidase, are expressed in the mouse bladder, as demonstrated by RT-PCR (Yu et al., 2011). However, the topology of these ecto-enzymes differs between species and among the various layers of the bladder wall. Using immunofluorescence confocal microscopy, we showed that the human urothelium exhibits NTPDase1, NTPDase2 and NTPDase3 in the apical plasma membrane of umbrella cells, whereas the intermediate layer stained positively with NTPDase1 and NTPDase2, but no NTPDase3 immunoreactivity was found (Correia-de Sá, 2010; Silva-Ramos et al., 2015b). The most expressed NTPDase2 is the main contributor to the extracellular catabolism of ATP leading to a preferential ADP accumulation with low adenosine formation at the luminal surface of the isolated human urothelium. Despite this, a role for ADP in the urothelium is still lacking. Interestingly, tissue elements at or below the basal layer of the urothelium (e.g., blood vessels, myofibroblasts and nerve fibers), as well as the detrusor smooth muscle layer, were positively stained with NTPDase1, NTPDase2 and ecto-5'-nucleotidase indicating that biosynthesis of adenosine from adenine nucleotides is positioned to favour a more important role of the nucleoside in the suburothelium and detrusor smooth muscle, namely regulating cholinergic nerve activity via inhibitory A_1 receptors (see above). Notwithstanding this, adenosine has been shown to negatively modulate stretch-induced ATP release from apical umbrella cells through the activation of A_1 receptors (Dunning-Davies et al., 2013). Taking into consideration that adenosine levels at the luminal site of the urothelium are 10-fold below those found beneath the basal layer, one may hypothesize that adenosine A_1 receptor-mediated facilitation of ATP release plays a minor role (if at all) in physiological conditions, yet it may contribute to bladder overactivity in disease states once its concentration becomes elevated, like in bladder ischemia-reperfusion and inflammatory cystitis.

Besides mechanical, chemical and purinergic stimulation, other compounds can elicit ATP release from urothelial cells. Notably, ACh has an important role in modulating this process. All 5 muscarinic receptors are present in urothelial cells. Stimulation of these receptors can trigger ATP release from urothelial cells in culture (Kullmann, et al., 2008). Likewise, intravesical infusion of high doses of the muscarinic agonist oxotremorine increased the voiding frequency in anesthetized rats, an effect that was blunted by blocking P2X receptors with PPADS applied into to bladder lumen (Kullmann et al., 2008). Carbachol and oxotremorine also favored the release of ATP from the human urothelium and the effects of these drugs were abolished by the muscarinic M_2 receptor antagonist, methoctramine (Sui et al., 2014). These results suggest that activation of muscarinic receptors located near the luminal surface of the bladder affects the voiding function by mechanisms involving ATP release, thus strengthening the concepts that antimuscarinic drugs used to treat OAB syndromes exert their effect at least in part through actions in the urothelium.

In the suburothelial layer, the recently discovered interstitial cells have become an exiting focus of research (Wiseman et al., 2003). These cells form a syncytium through extensive coupling via connexin 43-containing gap junctions in a similar manner to that described in the gastrointestinal tract. Through this arrangement signals initiated in a group of interstitial cells can travel considerable distances in the suburotelium and its information conveyed above to the urothelium and below to the detrusor smooth muscle layer. These cells are in close proximity to afferent nerves and elicit excitatory responses mediated by both purines and pyrimidines, such as ATP, ADP, UTP and UDP, via several P2Y receptor subtypes (Fry et al., 2007), including the most expressed $P2Y_6$ receptor (Sui et al., 2006).

ATP-Mediated Signals in OAB Patients

Most OAB patients, excluding some neurogenic cases, report an increase in bladder sensation. Whether this is a cause or a consequence of OAB remains to be elucidated. Anyway, there is a considerable amount of evidence showing that afferent inputs are increased in these patients.

The urothelium from patients with neurogenic or idiopathic detrusor overactivity, as well as with BOO, release more ATP than urothelial strips from control individuals (Kumar et al., 2010; Silva et al., 2015; Sun et al., 2002). Although the basal release of ATP from both neurogenic and control bladders was similar, it reached values that were 20-fold higher the control amounts in bladders from patients with idiopathic OAB, indicating different pathophysiological mechanisms underlying the two disease conditions (Kumar et al., 2010). While in neurogenic OAB the defect is predominantly in the central control of the micturition, in idiopathic OAB the urothelium may play a dominant role in its pathogenesis. This has been evidenced in a clinical study where we demonstrated that urinary ATP can be used as a dynamic biomarker of detrusor overactivity in women with OAB syndrome (Silva-Ramos et al., 2013). Likewise, in patients with BOO, both stretch and electric field stimulation (EFS) can trigger the release of ATP from the urothelium (Silva et al., 2015; Sun et al., 2002). EFS-induced ATP release from the urothelium was 5-fold higher in BOO patients compared to control; this difference can be attributed, at least partially, to an increase in the half-degradation time of ATP by ectonucleotidases confirming that these patients exhibit enhanced purinergic tone (Silva et al., 2015).

Moreover, patients with neurogenic detrusor overactivity possess higher P2X3 receptor amounts in suburothelial afferent sensory neurons compared to control individuals (Brady et al., 2004). It was also observed that the number of suburothelial sensory nerves is increased in patients with idiopathic detrusor overactivity (Moore et al., 1992; Smet et al., 1997). Notably, it was demonstrated that responders to the TRPV1 activator, resiniferatoxin, exhibit reduced expression of the P2X3 receptor after treatment, but this change was not observed in non-responders (Brady et al., 2004). The same group studied the effects of botulinum toxin A injection on P2X3 and TRPV1 receptors expression in patients with neurogenic and idiopathic detrusor overactivity; they found a decrease in the expression of both receptors in suburothelial nerve fibers after injection of the toxin (Apostolidis et al., 2005). Taken together these data indicate a role for ionotropic P2X3 receptors in the pathophysiology of detrusor overactivity.

Interestingly, the population of suburothelial interstitial cells is also increased in OAB patients (Roosen et al., 2009) and this is accompanied by increased expression of P2X2 receptor subunits demonstrated by immunofluorescence and Western blot analysis in female patients with OAB compared to controls (Meng et al., 2015) – see Figure 2. However, the same was not observed in male patients with BOO due to BPH (Silva et al., 2015). The immunoreactivity against P2X2 and P2X3 ionotropic receptor subunits localized respectively in vimentin-positive interstitial cells and suburothelial nerve afferents, as well as in the urothelium, almost disappeared in BPH patients submitted to surgery to relief BOO. Disappearance of the P2X2 immunostaining was not detected in suburothelial blood vessels from BPH patients. In contrast to the partial loss of ionotropic P2X receptors staining, immunoreactivity against the metabotropic $P2Y_6$ receptor was conserved in the urothelium of BPH patients compared to healthy controls. This receptor is abundantly expressed throughout the urothelial layer (including the more superficial umbrella cells), in suburothelial interstitial cells and in the detrusor smooth muscle; interestingly, the $P2Y_6$ staining accompanied the increase in the population of suburothelial interstitial cells observed in patients with BOO due BPH (Silva et al., 2015). These findings denote different purinoceptor arrangements depending on the underlying pathophysiological mechanism of OAB. P2X3 and the heterodimer P2X2/3 are fast desensitizing ionotropic receptors that are activated exclusively by ATP. Decreased activity of ectonucleotidases has been shown in OAB, leading to increased responses to ATP (Harvey et al., 2002; Silva et al., 2015), which might contribute to the loss of P2X2 and P2X3 receptor staining in BOO patients.

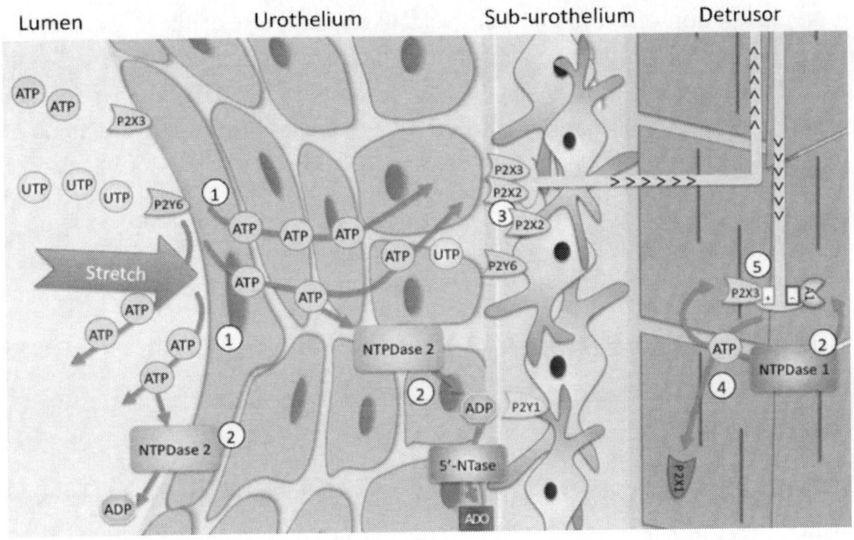

Figure 2. Mechanisms underlying enhanced purinergic tone in OAB. **(1)** The urothelium of OAB patients releases higher amounts of ATP; involvement of $P2Y_6$ receptors activation and ATP-induced ATP release operated by P2X3 and/or P2X2/3 receptors; **(2)** The extracellular ATP catabolism and adenosine formation by ectonucleotidases is deficient in OAB patients; NTPDase 2 predominates in the urothelium and lamina propria leading to preferential ADP formation; NTPDase1 is more abundant in the detrusor, whereas ecto-5'-nucleotidase is expressed predominantly beneath the basal layer of the urothelium resulting in adenosine formation. **(3)** Surplus ATP released from the uroepithelium activates suburothelial P2X3 receptors on sensory nerve afferents and P2X2 receptors on interstitial cells leading to increased sensation during bladder filling. **(4)** Atropine-resistant purinergic contractile responses are also potentiated in the detrusor of OAB patients, which may be due to overexpression of P2X1 receptors and/or deficient ATP inactivation by NTPDase1. **(5)** Patients with OAB exhibit cholinergic nerve hyperactivity due to excessive P2X3-mediated facilitation of acetylcholine release and/or to a deficient inhibitory tone mediated by prejunctional adenosine A_1 receptors.

PURINERGIC CONTROL OF CENTRAL BLADDER REFLEXES

Several disorders of the CNS are known to cause OAB. CNS disease conditions associated with detrusor overactivity are, for instance, cortical lesions secondary to cerebral vascular accidents, multiple sclerosis lesions in the pons and traumatic spinal cord injuries. There is, however, a gap in our knowledge about the role of purines in bladder overactivity secondary to CNS diseases. Nowadays, the role of ATP as a fast synaptic neurotransmitter is by far best characterized at peripheral neuro-effector junctions than in the CNS (Khakh & North, 2012). Nonetheless, activation of P2 receptors on two important CNS areas controlling micturition reflexes (peri-aqueductal grey matter and Barrington nucleus) triggered increases in bladder pressure and efferent pelvic nerve activity, suggesting a role in modulating parasympathetic bladder innervation (Rocha et al., 2001).

At the spinal cord level, there is also evidence of ATP signaling mediating bladder reflexes. ATP mediated responses may be partially responsible for detrusor overactivity induced by acetic acid, acrolein or cyclosphophamide in the rat (Masuda et al., 2005). Involvement of ionotropic P2X3 and P2X2/3 receptor subunits have been claimed, since intrathecal administration of the potent and selective antagonist of these receptors, AF-792, produced long lasting inhibition of micturition reflex contractions (Khakh & North, 2012). These data support a role for presynaptic P2X3 and P2X2/3 receptors in facilitating the micturition reflex at the spinal cord level. Following spinal cord injury, the amount of ATP released in the damaged tissue increases dramatically (Peng et al., 2009), as well as the expression of P2X2 and P2X3 receptor subunits increase in the bladder (Brady et al., 2004; Pannek et al., 2009).

PURINERGIC-BASED BIOMARKERS AND THERAPEUTIC TARGETS IN OAB PATIENTS

In the clinical setting diagnosing OAB is not always an easy task. Symptoms are subjective, patients do not always mean what they say and clinicians do not always get what patients mean. Therefore, there is a clinical need for a simple non-invasive test that could help diagnose OAB. In the last few years several urinary biomarkers for OAB have been investigated and proposed (Antunes-Lopes et al., 2011). Our group demonstrated that urinary ATP levels are significantly elevated in women with detrusor overactivity, rendering ATP as a biomarker candidate, possibly with a higher sensitivity for assessing detrusor overactivity in women with OAB syndrome compared to others previously proposed, like the urinary NGF (Silva-Ramos et al., 2013).

Targeting the purinergic system also seems a reasonable option for the treatment of several lower urinary tract dysfunctions. In fact, antimuscarinic drugs frequently used as a first-line therapeutic option for OAB lose efficacy with the time of treatment (Sears et al., 2010). Long-term exposure to anticholinergics is associated with downregulation of the postjunctional response to carbachol and with an upregulation of purinergic responses to ATP in experimental rats (Uvin et al., 2013), leading us to hypothesize that association with P2 receptor antagonists might be appropriate.

Here, we show that the detrusor smooth muscle from BOO patients due to BPH overexpresses P2X1 receptors and exhibits higher sensitivity to ATP when compared to healthy controls. Novel, potent and orally-active P2X3 antagonists have been developed and tested in lower urinary tract dysfunctions (Gever et al., 2010). The selective P2X3 antagonist, A317491, improved bladder function parameters in a rat model of spinal cord injury and in cyclophosphamide-induced cystitis; this drug effectively inhibited non-micturition contractions and increased inter-contraction intervals and bladder capacity (Ito et al., 2008; Lu et al., 2007). Likewise, AF-353 diminished the frequency of non-voiding contractions in spinal cord injured rats (Munoz et al., 2012). P2X3 antagonists, like AF-219, are being tested in clinical trials for chronic cough and interstitial cystitis/bladder pain syndrome (Abdulqawi et al., 2015; Moldwin, 2015). A phase 2 study recently presented, showed that AF-219 improved pain and related symptoms in patients with interstitial cystitis/bladder pain syndrome compared to placebo, with minor adverse events (Moldwin, 2015). Figure 2 shows the rationale for using selective P2X3 (or P2X2/3) antagonists in OAB syndromes, which may derive from their relevant role in urothelium-mediated pressure transducer signaling pathway involving excessive (1) ATP-induced ATP release from uroepithelial cells, (2) activation of suburothelial nerve afferents and interstitial cells by non-neuronal released ATP, and (3) facilitation of the micturition reflex at the spinal cord level. The P2X3 receptor may also be involved in cholinergic nerve hyperactivity in OAB patients, because the facilitatory effect of ATP on nerve-evoked ACh release increases significantly in these patients (unpublished observations from our group). The P2X3 receptor facilitation of transmitter release may operate unrestrained in the detrusor of OAB patients given that formation of adenosine via the ectonucleotidase pathway is significantly impaired and, thus, the A_1 receptor-mediated inhibitory tone (Silva-Ramos et al., 2015a). This led us to propose that inhibition of adenosine inactivation (via uptake and/or deamination) or activation of the inhibitory A_1 receptor can prevent cholinergic hyperactivity in cases of therapeutic failure with anti-muscarinic drugs. In this context, one may also speculate that decreased ADP formation from the extracellular catabolism of released ATP prevents detrusor relaxation via activation of $P2Y_1$ receptors on inhibitory PDGFRα^+ interstitial cells during urine storage. Activation of inhibitory $P2Y_1$ receptors may be of therapeutic value in addition to β_3 receptor agonists (e.g., mirabegron) to increase the bladder capacity for the treatment of OAB with persistent storage symptoms.

Another interesting finding from our work suggests that UDP-sensitive $P2Y_6$ receptors activation triggers the release of ATP from urothelial cells via pannexin-1 hemichannels (Carneiro et al., 2014; Timóteo et al., 2014), which result in increased release of the nucleotide in BOO patients (Silva et al., 2015). Thus, blocking the $P2Y_6$ receptor in the urothelium may constitute a novel therapeutic approach to control bladder overactivity and persistent storage symptoms in patients with BOO.

Botulinum toxin A (BTX-A) is clinically used to treat both neurogenic and idiopathic bladder overactivity when anti-muscarinic drugs fail (Cruz et al., 2011; Pinto et al., 2010). The actions of BTX-A are not restricted to suppression of ACh and norepinephrine release from autonomic nerves in the rat bladder, but, interestingly, it also diminishes the release of ATP (Khera et al., 2004; Smith et al., 2003). Reduction of ATP release by BTX-A may decrease the activation of sensory nerve afferents induced by bladder irritation with acetic acid (Chuang et al., 2004). Therefore, it appears that the clinical efficacy of BTX-A relies not only on the blockade of transmitter release from efferent nerves, but also on its action on urothelial sensory mechanisms.

All together, these data support a central role of ATP and its derivatives in the pathophysiology of OAB and foresee future drugs targeting the purinergic cascade, including ATP release sites, ectonuleotidases, and purinoceptors, for the treatment of OAB syndromes.

REFERENCES

Abdulqawi, R., Dockry, R., Holt, K., Layton, G., McCarthy, B. G., Ford, A. P., & Smith, J. A. (2015). P2X3 receptor antagonist (AF-219) in refractory chronic cough: a randomised, double-blind, placebo-controlled phase 2 study. *Lancet, 385*(9974), 1198-1205. doi:10.1016/S0140-6736(14)
61255-1.

Acevedo, C. G., Contreras, E., Escalona, J., Lewin, J., & Huidobro-Toro, J. P. (1992). Pharmacological characterization of adenosine A1 and A2 receptors in the bladder: evidence for a modulatory adenosine tone regulating non-adrenergic non-cholinergic neurotransmission. *Br J Pharmacol, 107*(1), 120-126. doi: 10.1111/j.1476-5381.1992.tb14473.x.

Afeli, S. A., Hristov, K. L., & Petkov, G. V. (2012). Do beta3-adrenergic receptors play a role in guinea pig detrusor smooth muscle excitability and contractility? *Am J Physiol Renal Physiol, 302*(2), F251-263. doi:10.1152/ajprenal.00378.2011.

Alexander, S. P., Benson, H. E., Faccenda, E., Pawson, A. J., Sharman, J. L., Spedding, M. et al. (2013a). The Concise Guide to PHARMACOLOGY 2013/14: G protein-coupled receptors. *Br J Pharmacol, 170*(8), 1459-1581. doi:10.1111/bph.12445.

Alexander, S. P., Benson, H. E., Faccenda, E., Pawson, A. J., Sharman, J. L., Spedding, M. et al. (2013b). The Concise Guide to PHARMACOLOGY 2013/14: ligand-gated ion channels. *Br J Pharmacol, 170*(8), 1582-1606. doi:10.1111/bph.12446.

Antunes-Lopes, T., Carvalho-Barros, S., Cruz, C. D., Cruz, F., & Martins-Silva, C. (2011). Biomarkers in overactive bladder: a new objective and noninvasive tool? *Adv Urol, 2011*, 382431. doi:10.1155/2011/382431.

Apostolidis, A., Popat, R., Yiangou, Y., Cockayne, D., Ford, A. P., Davis, J. B. et al. (2005). Decreased sensory receptors P2X3 and TRPV1 in suburothelial nerve fibers following intradetrusor injections of botulinum toxin for human detrusor overactivity. *J Urol, 174*(3), 977-982; discussion 982-973. doi:10.1097/01.ju.0000169481.42259.54.

Aronsson, P., Andersson, M., Ericsson, T., & Giglio, D. (2010). Assessment and characterization of purinergic contractions and relaxations in the rat urinary bladder. *Basic Clin Pharmacol Toxicol, 107*(1), 603-613. doi:PTO554 [pii]. 10.1111/j.1742-7843.2010.00554.x.

Birder, L. A., Kanai, A. J., Cruz, F., Moore, K., & Fry, C. H. (2010). Is the urothelium intelligent? *Neurourol Urodyn, 29*(4), 598-602. doi:10.1002/nau.20914.

Bodin, P., & Burnstock, G. (1996). ATP-stimulated release of ATP by human endothelial cells. *J Cardiovasc Pharmacol, 27*(6), 872-875. Retrieved from http://www.ncbi.nlm.nih.gov/entrez/query.fcgi?cmd=Retrieve&db=
PubMed&dopt=Citation&list_uids=8761855.

Brading, A. F., & Williams, J. H. (1990). Contractile responses of smooth muscle strips from rat and guinea-pig urinary bladder to transmural stimulation: effects of atropine and alpha,beta-methylene ATP. *Br J Pharmacol, 99*(3), 493-498. doi: 10.1111/j.1476-5381.1990.tb12956.x.

Brady, C. M., Apostolidis, A., Yiangou, Y., Baecker, P. A., Ford, A. P., Freeman, A. et al. (2004). P2X3-immunoreactive nerve fibres in neurogenic detrusor overactivity and the effect of intravesical resiniferatoxin. *Eur Urol, 46*(2), 247-253. doi:10.1016/j.eururo.2003.12.017.

Brown, C., Burnstock, G., & Cocks, T. (1979). Effects of adenosine 5'-triphosphate (ATP) and beta-gamma-methylene ATP on the rat urinary bladder. *Br J Pharmacol, 65*(1), 97-102. doi: 10.1111/j.1476-5381.1979.tb17337.x.

Brown, S. M., Bentcheva-Petkova, L. M., Liu, L., Hristov, K. L., Chen, M., Kellett, W. F. et al. (2008). Beta-adrenergic relaxation of mouse urinary bladder smooth muscle in the absence of large-conductance Ca2+-activated K+ channel. *Am J Physiol Renal Physiol, 295*(4), F1149-1157. doi:10.1152/ajprenal.00440.2007.

Burnstock, G. (1972). Purinergic nerves. *Pharmacol Rev, 24*(3), 509-581. Retrieved from http://www.ncbi.nlm.nih.gov/pubmed/4404211.

Burnstock, G. (2014). Purinergic signalling in the urinary tract in health and disease. *Purinergic Signal, 10*(1), 103-155. doi:10.1007/s11302-013-9395-y.

Burnstock, G., Cocks, T., Crowe, R., & Kasakov, L. (1978). Purinergic innervation of the guinea-pig urinary bladder. *Br J Pharmacol, 63*(1), 125-138. doi: 10.1111/j.1476-5381.1978.tb07782.x.

Burnstock, G., Cocks, T., Kasakov, L., & Wong, H. K. (1978). Direct evidence for ATP release from non-adrenergic, non-cholinergic ("purinergic") nerves in the guinea-pig taenia coli and bladder. *Eur J Pharmacol, 49*(2), 145-149. doi:0014-2999(78)90070-5 [pii].

Burnstock, G., Dumsday, B., & Smythe, A. (1972). Atropine resistant excitation of the urinary bladder: the possibility of transmission via nerves releasing a purine nucleotide. *Br J Pharmacol, 44*(3), 451-461. doi: 10.1111/j.1476-5381.1972.tb07283.x.

Carneiro, I., Timóteo, M. A., Silva, I., Vieira, C., Baldaia, C., Ferreirinha, F. et al. (2014). Activation of P2Y6 receptors increases the voiding frequency in anaesthetized rats by releasing ATP from the bladder urothelium. *Br J Pharmacol, 171*(14), 3404-3419. doi:10.1111/bph.12711.

Chopra, B., Gever, J., Barrick, S. R., Hanna-Mitchell, A. T., Beckel, J. M., Ford, A. P., & Birder, L. A. (2008). Expression and function of rat urothelial P2Y receptors. *Am J Physiol Renal Physiol, 294*(4), F821-829. doi:10.1152/ajprenal.00321.2006.

Chua, W. C., Liu, L., Mansfield, K. J., Vaux, K. J., Moore, K. H., Millard, R. J., & Burcher, E. (2007). Age-related changes of P2X(1) receptor mRNA in the bladder detrusor from men with and without bladder outlet obstruction. *Exp Gerontol, 42*(7), 686-692. doi:S0531-5565(07)00034-4 [pii].10.1016/j.exger.2007.02.003.

Chuang, Y. C., Yoshimura, N., Huang, C. C., Chiang, P. H., & Chancellor, M. B. (2004). Intravesical botulinum toxin a administration produces analgesia against acetic acid induced bladder pain responses in rats. *J Urol, 172*(4 Pt 1), 1529-1532. doi:10.1097/01.ju.0000137844.77524.97.

Cockayne, D. A., Dunn, P. M., Zhong, Y., Rong, W., Hamilton, S. G., Knight, G. E. et al. (2005). P2X2 knockout mice and P2X2/P2X3 double knockout mice reveal a role for the

P2X2 receptor subunit in mediating multiple sensory effects of ATP. *J Physiol, 567*(Pt 2), 621-639. doi:jphysiol.2005.088435 [pii]. 10.1113/jphysiol.2005.088435.

Cockayne, D. A., Hamilton, S. G., Zhu, Q. M., Dunn, P. M., Zhong, Y., Novakovic, S. et al. (2000). Urinary bladder hyporeflexia and reduced pain-related behaviour in P2X3-deficient mice. *Nature, 407*(6807), 1011-1015. doi:10.1038/35039519.

Correia-de-Sá, P. (2010). Pathophysiological significance of nucleotide hydrolyzing enzymes in urologic disorder. *Purinergic Signal, 6*(Suppl 2), S13.13. ISSN: 1573-9538 (Print) 1573-9546 (Online).

Cruz, F., Herschorn, S., Aliotta, P., Brin, M., Thompson, C., Lam, W. et al. (2011). Efficacy and safety of onabotulinumtoxinA in patients with urinary incontinence due to neurogenic detrusor overactivity: a randomised, double-blind, placebo-controlled trial. *Eur Urol, 60*(4), 742-750. doi:10.1016/j.eururo.2011.07.002.

D'Agostino, G., Condino, A. M., Calvi, V., Boschi, F., Gioglio, L., & Barbieri, A. (2012). Purinergic P2X3 heteroreceptors enhance parasympathetic motor drive in isolated porcine detrusor, a reliable model for development of P2X selective blockers for detrusor hyperactivity. *Pharmacol Res, 65*(1), 129-136. doi:S1043-6618(11)00276-3 [pii]. 10.1016/j.phrs. 2011.10.002.

Duarte-Araujo, M., Nascimento, C., Timoteo, M. A., Magalhaes-Cardoso, M. T., & Correia-de-Sa, P. (2009). Relative contribution of ecto-ATPase and ecto-ATPDase pathways to the biphasic effect of ATP on acetylcholine release from myenteric motoneurons. *Br J Pharmacol, 156*(3), 519-533. doi:BPH058 [pii]. 10.1111/j.1476-5381.2008.00058.x.

Dunning-Davies, B. M., Fry, C. H., Mansour, D., & Ferguson, D. R. (2013). The regulation of ATP release from the urothelium by adenosine and transepithelial potential. *BJU Int, 111*(3), 505-513. doi:10.1111/j.1464-410X.2012.11421.x.

Elneil, S., Skepper, J. N., Kidd, E. J., Williamson, J. G., & Ferguson, D. R. (2001). Distribution of P2X(1) and P2X(3) receptors in the rat and human urinary bladder. *Pharmacology, 63*(2), 120-128. doi: 10.1159/000056122.

Ferguson, D. R., Kennedy, I., & Burton, T. J. (1997). ATP is released from rabbit urinary bladder epithelial cells by hydrostatic pressure changes--a possible sensory mechanism? *J Physiol, 505 (Pt 2)*, 503-511. doi: 10.1111/j.1469-7793.1997.503bb.x.

Ford, A. P., & Cockayne, D. A. (2011). ATP and P2X purinoceptors in urinary tract disorders. *Handb Exp Pharmacol*(202), 485-526. doi:10.1007/978-3-642-16499-6_22.

Fredholm, B. B., AP, I. J., Jacobson, K. A., Linden, J., & Muller, C. E. (2011). International Union of Basic and Clinical Pharmacology. LXXXI. Nomenclature and classification of adenosine receptors--an update. *Pharmacol Rev, 63*(1), 1-34. doi:10.1124/pr.110.003285.

Fry, C. H., Sui, G. P., Kanai, A. J., & Wu, C. (2007). The function of suburothelial myofibroblasts in the bladder. *Neurourol Urodyn, 26*(6 Suppl), 914-919. doi:10.1002/nau.20483.

Fry, C. H., Young, J. S., Jabr, R. I., McCarthy, C., Ikeda, Y., & Kanai, A. J. (2012). Modulation of spontaneous activity in the overactive bladder: the role of P2Y agonists. *Am J Physiol Renal Physiol, 302*(11), F1447-1454. doi:10.1152/ajprenal.00436.2011.

Gever, J. R., Soto, R., Henningsen, R. A., Martin, R. S., Hackos, D. H., Panicker, S. et al. (2010). AF-353, a novel, potent and orally bioavailable P2X3/P2X2/3 receptor antagonist. *Br J Pharmacol, 160*(6), 1387-1398. doi:BPH796 [pii]. 10.1111/j.1476-5381.2010.00796.x.

Harvey, R. A., Skennerton, D. E., Newgreen, D., & Fry, C. H. (2002). The contractile potency of adenosine triphosphate and ecto-adenosine triphosphatase activity in guinea pig detrusor and detrusor from patients with a stable, unstable or obstructed bladder. *J Urol, 168*(3), 1235-1239. doi:10.1097/01.ju.0000024391.74486.f1. S0022-5347(05)64632-0 [pii].

Hegde, S. S., Mandel, D. A., Wilford, M. R., Briaud, S., Ford, A. P., & Eglen, R. M. (1998). Evidence for purinergic neurotransmission in the urinary bladder of pithed rats. *Eur J Pharmacol, 349*(1), 75-82. doi:10.1016/S0014-2999(98)00173-3.

Igawa, Y., Mattiasson, A., & Andersson, K. E. (1993). Functional importance of cholinergic and purinergic neurotransmission for micturition contraction in the normal, unanaesthetized rat. *Br J Pharmacol, 109*(2), 473-479. doi: 10.1111/j.1476-5381.1993.tb13593.x.

Ito, K., Iwami, A., Katsura, H., & Ikeda, M. (2008). Therapeutic effects of the putative P2X3/P2X2/3 antagonist A-317491 on cyclophosphamide-induced cystitis in rats. *Naunyn Schmiedebergs Arch Pharmacol, 377*(4-6), 483-490. doi:10.1007/s00210-007-0197-z.

Khakh, B. S., & North, R. A. (2012). Neuromodulation by extracellular ATP and P2X receptors in the CNS. *Neuron, 76*(1), 51-69. doi:10.1016/ j.neuron.2012.09.024.

Khera, M., Somogyi, G. T., Kiss, S., Boone, T. B., & Smith, C. P. (2004). Botulinum toxin A inhibits ATP release from bladder urothelium after chronic spinal cord injury. *Neurochem Int, 45*(7), 987-993. doi:10.1016/j.neuint.2004.06.001. S0197018604001111 [pii].

King, B. F., Knowles, I. D., Burnstock, G., & Ramage, A. G. (2004). Investigation of the effects of P2 purinoceptor ligands on the micturition reflex in female urethane-anaesthetized rats. *Br J Pharmacol, 142*(3), 519-530. doi:10.1038/sj.bjp.0705790. 0705790 [pii].

King, J. A., Huddart, H., & Staff, W. G. (1997). Purinergic modulation of rat urinary bladder detrusor smooth muscle. *Gen Pharmacol, 29*(4), 597-604. doi:S0306362396005733 [pii].

Kullmann, F. A., Artim, D., Beckel, J., Barrick, S., de Groat, W. C., & Birder, L. A. (2008). Heterogeneity of muscarinic receptor-mediated Ca2+ responses in cultured urothelial cells from rat. *Am J Physiol Renal Physiol, 294*(4), F971-981. doi:00313.2007 [pii]. 10.1152/ajprenal. 00313.2007.

Kullmann, F. A., Artim, D. E., Birder, L. A., & de Groat, W. C. (2008). Activation of muscarinic receptors in rat bladder sensory pathways alters reflex bladder activity. *J Neurosci, 28*(8), 1977-1987. doi:28/8/1977 [pii].10.1523/JNEUROSCI.4694-07.2008.

Kumar, V., Chapple, C. R., Rosario, D., Tophill, P. R., & Chess-Williams, R. (2010). In vitro release of adenosine triphosphate from the urothelium of human bladders with detrusor overactivity, both neurogenic and idiopathic. *Eur Urol, 57*(6), 1087-1092. doi:S0302-2838(09)01204-4 [pii].10.1016/j.eururo.2009.11.042.

Lee, H., Koh, B. H., Peri, L. E., Sanders, K. M., & Koh, S. D. (2014). Purinergic inhibitory regulation of murine detrusor muscles mediated by PDGFRalpha+ interstitial cells. *J Physiol, 592*(Pt 6), 1283-1293. doi:10.1113/jphysiol.2013.267989.

Lee, H. Y., Bardini, M., & Burnstock, G. (2000). Distribution of P2X receptors in the urinary bladder and the ureter of the rat. *J Urol, 163*(6), 2002-2007. doi:10.1016/S0022-5347(05)67618-5.

Lu, S. H., Groat, W. C., Lin, A. T., Chen, K. K., & Chang, L. S. (2007). Evaluation of purinergic mechanism for the treatment of voiding dysfunction: a study in conscious spinal cord-injured rats. *J Chin Med Assoc, 70*(10), 439-444. doi:S1726-4901(08)70035-2 [pii].

Lukacsko, P., & Krell, R. D. (1982). Response of the guinea-pig urinary bladder to purine and pyrimidine nucleotides. *Eur J Pharmacol, 80*(4), 401-406. doi:10.1016/0014-2999(82)90086-3.

Masuda, H., Chancellor, M.B., Kihara, K., de Groat, W,C., & Yoshimura, N. (2005). Evidence for the involvement of spinal endogenous ATP and P2X receptors in detrusor overactivity caused by acetic acid, acrolein or cyclophosphamide. *Neurourol Urodyn, 24*(5-6). doi:10.1002/nau.20173.

McMurray, G., Dass, N., & Brading, A. F. (1998). Purinoceptor subtypes mediating contraction and relaxation of marmoset urinary bladder smooth muscle. *Br J Pharmacol, 123*(8), 1579-1586. doi:10.1038/sj.bjp.0701774.

Meng, M., Zheng, J., Yan, J., Li, Q., Fang, Q., & Li, W. (2015). P2X and P2X Receptors Mediate Bladder Hyperesthesia in ICC in Female Overactive Bladder. *Cell Biochem Biophys*. doi:10.1007/s12013-014-0471-x.

Moldwin, R., Kitt, M., Mangel, J., Beyer, R., Hanno, P., Butera, P., & Ford, A. (2015). A phase 2 study in women with interstitial cystitis/bladder pain syndrome (IC/PBS) of the novel P2X3 antagonist AF-219. *Neurourol Urodyn, 34*(S3), S50.

Moore, K. H., Gilpin, S. A., Dixon, J. S., Richmond, D. H., & Sutherst, J. R. (1992). Increase in presumptive sensory nerves of the urinary bladder in idiopathic detrusor instability. *Br J Urol, 70*(4), 370-372. Retrieved from http://www.ncbi.nlm.nih.gov/pubmed/1450843.

Munoz, A., Somogyi, G. T., Boone, T. B., Ford, A. P., & Smith, C. P. (2012). Modulation of bladder afferent signals in normal and spinal cord-injured rats by purinergic P2X3 and P2X2/3 receptors. *BJU Int, 110*(8 Pt B), E409-414. doi:10.1111/j.1464-410X.2012.11189.x.

Namasivayam, S., Eardley, I., & Morrison, J. F. (1999). Purinergic sensory neurotransmission in the urinary bladder: an in vitro study in the rat. *BJU Int, 84*(7), 854-860. Retrieved from http://www.ncbi.nlm.nih.gov/ pubmed/10532986.

Nicholls, J., Hourani, S. M., & Kitchen, I. (1992). Characterization of P1-purinoceptors on rat duodenum and urinary bladder. *Br J Pharmacol, 105*(3), 639-642. doi: 10.1111/j.1476-5381.1992.tb09032.x.

O'Reilly, B. A., Kosaka, A. H., Chang, T. K., Ford, A. P., Popert, R., & McMahon, S. B. (2001). A quantitative analysis of purinoceptor expression in the bladders of patients with symptomatic outlet obstruction. *BJU Int, 87*(7), 617-622. doi:bju179 [pii].

Palea, S., Corsi, M., Pietra, C., Artibani, W., Calpista, A., Gaviraghi, G., & Trist, D. G. (1994). ADP beta S induces contraction of the human isolated urinary bladder through a purinoceptor subtype different from P2X and P2Y. *J Pharmacol Exp Ther, 269*(1), 193-197. Retrieved from http://www.ncbi.nlm.nih.gov/entrez/query.fcgi?cmd=Retrieve& db=PubMed&dopt=Citation&list_uids=8169824.

Pannek, J., Janek, S., Sommerer, F., & Tannapfel, A. (2009). Expression of purinergic P2X2-receptors in neurogenic bladder dysfunction due to spinal cord injury: a preliminary immunohistochemical study. *Spinal Cord, 47*(7), 561-564. doi:10.1038/sc.2008.165.

Peng, W., Cotrina, M. L., Han, X., Yu, H., Bekar, L., Blum, L. et al. (2009). Systemic administration of an antagonist of the ATP-sensitive receptor P2X7 improves recovery after spinal cord injury. *Proc Natl Acad Sci U S A, 106*(30), 12489-12493. doi:10.1073/pnas.0902531106.

Pinto, R., Lopes, T., Frias, B., Silva, A., Silva, J. A., Silva, C. M. et al. (2010). Trigonal injection of botulinum toxin A in patients with refractory bladder pain syndrome/interstitial cystitis. *Eur Urol, 58*(3), 360-365. doi:10.1016/ j.eururo. 2010.02.031.

Rocha, I., Burnstock, G., & Spyer, K. M. (2001). Effect on urinary bladder function and arterial blood pressure of the activation of putative purine receptors in brainstem areas. *Auton Neurosci, 88*(1-2), 6-15. doi:10.1016/S1566-0702(00)00284-8.

Roosen, A., Datta, S. N., Chowdhury, R. A., Patel, P. M., Kalsi, V., Elneil, S. et al. (2009). Suburothelial myofibroblasts in the human overactive bladder and the effect of botulinum neurotoxin type A treatment. *Eur Urol, 55*(6), 1440-1448. doi:S0302-2838(08)01314-6 [pii].10.1016/
j.eururo.2008.11.009.

Rubinstein, R., Shalev, M., Nissenkorn, I., & Cohen, S. (1998). Effect of exogenous adenosine and its monophosphate on the contractile response to acetylcholine in the human isolated detrusor muscle strips. *J Auton Pharmacol, 18*(2), 99-104. doi: 10.1046/j.1365-2680.1998.1820099.x.

Ruggieri, M. R., Sr. (2006). Mechanisms of disease: role of purinergic signaling in the pathophysiology of bladder dysfunction. *Nat Clin Pract Urol, 3*(4), 206-215. doi:10.1038/ncpuro0456.

Sears, C. L., Lewis, C., Noel, K., Albright, T. S., & Fischer, J. R. (2010). Overactive bladder medication adherence when medication is free to patients. *J Urol, 183*(3), 1077-1081. doi:10.1016/j.juro.2009.11.026.

Shabir, S., Cross, W., Kirkwood, L. A., Pearson, J. F., Appleby, P. A., Walker, D. et al. (2013). Functional expression of purinergic P2 receptors and transient receptor potential channels by the human urothelium. *Am J Physiol Renal Physiol, 305*(3), F396-406. doi:10.1152/ajprenal.00127.2013.

Silva, I., Ferreirinha, F., Magalhães-Cardoso, M. T., Silva-Ramos, M., & Correia-de-Sá, P. (2015). Activation of P2Y6 Receptors Facilitates Nonneuronal Adenosine Triphosphate and Acetylcholine Release from Urothelium with the Lamina Propria of Men with Bladder Outlet Obstruction. *J Urol, 194*(4), 1146-1154. doi:10.1016/j.juro.2015.05.080.

Silva-Ramos, M., Silva, I., Duarte-Araújo, M., Magalhães-Cardoso, T., Lafuente-de-Carvalho, J., & Correia-de-Sá, P. (2010). Loss of balance between excitatory P2X3 and inhibitory A1 receptors contribute to cholinergic hyperactivity in obstructed human bladder. *Basic Clin Pharmacol Toxicol, 107* (supplement s1), Abstract n 2397.

Silva-Ramos, M., Silva, I., Faria, M., Magalhães-Cardoso, M. T., Correia, J., Ferreirinha, F., & Correia-de-Sá, P. (2015a). Impairment of ATP hydrolysis decreases adenosine A1 receptor tonus favoring cholinergic nerve hyperactivity in the obstructed human urinary bladder. *Purinergic Signal, 11*(4), 595-606. doi:10.1007/s11302-015-9478-z.

Silva-Ramos, M., Silva, I., Faria, M., Magalhães-Cardoso, M. T., & Correia-de-Sá, P. (2015b). Urinary bladder disorders: Is adenosine friend or foe? In K. Warrick (Ed.), *Adenosine receptors: Pharmacology, functions and therapeutic aspects* (1st ed., pp. 115-142). Hauppauge, NY: Nova Science Publishers Inc.. ISBN: 978-1-63463-454-0.

Silva-Ramos, M., Silva, I., Oliveira, O., Ferreira, S., Reis, M. J., Oliveira, J. C., & Correia-de-Sá, P. (2013). Urinary ATP may be a dynamic biomarker of detrusor overactivity in women with overactive bladder syndrome. *PLoS One, 8*(5), e64696. doi:10.1371/journal.pone.0064696.

Smet, P. J., Moore, K. H., & Jonavicius, J. (1997). Distribution and colocalization of calcitonin gene-related peptide, tachykinins, and vasoactive intestinal peptide in normal and idiopathic unstable human urinary bladder. *Lab Invest, 77*(1), 37-49. Retrieved from http://www. ncbi.nlm.nih.gov/pubmed/9251677.

Smith, C. P., Franks, M. E., McNeil, B. K., Ghosh, R., de Groat, W. C., Chancellor, M. B., & Somogyi, G. T. (2003). Effect of botulinum toxin A on the autonomic nervous system of the rat lower urinary tract. *J Urol, 169*(5), 1896-1900. doi:10.1097/01. ju.0000049202.56189.54. S0022-5347(05)63710-X [pii].

Sperlagh, B., & Vizi, E. S. (1991). Effect of presynaptic P2 receptor stimulation on transmitter release. *J Neurochem, 56*(5), 1466-1470. doi: 10.1111/j.1471-4159.1991.tb02039.x.

Sui, G., Fry, C. H., Montgomery, B., Roberts, M., Wu, R., & Wu, C. (2014). Purinergic and muscarinic modulation of ATP release from the urothelium and its paracrine actions. *Am J Physiol Renal Physiol, 306*(3), F286-298. doi:10.1152/ajprenal.00291.2013.

Sui, G. P., Wu, C., & Fry, C. H. (2006). Characterization of the purinergic receptor subtype on guinea-pig suburothelial myofibroblasts. *BJU Int, 97*(6), 1327-1331. doi:BJU6200 [pii]. 10.1111/j.1464-410X.2006.06200.x.

Sun, Y., & Chai, T. C. (2006). Augmented extracellular ATP signaling in bladder urothelial cells from patients with interstitial cystitis. *Am J Physiol Cell Physiol, 290*(1), C27-34. doi:00552.2004 [pii].10.1152/ ajpcell.00552.2004.

Sun, Y., MaLossi, J., Jacobs, S. C., & Chai, T. C. (2002). Effect of doxazosin on stretch-activated adenosine triphosphate release in bladder urothelial cells from patients with benign prostatic hyperplasia. *Urology, 60*(2), 351-356. doi:S0090429502017107 [pii].

Suzuki, H., & Kokubun, S. (1994). Subtypes of purinoceptors in rat and dog urinary bladder smooth muscles. *Br J Pharmacol, 112*(1), 117-122. doi: 10.1111/j.1476-5381.1994.tb13039.x.

Timóteo, M. A., Carneiro, I., Silva, I., Noronha-Matos, J. B., Ferreirinha, F., Silva-Ramos, M., & Correia-de-Sá, P. (2014). ATP released via pannexin-1 hemichannels mediates bladder overactivity triggered by urothelial P2Y6 receptors. *Biochem Pharmacol, 87*(2), 371-379. doi:10.1016/ j.bcp.2013.11.007.

Truschel, S. T., Wang, E., Ruiz, W. G., Leung, S. M., Rojas, R., Lavelle, J. et al. (2002). Stretch-regulated exocytosis/endocytosis in bladder umbrella cells. *Mol Biol Cell, 13*(3), 830-846. doi:10.1091/mbc.01-09-0435.

Uvin, P., Boudes, M., Menigoz, A., Franken, J., Pinto, S., Gevaert, T. et al. (2013). Chronic administration of anticholinergics in rats induces a shift from muscarinic to purinergic transmission in the bladder wall. *Eur Urol, 64*(3), 502-510. doi:10.1016/j.eururo.2013.05.031.

Vial, C., & Evans, R. J. (2000). P2X receptor expression in mouse urinary bladder and the requirement of P2X(1) receptors for functional P2X receptor responses in the mouse urinary bladder smooth muscle. *Br J Pharmacol, 131*(7), 1489-1495. doi:10.1038/sj.bjp.0703720.

Vlaskovska, M., Kasakov, L., Rong, W., Bodin, P., Bardini, M., Cockayne, D. A. et al. (2001). P2X3 knock-out mice reveal a major sensory role for urothelially released ATP. *J Neurosci, 21*(15), 5670-5677. doi:21/15/5670 [pii].

Wang, E. C., Lee, J. M., Ruiz, W. G., Balestreire, E. M., von Bodungen, M., Barrick, S. et al. (2005). ATP and purinergic receptor-dependent membrane traffic in bladder umbrella cells. *J Clin Invest, 115*(9), 2412-2422. doi:10.1172/JCI24086.

Wiseman, O. J., Fowler, C. J., & Landon, D. N. (2003). The role of the human bladder lamina propria myofibroblast. *BJU Int, 91*(1), 89-93. doi: 10.1046/j.1464-410X.2003.03802.x.

Wu, C., Bayliss, M., Newgreen, D., Mundy, A. R., & Fry, C. H. (1999). A comparison of the mode of action of ATP and carbachol on isolated human detrusor smooth muscle. *J Urol, 162*(5), 1840-1847. doi:10.1016/S0022-5347(05)68248-1.

Yu, W., Robson, S. C., & Hill, W. G. (2011). Expression and distribution of ectonucleotidases in mouse urinary bladder. *PLoS One, 6*(4), e18704. doi:10.1371/journal.pone.0018704.

Yu, W., Sun, X., Robson, S. C., & Hill, W. G. (2013). Extracellular UDP enhances P2X-mediated bladder smooth muscle contractility via P2Y(6) activation of the phospholipase C/inositol trisphosphate pathway. *FASEB J, 27*(5), 1895-1903. doi:10.1096/fj.12-219006.

Yu, W., Sun, X., Robson, S. C., & Hill, W. G. (2014). ADP-induced bladder contractility is mediated by P2Y12 receptor and temporally regulated by ectonucleotidases and adenosine signaling. *FASEB J, 28*(12), 5288-5298. doi:10.1096/fj.14-255885.

Biographical Sketch

Paulo Correia-de-Sá, MD, PhD

Laboratório de Farmacologia e Neurobiologia
Departamento de Imuno-Fisiologia e Farmacologia
Center for Drug Discovery and Innovative Medicines (MedInUP)
ICBAS - Universidade do Porto
L. Prof. Abel Salazar, 2
4099-003 Porto
PORTUGAL

Tel: 351 22 0428 212	Fax: 351 22 0428 090
E-Mail (particular):	pcorreiasa@mail.telepac.pt
E-Mail (ICBAS):	farmacol@icbas.up.pt

Portuguese nationality, born on the 24th April 1963, in Lourenço Marques - Mozambique. Married.

Medical Doctor (MD) graduation - Biomedical Sciences Institute of Abel Salazar - University of Oporto (PORTUGAL) (1988).

Philosophy Doctor (PhD) graduation in Biomedical Sciences (Pharmacology) - Biomedical Sciences Institute of Abel Salazar - University of Oporto (PORTUGAL) (1995).

PhD Thesis: *Presynaptic adenosine receptors at neuromuscular junction.*

Supervisor: Prof. J. Alexandre Ribeiro.

Academic activity

Full Professor of Pharmacology and Neurosciences, ICBAS-UP (October, 2007).

Associate Professor of Pharmacology and Therapeutics, ICBAS/UP (April, 2004 – September, 2007).

Assistant Professor of Pharmacology and Therapeutics, ICBAS/UP (October, 1997 – March, 2004).

Young Research Fellow at the Laboratory of Pharmacology, ICBAS/UP (September, 1986 – September, 1989).

Head of the Department of Immuno-Physiology and Pharmacology, ICBAS/UP (January, 2000 -).

Head of the Laboratory of Pharmacology and Neurobiology, ICBAS/UP (April, 1999 -).

President of the Portuguese Society for Pharmacology (February 2013 -).

President of the Unit for Multidisciplinary Investigation in Biomedicine (UMIB), FCT - Programa de Financiamento Plurianual de Unidades de I&D (January, 2004-14).

Vice-President of the Scientific Council, ICBAS/UP (January, 2002 – December, 2003).

Main Research Interests

Investigate the pathophysiological role of purines (ATP and its metabolites) in human cells signaling and in animal models of human diseases, searching for new targets for therapeutic intervention.

Ongoing Research Topics and collaborations

Origin and fate of extracellular purines regulating bone formation and neuron-fibroblast interaction using human cells in culture (Collab. Depart. Orthopedics and Maxillofacial Surgery – HGSA-CHPorto and CHVNGaia) - Integrative activities with GCR/UMIB) + 3 PhD students (JBNM, ARP, MC).

Pharmacological aspects of purinergic signaling of overactive human bladders in situ, in vitro and in the rat in vivo (Collab. Depart. Urology - HGSA-CHPorto) - Integrative activities with GCR/UMIB) + 2 PhD students (MSR, IS).

Purinergic modulation of cavernosal vessel tonus in men with vasculogenic erectile dysfunction (Collab. Depart. Urology – HGSA-CHPorto; Inst. Andrologia (Madrid, Spain); Hosp. Ramon y Cajal (Madrid, Spain) - Integrative activities with GCR/UMIB) + 1 PhD student (NL).

Functional status of the purinergic system and the neuron-glial interaction in patients with pharmaco-resistant Mesial Temporal Lobe Epilepsy (Depart. Neurosciences – HGSA-CHPorto, INML and INSA Dr Ricardo Jorge; Fac. Pharmacy UP) - Integrative activities with IGIA/UMIB + 2 PhD students (ABB, BGL).

Pathophysiological role of subtype-specific ecto-NTPDases in human diseases (Collab. Centre de Recherche en Rhumatologie et Immunologie (Jean Sévigny, Laval, Quebec, Canada).

Intracellular calcium signature in programmed cell death (Neurospora crassa) – involvement of mitochondrial proteins (Collab. Depart. Molecular Biology – ICBAS, Prof. Arnaldo Videira) + 1 Post-Doc (JMC).

Animal-based research studies on the role of purines as potential targets for therapeutic intervention:

- Myasthenic syndromes (Collab. Depart. Neurosciences – HGSA; Univ. Estadual de Maringá (Paraná, Brasil); UT Southwestern Med. Center (Steven Vernino, Dallas, USA); Weatheral Inst. Mol. Med., John Radcliffe Hosp. (M. Isabel Leite, Oxford, UK). - Integrative activities with GCR/UMIB) + 1 FCT Project (PTDC/NEU-NMC/0237/2012, in collaboration with ICETA-Porto/UP, UCL-London and REQUIMTE).
- Inflammatory instestinal diseases (Collab. Depart. of General Surgery – HGSA); Nestlé Research Centre (Lausanne, Switzerland) and Inst. Ciências Biomédicas, USP (Patrícia Castelucci, S. Paulo, Brazil). 2 PhD students (CV, IS).
- Involvement of purines in heart failure and pulmonary hypertension (Depart. of Physiology – FMUP (Porto, Portugal) + 1 PhD student (BB) + 1 FCT Project (PTDC/DTP-FTO/0802/2012).

Facilities and Technical Resources of the Research Group

The group headed by PCS provides an attractive environment, grounded in cutting-edge pieces of equipment, for molecular biology (e.g., real-time PCR, laser-microdissection system, flow cytometry), life-cell and tissue imaging (e.g., spectral laser-scanning confocal microscope, laser microdissection, single-cell calcium imaging), and functional studies (e.g., liquid scintillation counter, electrophysiology equipment, in vivo experimental setups). Metabolite identification potential was recently upgraded from HPLC to UPLC in tandem with mass spectrometry.

Scientific Research Projects (funded)

Adenosine and ^{3}H-acetylcholine release from rat phrenic nerve endings
P. Correia-de-Sá, J.L. Fougo & J.A. Ribeiro (1987) - University of Porto.

Characterization of neuromodulatory role of adenosine in mammalia
J.A. Ribeiro et al. (1990-93) - JNICT, Proj. I & D, PMCT/C/SAU/792/90.

Presynaptic adenosine receptors at rat neuromuscular junction
P. Correia-de-Sá (Ph. D Thesis) (1991-93) - JNICT Ph. D Studentship, BD/721/90-ID.

Microlabs for pharmacologists
Henk van Wilgenburg et al. (1990-93) - EC, COMETT Project

Cholinergic and peptidergic modulation of evoked transmitter release from rat motor nerve terminals: Influence of adenosine
P. Correia-de-Sá, M.A. Timóteo & J.A. Ribeiro (1994-).
Unit Multidisciplinar of Investigation in Biomedicine (UMIB)

Nuno R. Grande et al. (1994-).
Lab. of Macroscopic Anatomy, Lab. of Cell Biology, Lab. of Molecular Genetics & Lab. of Pharmacology (ICBAS) - JNICT.

E.C. Concerted Action ADEURO
Dept. of Chemistry (Camerino-Italy), Rega Instituut (Leuven-The Netherlands), Dept. of Medicinal Chemistry (Leiden-The Netherlands), Dept. of Organic Pharmaceutical Chemistry (Uppsala-The Netherlands), Lab. for Molecular Biology (München-Germany), Inst. of Pharmacology (Vienna-Austria), Dept. of Pharmacology (Heidelberg-Germany), Dept. of Pharmacology (Milan-Italy), Dept. of Pharmacology (Florence-Italy), Dept. of Pharmacology (Leiden-The Netherlands), Inst. for Histology and Neurobiology (Stockholm-Sweden), Dept. of Pharmacology (Stockholm-Sweden), Dept. of Pharmacology (IGC-Oeiras/ICBAS-Porto-Portugal) (1994-96) - EC, ADEURO Project.

Interactions between adenosine and neuropeptides on neurotransmitter release
A.M. Sebastião et al. (1996-99) - JNICT, PRAXIS XXI/2/2.1/BIA/137/94.

Role of adenosine in neurotransmitter release and synaptic activity from myoneural, vascular and hippocampal synapses: Influence of calcium and of the stimulation paradigm
P. Correia-de-Sá et al. (2001-04) - FCT, SAPIENS Project POCTI/FCB/36545/2000.

Neuronal release of nucleotidases and their role in purinergic modulation of synaptic transmission
P. Correia-de-Sá et al. (2003-05) - FCT, SAPIENS Project POCTI/FCB/45549/2002.

Amplification of neuromuscular transmission by adenosine in mammals: New insight for treating myasthenic syndromes
P. Correia-de-Sá et al. (2004-06) - FCT, SAPIENS Project POCTI/CVT/43368/2001.

Purinergic modulation of cavernousal tissue from man with erectile dysfunction
P. Correia-de-Sá et al. (2004) – University of Porto/Ilídio Pinho's Foundation.
Pre-graduation Programme for Scientific Research.

HPLC analysis of the adenine nucleotides catabolism into adenosine regulating the release of neurotransmitters: Functional role of secreted nucleotidases
P. Correia-de-Sá et al. (2004) - FCT, Health Sciences - CONC-REEQ/1168/2001.
Programme for Scientific Re-equipment of National Laboratories.

Applications of confocal laser scanning microscopy to morphofunctional cell dynamics
P. Correia-de-Sá et al. (2004) - FCT, Health Sciences - CONC-REEQ/1264/2001.
Programme for Scientific Re-equipment of National Laboratories.

Origin and fate of extacellular purines regulating human bone formation
P. Correia-de-Sá et al. (2008-10)
Supported by FCT, Project PTDC/SAU-OSM/73576/2006.

Enteric purines as potential therapeutic targets for inflammatory bowel diseases

P. Correia-de-Sá et al. (2008-10)

Supported by FCT, Project PTDC/CVT/74462/2006.

Liquid crystal biosensors for endogenous cathecolamines

Carlos Manuel Melo Pereira & P. Correia-de-Sá (2008-10)

Collaborative: Centro de Investigação em Química (CIQ/FCUP) and Laboratório de Farmacologia e Neurobiologia (ICBAS/UP)

Supported by FCT, Project PTDC/QUI/69685/2006.

Relevance of HHV-6B in meso-temporal lobe epilepsy (MTLE) with hippocampal sclerosis: prevention and treatment

M. Berta Silva & P. Correia de Sá (2008-11).

Collaborative: Laboratório de Imunogenética and Laboratório de Farmacologia e Neurobiologia (ICBAS/UP), Hospital Geral de Santo António (HGSA), Instituto Nacional de Medicina Legal (INML) e Instituto Nacional de Saúde Dr. Ricardo Jorge (INSARJ).

Suported by FCT, Project PIC/IC/83297/2007.

Pathophysiological role of purines (ATP and adenosine) in the human bladder hyperactivity

P. Correia-de-Sá et al. (2010-12)

Supported by FCT, Project PTDC/SAU-OSM/104369/2008.

Fibroblasts as mechano-sensory signaling intermediates between epithelia and primary afferent neurons: Role of extracellular ATP, purinoceptors and $[Ca^{2+}]_i$ waves

P. Correia-de-Sá et al. (2010-12)

Supported by FCT, Project PTDC/SAU-FCF/108263/2008.

Is there a place for adenosine mediating impairment of both neuromuscular and immunological synapses in myasthenics?

Laura Oliveira & P. Correia-de-Sá (2010-12)

Supported by FCT, Project PTDC/SAU-FCF/108462/2008.

Toxin-induced myasthenia gravis and in vitro assays to characterize neuromuscular impairment: crosstalk between presynaptic adenosine and cholinergic receptors

P. Correia-de-Sá et al. (2010-11)

Collaborative: Laboratório de Farmacologia e Neurobiologia (ICBAS/UP), Steven Vernino (MD, PhD, Associate Professor of Neurology, Neurology Residency Program Director, UT Southwestern Medical Center at Dallas, USA) e M. Isabel Leite (MD, PhD, Neurosciences Group, Weatheral Institute of Molecular Medicine, John Radcliffe Hospital, Headington, Oxford OX3 9DU, UK).

Supported by Universidade do Porto/Banco Santander Totta – Starting research grant.

Astrocyte-microglia crosstalk in astrogliosis: modulation by P2 receptors

Glória Queiroz & P. Correia-de-Sá (2010-12)

Collaborative: Instituto de Ciências e Tecnologias Agrárias e Agro-Alimentares - Porto (ICETA-Porto/UP), REQUIMTE (Rede de Química e Tecnologia) - Laboratório Associado para a Química Verde (REQUIMTE) e Laboratório de Farmacologia e Neurobiologia (ICBAS/UP)

Supported by FCT, Project PTDC/SAU-TOX/115597/2009.

Unit for Multidisciplinary Investigations in Biomedicine (UMIB)

P. Correia-de-Sá et al. (2011-13) – Scientific Coordination

Supported by FCT, Projet PEst-OE/SAU/UI0215/2011.

On the role of adenosine signaling in the progression of pulmonary hypertension to heart failure

Ana Patrícia Fontes Sousa & P. Correia-de-Sá (2013-15)

Supported by FCT, Project PTDC/DTP-FTO/0802/2012.

KDAC inhibition and intracellular dynamics: impact on neuronal development, survival and transmission

Jorge Oliveira & P. Correia-de-Sá (2013-15)

Collaborative: Instituto de Ciências e Tecnologias Agrárias e Agro-Alimentares - Porto (ICETA-Porto/UP), Instituto de Ciências Biomédicas Abel Salazar (ICBAS/UP), Unidade Multidisciplinar de Investigação Biomédica (UMIB/ICBAS/UP), University College London (UCL), REQUIMTE - Rede de Química e Tecnologia - Associação (REQUIMTE-P) e Faculdade de Farmácia da Universidade do Porto (FF/UP).

Supported by FCT, Projecto PTDC/NEU-NMC/0237/2012.

Unit for Multidisciplinary Investigations in Biomedicine (UMIB)

P. Correia-de-Sá et al. (2011-13) – Scientific Coordination

Supported by FCT, Projeto PEst-OE/SAU/UI0215/2014.

Center for Drug Discovery and Innovative Medicines – University of Porto (MedInUP)

P. Correia-de-Sá et al. (2015) – Scientific Executive Committee

Supported by UP/Banco Santander.

Peer-Reviewed Publications (last three years)

- **Role of ecto-NTPDases on UDP-sensitive P2Y$_6$ receptor activation during osteogenic differentiation of primary bone marrow stromal cells from postmenopausal women.**
  J.B. Noronha-Matos, M.A. Costa, M.T. Magalhães-Cardoso, F. Ferreirinha, R. Freitas, J.M. Neves, J. Sévigny & P. Correia-de-Sá
  J. Cell. Physiol. (2012) 227, 2694-2709.
- **Synthesis of new chiral xanthone derivatives acting as nerve conduction blockers in the rat sciatic nerve.**
  C. Fernandes§, L. Oliveira§, M.E. Tiritan, L. Leitao, A. Pozzi, J.B. Noronha-Matos, P. Correia-de-Sá & M. Pinto.
  Eur. J. Med. Chem. (2012) **55**, 1-11.

- **Adenosine A2A receptor antagonists are broad facilitators of antinicotinic neuromuscular blockade monitored either with 2-Hz train-of-four or 50-Hz tetanic stimuli.**
  M.W. Pereira, P. Correia-de-Sá & W. Alves-Do-Prado
  Clin. Exp. Pharmacol. Physiol. (2012) **39**, 869-877.
- **Bothropstoxin-I reduces evoked acetylcholine release from rat motor nerve terminals: radiochemical and real-time video-microscopy studies.**
  P. Correia-de-Sá, J.B. Noronha-Matos, M.A. Timóteo, F. Ferreirinha, P. Marques, A.M. Soares, C. Carvalho, W.L.G. Cavalcante & M. Gallacci
  Toxicon (2013) **61**, 16-25, http://dx.doi.org/10.1016/j.toxicon.2012. 10.014.
- **Doxorubicin decreases paraquat accumulation and toxicity in Caco-2 cells.**
  R. Silva, H. Carmo, V. Vilas-Boas, P. Guedes de Pinho, R. Dinis-Oliveira, F. Carvalho, I. Silva, P. Correia-de-Sá, M.L. Bastos & F. Remião
  Toxicol. Lett. (2013) **217**, 34–41. http://dx.doi.org/10.1016/j.toxlet2012. 11.028.
- **Urinary ATP may be a dynamic biomarker of detrusor overactivity in women with overactive bladder syndrome.**
  M. Silva-Ramos*, I. Silva*, O. Oliveira, S. Ferreira, M.J. Reis, J.C. Oliveira & P. Correia-de-Sá
  PLoS ONE (2013) **8**, e64696. doi:10.1371/journal.pone.0064696.
- **Histamine induces ATP release from human subcutaneous fibroblasts, via pannexin-1 hemichannels, leading to Ca^{2+} mobilization and cell proliferation.**
  A.R. Pinheiro, D. Paramos-de-Carvalho, M. Certal, M.A. Costa, A.C. Costa, M.T. Magalhães-Cardoso, F. Ferreirinha, J. Sévigny & P. Correia-de-Sá
  J. Biol. Chem. (2013) **288**, 27571–27583. doi: 10.1074/jbc.M113.460865.
- **Bradykinin Ca2+ signaling in human subcutaneous fibroblasts involves ATP release via hemichannels and P2Y12 receptors activation.**
  A.R. Pinheiro, D. Paramos-de-Carvalho, M. Certal, C. Costa, M.T. Magalhães-Cardoso, M.A. Costa & P. Correia-de-Sá
  Cell Commun. Signal. (2013) **11**, 70. doi:10.1186/1478-811X-11-70.
- **For women with overactive bladder syndrome, urinary ATP may be a dynamic biomarker of detrusor overactivity.**
  M. Silva-Ramos & P. Correia-de-Sá
  UroToday "Beyond the Abstract" (2013) Commentary published on 08 November 2013 in UroToday.com.
- **Paradoxical neostigmine-induced TOF_{fade}: on the role of presynaptic cholinergic and adenosine receptors.**
  E. Paula-Ramos, M.B. Antônio, C.R. Ambiel, P. Correia-de-Sá & W. Alves-do-Prado
  Eur. J. Pharmacol. (2014) **723**, 389-396. doi: 10.1016/j.ejphar. 2013.11.001.
- **ATP released via pannexin-1 hemichannels mediates bladder overactivity triggered by urothelial $P2Y_6$ receptors.**
  M.A. Timóteo*, I. Carneiro*, I. Silva, J.B. Noronha-Matos, F. Ferreirinha, M. Silva-Ramos & P. Correia-de-Sá
  Biochem Pharmacol. (2014) 87, 371-379. doi: 10.1016/j.bcp.2013.11.007.
- **Activation of $P2Y_6$ receptors increases the voiding frequency in anaesthetized rats by releasing ATP from the bladder urothelium.**

I. Carneiro*, M.A. Timóteo*, I. Silva, C. Vieira, C. Baldaia, F. Ferreirinha, M. Silva-Ramos & P. Correia-de-Sá
Br. J. Pharmacol. (2014) **171**, 3404-3419. doi: 10.1111/bph.12711.

- **Activation of a TRP-like channel and intracellular calcium dynamics during phospholipase C-mediated cell death.**
A.P. Gonçalves*, J.M. Cordeiro*, J. Monteiro, A. Muñoz, P. Correia-de-Sá, N.D. Read & A. Videira
J. Cell Science (2014) **127**, 3817-3829. doi: 10.1242/jcs.152058.
- **Extracellular calcium triggers unique transcriptional programs and modulates staurosporine-induced cell death in *Neurospora crassa*.**
A.P. Gonçalves, J. Monteiro, C. Lucchi, D.J. Kowbel, J.M. Cordeiro, P. Correia-de-Sá, D.J. Rigden, N. Louise Glass & A. Videira
Microbial Cell (2014) **1**, 289-302. doi: 10.15698/mic2014.09.165.
- **Feed-forward inhibition of CD73 and upregulation of adenosine deaminase contribute to the loss of adenosine neuromodulation in postinflammatory ileitis**
C. Vieira, M.T. Magalhães-Cardoso, F. Ferreirinha, I. Silva, A.S. Dias, J. Pelletier, J. Sévigny & P. Correia-de-Sá
Mediators Inflamm. (2014) **2014**, 254640. doi: 10.1155/2014/254640.
- **Lack of endogenous adenosine tonus on vascular sympathetic neurotransmission in spontaneously hypertensive rat mesenteric artery.**
J.B. Sousa, M.S. Vieira-Rocha, C. Sá, F. Ferreirinha, P. Correia-de-Sá, P. Fresco & C. Diniz
PLoS One (2014) **9(8)**:e105540. doi: 10.1371/journal.pone.0105540. eCollection 2014.
- **P2X7-induced zeiosis promotes osteogenic differentiation and mineralization of postmenopausal bone marrow-derived mesenchymal stem cells.**
J.B. Noronha-Matos, J. Coimbra, A. Sá-e-Sousa, R. Rocha, J. Marinhas, R. Freitas, S. Guerra-Gomes, F. Ferreirinha, M.A. Costa & P. Correia-de-Sá
FASEB J. (2014) **28(12)**, 5208-5222. doi: 10.1096/fj.14-257923.
- **Attenuated aortic vasodilation and sympathetic prejunctional facilitation in epinephrine-deficient mice: selective impairment of β_2-adrenoceptors responses.**
M. Moreira-Rodrigues, A. Graça, M. Ferreira, J. Afonso, P. Serrão, M. Morato, F. Ferreirinha, P. Correia-de-Sá, S. Ebert & D. Moura
J. Pharmacol. Exp. Therap. (2014) **351**, 243-249. doi: 10.1124/ jpet.114.217281.
- **Real-time video exocytosis in rat neuromuscular junction: a powerful live cell imaging technique.**
J.B. Noronha-Matos & P. Correia-de-Sá
In *Microscopy: Advances in Scientific Research and Education* (2014). Ed. A. Méndez-Vilas, Microscopy Book Series No. 6, Vol. 2, pp 752-760.
- **Urinary Bladder Disorders: Is Adenosine Friend or Foe?**
M. Silva-Ramos*, I. Silva*, M. Faria, M.T. Magalhães-Cardoso and P. Correia-de-Sá
In *Adenosine Receptors: Pharmacology, Functions and Therapeutic Aspects* (2015).
Ed. K. Warrick, Nova Science Publishers, Inc (USA). ISBN: 978-1-63463-471-7.
- **Amplification of neuromuscular transmission by methylprednisolone involves activation of presynaptic facilitatory adenosine A_{2A} receptors and redistribution of synaptic vesicles.**

L. Oliveira, A.C. Costa, J.B. Noronha-Matos, I. Silva, W.L. Cavalcante, M.A. Timóteo, A.P. Corrado, C.A. Dal Belo, C. Ambiel, W. Alves-do-Prado & P. Correia-de-Sá
Neuropharmacol. (2015) **89**, 64-76. doi: 10.1016/j.neuropharm. 2014.09.004.

- **Deficits in endogenous adenosine formation by ecto-5'-nucleotidase/CD73 impair neuromuscular transmission and immune competence in experimental autoimmune *Myasthenia gravis*.**
  L. Oliveira, A. Correia, A.C. Costa, S. Guerra-Gomes, F. Ferreirinha, M.T. Magalhães-Cardoso, M. Vilanova & P. Correia-de-Sá
  Mediators Inflamm. (2015) **2015**, 460610. doi: 10.1155/2015/460610.
- **Involvement of mitochondrial proteins in calcium signaling and cell death induced by staurosporine in *Neurospora crassa*.**
  A.P. Gonçalves, J.M. Cordeiro, J. Monteiro, C. Lucchi, P. Correia-de-Sá & A. Videira
  Biochimica et Biophysica Acta - Bioenergetics (2015) **1847**, 1064-1074.
  doi: 10.1016/j.bbabio.2015.05.011.
- **Impact of ectonucleotidases in autonomic nervous functions.**
  A.M. Cardoso, M.R.C. Schetinger, P. Correia-de-Sá & J. Sévigny
  Autonom. Neuroscience: Basic and Clinical (2015) **191**, 25-38.
  doi: 10.1016/j.autneu.2015.04.014 (Review Paper).
- **The effect of ischemia and reperfusion on enteric glial cells and contractile activity in the ileum.**
  C.E. Mendes, K. Palombit, C. Vieira, I. Silva, P. Correia-de-Sá & P. Castelucci
  Digestive Diseases and Sciences (2015) **60**, 2677-2689.
  doi: 10.1007/s10620-015-3663-3.
- **Activation of $P2Y_6$ receptors facilitates non-neuronal ATP and acetylcholine release from urothelium with the lamina propria of men with bladder outlet obstruction.**
  I. Silva, F. Ferreirinha, M.T. Magalhães-Cardoso, M. Silva-Ramos & P. Correia-de-Sá
  J. Urol. (2015) 194, 1146-1154.
  doi: 10.1016/j.juro.2015.05.080.
  Research Highlight – BPH – $P2Y_6$ blockade might help control bladder storage symptoms by Rebecca Kelsey in *Nature Reviews Urology* (2015) 12 358.
  doi: 10.1038/nrurol.2015.134.
- **P2X7 receptor activation downmodulates Na^+-dependent high-affinity GABA and glutamate transport into rat brain cortex synaptosomes.**
  A.R. Barros-Barbosa, M.G. Lobo, F. Ferreirinha, P. Correia-de-Sá* & J.M. Cordeiro*
  Neuroscience (2015) 306, 74–90.
  doi: 10.1016/j.neuroscience.2015.08.026.
- **Calcium signalling and the novel anti-proliferative effect of the UTP-sensitive $P2Y_{11}$ receptor in rat cardiac myofibroblasts**
  M. Certal, A. Vinhas, A.R. Pinheiro, F. Ferreirinha, A. Barros-Barbosa, I. Silva, M.A. Costa & P. Correia-de-Sá
  Cell Calcium (2015) 58, 518-533.
  doi: 10.1016/j.ceca.2015.08.004.
- **Impairment of ATP hydrolysis decreases adenosine A_1 receptor tonus favoring cholinergic nerve hyperactivity in the obstructed human urinary bladder.**

M. Silva-Ramos*, I. Silva*, M. Faria, M.T. Magalhães-Cardoso, J. Correia, F. Ferreirinha & P. Correia-de-Sá
Purinergic Signalling (2015) 11, 595-606.
doi: 10.1007/s11302-015-9478-z.

- **Up-regulation of P2X7 receptor-mediated inhibition of GABA uptake by nerve terminals of the human epileptic neocortex.**
  A.R. Barros-Barbosa, A. Fonseca, S. Guerra-Gomes, F. Ferreirinha, A. Santos, R. Rangel, M.G. Lobo, P. Correia-de-Sá* & J.M. Cordeiro*
  Epilepsia (2016) 57, 99-110.
  doi: 10.1111/epi.13263.
- **Inverse gradient of nitrergic and purinergic inhibitory co-transmission in the mouse colon.**
  N. Mañé*, R. Viais*, M. Martínez-Cutillas, D. Gallego, P. Correia-de-Sá & M. Jimenez
  Acta Physiologica (Oxf) (2016) **216**, 120-131.
  doi: 10.1111/apha.12599.
- **Mesenchymal stem cells: targeting the "purinome" to promote osteogenic differentiation and bone repair.**
  J.B. Noronha-Matos & P. Correia-de-Sá
  J. Cell. Physiol. (2016, *Epub ahead of print* JCP-15-0689, "Mini-review") Jan 11.
  doi: 10.1002/jcp.25303.

In: Overactive Bladder (OAB)
Editor: Elvira Larson

ISBN: 978-1-63485-033-9

Chapter 7

MIRABEGRON FOR THE TREATMENT OF OVERACTIVE BLADDER

Federica Laraud[1,2], Simone Ferrero[1,2*], and Umberto Leone Roberti Maggiore[1,2]

[1]Academic Unit of Obstetrics and Gynaecology, IRCCS AOU San Martino IST, Genoa, Italy

[2]Department of Neurosciences, Rehabilitation, Ophthalmology, Genetics, Maternal and Child Health (DiNOGMI), University of Genoa, Italy

ABSTRACT

Mirabegron is used for the treatment of symptoms caused by overactive bladder (OAB) syndrome. It is a $ß_3$-adrenoreceptor agonist that relaxes the detrusor muscle, thus improving the urine storage during the filling phase. Several double-blind, randomized-controlled trials demonstrated the efficacy of mirabegron for the treatment of OAB. The majority of these trials compared various doses of mirabegron with placebo and/or tolterodine extended-release. Mirabegron improved the number of micturition per 24 hours and the number of incontinence episodes per 24 hours. Mirabegron is well tolerated; the most common adverse events observed with mirabegron in clinical trials were hypertension, nasopharyngitis, and urinary tract infection. The incidence of dry mouth was similar to placebo and was lower than for tolterodine extended release. Since dry mouth is the most common adverse event reported with antimuscarinics and one of the main causes of discontinuation of treatment, mirabegron may be a valuable treatment option for these patients. Future research should focus on the assessment of mirabegron concentrations in the central nervous system and on the evaluation of the potential of the combination of mirabegron with antimuscarinics

Keywords: antimuscarinics, efficacy, mirabegron, overactive bladder, safety, tolerability, urgency

[*] Corresponding author: Simone Ferrero, PhD, Academic Unit of Obstetrics and Gynaecology, IRCCS AOU San Martino – IST, Largo R. Benzi 10, 16132 Genoa, Italy. Department of Neurosciences, Rehabilitation, Ophthalmology, Genetics, Maternal and Child Health (DiNOGMI), University of Genoa, Italy. Telephone - 01139 010 511525, Mobile - 01139 3477211682, Fax - 01139 010511525, E-mail: simone.ferrero@unige.it.

INTRODUCTION

The overactive bladder syndrome (OAB) is a symptom complex consisting of urinary urgency with or without urgency urinary incontinence (UUI), often associated with nocturia and frequency (Haylen et al., 2010). The overall prevalence of this condition is of about 12% of men and women(Irwin et al., 2006), and it consistently impairs quality of life (QoL) of these patients(Coyne et al., 2008).

The management of OAB is multimodal and it includes both non-pharmacological and pharmacological therapeutic strategies. Bladder and pelvic floor retraining, lifestyle and dietary modifications are considered first-line options for the treatment of OAB. However, when these strategies fail, pharmacotherapy should be considered. Antimuscarinics (AMs) are the mainstay of pharmacological treatment of OAB and represent the most commonly prescribed drugs for this condition(Leone Roberti Maggiore et al., 2012). Other drugs including vasopressin analogues, antidepressants, a-adrenoceptor antagonists and ß-adrenergic receptor (AR) agonists are used to treat OAB.

Mirabegron (YM178, Myrbetriq™, Betanis®, Betmiga®) (Box 1) is the first $ß_3$-AR agonist approved for use in OAB(Leone Roberti Maggiore et al., 2014).

This chapter summarizes the literature regarding mirabegron in the treatment of OAB, offering the reader an overview of the mechanism of action, clinical efficacy, safety and tolerability of this compound.

METHODS

A literature search was performed to detect all the published studies investigating the use of mirabegron in treating OAB from inception until December 2015. The following electronic databases were used: PubMed and Medline. The following search terms, alone or in combination, were used: mirabegron, adverse events, efficacy, overactive bladder, safety and tolerability. All pertinent articles were carefully examined and their reference lists were assessed in order to find other manuscripts that could be included in this review. Case reports and letters to the editor were excluded from the review. Only articles in English were considered for this chapter. Two independent researchers (SF and ULRM) screened the studies originally identified from the literature search; disagreement about inclusion/exclusion was resolved by consensus. The reviewers were not blinded to the names of investigators or sources of publication.

β3-Adrenergic Receptors

β-adrenergic receptors (ARs) belong to the family of G-protein coupled receptors. Stimulation of β- ARs by catecholamines is realized via the β-adrenoceptor-adenylylcyclase-protein kinase A cascade (Wallukat, 2002).

Recent advances in the understanding of the physiopathology of overactive bladder (OAB) have identified three subtypes of β- ARs, β1, β2, and β3 in the detrusor muscle and urothelium (Andersson & Arner, 2004; Michel & Vrydag, 2006; Otsuka, Shinbo, Matsumoto,

Kurita, & Ozono, 2008). β3-ARs predominate, accounting for 97% of total β-ARs messenger (m)RNA (Yamaguchi, 2002) and are thought to be the main subtype mediating relaxation of the detrusor in humans (Wuest et al., 2009). In the urinary bladder under physiological circumstances, noradrenaline, acting mainly on β3-ARs in the detrusor muscle and on α_1-ARs in the bladder outflow tract, promotes urine storage, whereas neuronally released acetylcholine acting mainly on M_3 receptors promotes bladder emptying (Ochodnicky, Uvelius, Andersson, & Michel, 2013). In addition, β3-ARs are also suggested to inhibit sensory nerve activation, including activity in mechanosensitive A-δ fibers, and also reducing autonomous nonvoiding contraction. Finally, β3- ARs activation can elicit release of nitric oxide by urothelium, giving a potential indirect mechanism which could further contribute to bladder relaxation (Vij & Drake, 2015).

Mirabegron

Mirabegron owns high intrinsic activity for β3-ARs and very low intrinsic activity for β1 and β2-ARs. It is the first β3-ARs agonist to be approved for the treatment of OAB symptoms (urgency, increased micturition frequency and/or urgency urinary incontinence) in Japan, the USA, Europe, and Canada. Other selective β3-ARs agonist (e.g., solabegron, rafabegron, vibegron) are currently in development (Edmondson et al., 2015; Ellsworth & Fantasia, 2015; Otsuka, Shinbo, Hasebe, Matsumoto, & Ozono, 2008).

Mirabegron offers an alternative pharmacological option to the well-established treatment with AMs. Mirabegron mediates relaxation of the detrusor muscle during the storage phase of the micturition cycle, thus increasing bladder storage capacity, whereas, AMs mainly exert their action by decreasing bladder contraction through antagonism of M_3 receptors (Andersson, 2009; Takasu et al., 2007).

Mirabegron (25mg/day and 50 mg/day) for the treatment of OAB has been approved in Japan in 2010, in the USA and Canada in 2012 and, by the European authorities in 2013.

Mechanism of Action

Detrusor smooth muscle relaxation is crucial to guarantee bladder compliance and to mainatain low intravesical pressure in the bladder filling phase while the urethral sphincter is closed. Bladder relaxation is achieved by the activation of β3-ARs and consequent activation of adenylyl cyclase, which leads to cAMP synthesis. In addition, recent researches suggest a possible role of potassium (K+) channels, and particularly, big potassium channels, in the β-ARs-mediated bladder relaxation independently of cAMP (Frazier, Peters, Braverman, Ruggieri, & Michel, 2008; Hristov et al., 2008; Takemoto et al., 2008; Uchida, Shishido, Nomiya, & Yamaguchi, 2005).

Table 1. Primary and main secondary endpoints of available phase III randomized control trials

Reference	Drug and dose (number of case)	Treatment duration, weeks	Primary endpoints		Main secondary endpoints	
			Mean (SD) change in incontince episodes/24h	Mean (SD) change in micturitions/24h	Mean (SD) change in volume voided/micturition mL	Mean (SD) change in urgency episodes/24h
Nitti et al., 2013 (Nitti, Auerbach, et al., 2013)	Mirabegron 50 mg (442)	12	-1,47 (0,11)*	-1,66 (0,13)*	18,2 (2,44)*	NR
	Mirabegron 100 mg (433)		-1,63 (0,12)*	-1,75 (0,14)*	18,0 (2,47)*	NR
	Placebo (453)		-1,13 (0,11)*	-1,05 (0,13)*	7,0 (2,41)	NR
Khullar et al., 2013 (Khullar, Amarenco, et al., 2013)	Mirabegron 50 mg (493)	12	-1,62 (0,137) *	-1,94 (0,116)*	24,2 (2,01)*	-2,25 (0,15)*
	Mirabegron 100 mg (496)		-1,51 (0,128)*	-1,75 (0,110)*	25,6 (2,00)*	-1,96 (0,15)
	Tolterodine ER 4mg (475)		-1,21 (0,137)	-1,57 (0,123)	25,0 (2,00)	-2,07 (0,15)
	Placebo (494)		-1,13 (0,126)*	-1,37 (0,115)	12,3 (1,99)	-1,65 (0,15)
Chapple et al., 2013 (Chapple, Kaplan, et al., 2013)	Mirabegron 50 mg (812)	52	-1,01	-1,27	17,5	NR
	Mirabegron 100 mg (820)		-1,24	-1,41	21,5	NR
	Tolterodine ER 4mg (812)		-1,26	-1,39	18,1	NR
Herschorn et al., 2013 (Herschorn et al., 2013)	Mirabegron 25 mg (432)	12	-1,36 (0,12)	-1,65 (0,13)*	12,8 (2,2)	-1,68 (0,16)
	Mirabegron 50 mg (440)		-1,38 (0,12)	-1,60 (0,12)*	20,7 (2,2)*	-1,94(0,15)
Yamaguchi et al., 2014 (Yamaguchi et al., 2014)	Mirabegron 50 mg (380)	16	-1,12 (1,47)*	-1,67 (2,21)*	24,3 (35,47)*	-1,85 (2,55)*
	Tolterodine ER 4mg (378)		NR	-1,40 (2,17)	NR	NR
	Placebo (381)		-0,66 (1,86)	-0,86 (2,35)*	9,71 (29,08)*	-1,37 (3,91)*

Table 1 NR, not reported; *Statistically significantly superior compared with placebo at the 0.05 level.

Table 2. Phase III studies: main adverse events

Reference	Drug and dose (number of case)	Phase III studies: main adverse events (%)				
		Overall	Cardiac	Hypertension	Headache	Dry mouth
Nitti et al., 2013 (Nitti, Auerbach, et al., 2013)	Mirabegron 50 mg (442)	NR	NR	6,1	3,2	0, 5
	Mirabegron 100 mg (433)	NR	NR	4,9	3,0	2,1
	Placebo (453)	NR	NR	6,6	2,0	1,5
Khullar et al.,2013 (Khullar, Amarenco, et al., 2013)	Mirabegron 50 mg (493)	42,8	2,6	5,9	3,7	2,8
	Mirabegron 100 mg (496)	40,1	2,2	5,4	1,8	2,8
	Tolterodine ER 4mg (475)	46,7	4,6	8,1	3,6	10,1
	Placebo (494)	43,3	1,2	7,7	2,8	2,6
Chapple et al., 2013 (Chapple, Kaplan, et al., 2013)	Mirabegron 50 mg (812)	59,7	4,3	9,2	4,1	2,8
	Mirabegron 100 mg (820)	61,3	4,3	9,8	3,2	2,3
	Tolterodine ER 4mg (812)	62,6	6,4	9,6	2,5	8,6
Herschorn et al., 2013 (Herschorn et al., 2013)	Mirabegron 25 mg (432)	48,6	NR	11,3	2,1	1,9
	Mirabegron 50 mg (440)	47,3	NR	10,7	2,7	1,6
	Placebo (433)	50,1	NR	8,5	4,4	2,1
Yamaguchi et al., 2014 (Yamaguchi et al., 2014)	Mirabegron 50 mg (380)	24,5	1,9	0,3	NR	2,9
	Tolterodine ER 4mg (378)	34,9	1,4	0,8	NR	2,6
	Placebo (381)	24,0	0,8	0	NR	13,3
Hann-Chorng Kuo et al., 2015 (Kuo et al., 2015)	Mirabegron 50 mg (311)	28,7	1,1	0,5	NR	4,9
	Tolterodine ER 4mg (310)	34,5	2,2	1,1	NR	8,1
	Placebo (300)	33,9	2,2	0,3	NR	4,9
Jose E. Batista et al., 2015 (Batista et al., 2015)	Mirabegron 50 mg (943)	29,3	3,0	1,1	3,0	3,1
	Solifenacin 5 mg (944)	30,2	3,3	1,5	2,4	5,8

Table 2 NR, not reported.

In a rat study activation of β3-ARs by isoproterenol in urothelial cells can bring to the release nitric oxide (NO) by increasing the intracellular Ca2+ through cAMP accumulation. The activation of β3-ARs not only causes relaxation by releases NO but also inhibits detrusor muscle contraction by releasing an urothelial derived inhibiting factor (Birder et al., 2002; Murakami, Chapple, Akino, Sellers, & Chess-Williams, 2007). Other animal studies showed that β3-AR agonists promote an increase of bladder capacity without modifications in micturition pressure or residual volume(Gillespie et al., 2012; Hatanaka et al., 2013; Takasu et al., 2007).

Therefore, mirabegron in patients with OAB allow to obtain to an increase in bladder capacity and to the consequent reduced frequency of micturition (Sanford, 2013).

Furthermore, mirabegron, in anesthetized rat model, has shown also a possible additional action that involves the afferent nerves causing a reduction of the mechanosensitive afferent activity of both Aδ -fiber and C-fiber in a dose-dependent way (Aizawa, Homma, & Igawa, 2012).

Phase III Studies - Clinical Efficacy

The efficacy, safety and tolerability in patients with OAB were firstly investgated in three main researches (Herschorn et al., 2013; Khullar, Amarenco, et al., 2013; Nitti, Auerbach, et al., 2013). Herschorn et al. conducted a randomized, parallel-group, placebo-controlled, doubleblind, multicenter, multinational study to evaluate the efficacy and safety or tolerability of mirabegron 25 mg and 50 mg QD versus placebo in patients with OAB (Herschorn et al., 2013). A total of 1306 patients ≥ 18 years with OAB symptoms for ≥ 3 months who were enrolled in a 2-week, single-blind, placebo run-in. After fulfilling a 3-day micturition diary, patients with a ≥ 8 micturitions per 24 h and ≥ 3 urgency episodes, with or without incontinence, were randomly assigned to QD treatment with mirabegron 25 mg, mirabegron 50 mg, or placebo for 12 weeks. Both mirabegron 25 mg and mirabegron 50 mg caused significant improvements in changes from baseline to final visit in mean number of incontinence episodes and micturitions per 24 h versus placebo. Furthermore, mirabegron 50 mg caused significantly higher improvements versus placebo in the change to final visit in mean volume voided per micturition and change to week 4 in mean number of incontinence episodes per 24 h (Herschorn et al., 2013).

Another 12-week multinational and multicenter randomized double-blind, parallel-group placebo- and active controlled trial conducted in 27 countries in Europe and Australia in 1978 patients ≥ 18 years of age with symptoms of OAB for ≥3 months investigated the efficacy and tolerability of mirabegron versus placebo in treating OAB. After a 2-week single-blind placebo run-in period, patients were randomized to placebo, mirabegron 50 mg, mirabegron 100 mg, or tolterodine extended release (ER) 4 mg orally QD for 12 weeks. Significant ameliorations at the final visit in the number of incontinence episodes per 24 h and number of micturitions per 24 h were reported in patients treated with mirabegron 50 and 100 mg. In addition, a significant reduction in the number of incontinence episodes and micturitions per 24 h were observed at week 4 with mirabegron (both dosages) versus placebo, which was maintained at either week 8 or 12. A significant improvement from baseline to final visit in mean volume voided per micturition was achieved in both mirabegron groups compared with placebo and in mirabegron 50 mg group in the mean number of episodes of urgency. Finally, all patients treated with drug reporteed improvement in QoL outcomes assessed by using the OAB Questionnaire (OAB-q), the Patient Perception of Bladder Condition (PPBC), and the Treatment Satisfaction-Visual Analog Scale (TS-VAS) (Khullar, Amarenco, et al., 2013).

A Phase III, randomized, parallel group, double-blind, placebo-controlled, multicenter study in the USA and Canada, which enrolled a total of 1329 patients with an average of ≥8 micturitions per 24 h and ≥3 urgency episodes with or without incontinence during a 3-day period assessed the efficacu of mirabegron 50 mg, mirabegron 100 mg versus placebo for 12 weeks. Compared with placebo, both mirabegron groups had higher decreases from baseline for incontinence episodes and micturitions per 24 h. Furthermore, patients actively treated experienced significantly greater amelioration from baseline to final visit than placebo in OAB-q symptom bother and total health-related QoL scores (Nitti, Auerbach, et al., 2013).

Chapple et al. evaluated the long-term (12 months) efficacy and safety of mirabegron in OAB treatment. After a 2-week single-blind placebo run-in, patients with ≥ 8 micturitions per 24 h and ≥3 urgency episodes in a 3-day micturition diary were randomized 1:1:1 to receive QD mirabegron 50 mg, mirabegron 100 mg, or tolterodine ER 4 mg for 12 months. Efficacy end points consisted of modifications in key OAB symptoms recorded in the 3-day micturition diary and in patient-reported outcomes assessed using the OAB-q, PPBC and the TS-VAS. Improvements in efficacy end points were observed from the first month and were maintained until 12-month follow-up. (Chapple, Kaplan, et al., 2013).

Yamaguchi et al. (Yamaguchi et al., 2014) conducted a phase III randomized control trials evaluating the efficacy and safety of mirabegron 50 mg in a Japanese population with OAB. A total of 1139 patients were randomised to receive placebo, mirabegron 50 mg or Tolterodine 4 mg for 16 weeks. Mirabegron 50 mg once daily caused significant improvements vcompared with placebo in the mean number of micturitions/24 h, incontinence episodes/24 h and volume voided/micturition. Apost hoc, subgroup analysis of the European-Australian study aimed to assess the efficacy of mirabegron in the subgroups of patients who had not previously received AMs (treatment-naive) and in those who discontinued prior AM therapy because of insufficient efficacy or poor tolerability (Khullar, Cambronero, et al., 2013). Both dosages of mirabegron were associated with similar amelioration in the number of incontinence episodes and micturitions in patients with OAB who were AMs-naive and who had discontinued prior AMs therapy. In AM treatment-naive group, mirabegron 50 mg and 100 mg caused improvement versus placebo in the mean number of micturitions/24 h from baseline to final visit. In patients previously treated with AMs, active treatment ameliorated in the number of micturition episodes compared with placebo. Furthermore, mirabegron caused a decrease of incontinence and micturition frequency in patients who had discontinued prior AMs therapy due to insufficient efficacy, whereas, the efficacy of tolterodine was similar to that of placebo (Khullar, Cambronero, et al., 2013).

Otsuki et al. examined the safety and efficacy of mirabegron for patients with OAB that is unresponsive to AMs or is related to benign prostatic hyperplasia. This 8-week prospective study enrolled 52 newly diagnosed patients with OAB and 45 patients with OAB previously treated without success with AMs. Patients in both study groups received with mirabegron 50 mg QD. Controls consisted in 27 newly diagnosed patients with OAB treated with AMs (tolterodine, solifenacin, propiverine, or imidafenacin). The efficacy of mirabegron was demonstrated in 85.2% of patients with newly diagnosed OAB. An improvemet in all domains of OAB symptom score was reported, without any significant difference with AMs.

In patients with OAB unresponsive to AMs, the efficacy of mirabegron was 61.6% and significant reducrtions in OAB symptom score and international prostate symptom score QoL were recorded. Moreover voiding symptoms improved both in men with new diagnosis of OAB and in those with OAB unresponsive to AMs (Otsuki et al., 2013).

Kuo et al., in a 12-week multinational, randomized, double-blind, parallel-group placebo- and active-controlled trial, evaluated the efficacy and safety of mirabegron 50 mg once daily compared with placebo and the active control, tolterodine ER 4 mg once daily, in patients with symptoms of OAB in Taiwan, Korea, China, and India. A statistically significant amelioration in mean number of micturitions/24 hr was reported with mirabegron 50 mg in comparison with placebo. No difference between treatment groups was observed for other secondary outcome measures (mean number of urgency episodes, incontinence episodes and urge incontinence episodes/24 hr, mean number of nocturia episodes per night, and QoL scores as assessed by the King's Health Questionnaire) except volume voided per micturition(Kuo et al., 2015).

A recent randomized, double-blind, phase IIIb, noninferiority study compared the efficacy and safety of mirabegron 50 mg and solifenacin 5 mg in OAB patients dissatisfied with previous AM treatment due to lack of efficacy. This study demonstrated that for the primary variable, adjusted mean treatment difference in mean number of micturitions/24 h was −0.18 (−0.42, 0.06) and therefore noninferiority of mirabegron to solifenacin was not shown. However, both treatments caused clinically meaningful reductions in secondary efficacy variables (change from baseline in mean number of incontinence episodes/24 h, urgency incontinence episodes/24 h, urgency episodes/24 h and nocturia episodes/24 h)(Batista et al., 2015).

Phase III Studies – General Safety and Tolerability

Herschorn et al. evaluated the efficacy and safety of mirabegron at different dosages (25 and 50 mg) versus placebo. This research demonstrated that mirabegron was well tolerated at both dosages and the overall incidence of treatment-emergent AEs between the three groups was not different (48.6% in the mirabegron 25 mg group, 47.3% in the mirabegron 50 mg group, and 50.1% in the placebo group). The majority of treatment-emergent AEs were mild or moderate and the rate of severe treatment-emergent AEs was superior in the placebo group (3.7%) than in the mirabegron 25 mg (1.9%) and 50 mg groups (1.8%) (Herschorn et al., 2013). A multicenter randomized double-blind, parallel-group placebo- and active-controlled trial conducted in Europe and Australia investigated safety and tolerability of mirabegron. The incidence of treatment-emergent AEs was similar between the placebo, mirabegron 50 mg and 100 mg and tolterodine ER 4 mg groups. Most treatment-emergent AEs were mild or moderate in all study groups. The percentage of patients interrupting study drug due to an AE was 2.6, 4.9, 3.2 and 4.4% for placebo, mirabegron 50 mg, mirabegron 100 mg and tolterodine ER 4 mg groups, respectively. Interestingly dry mouth was experienced by patients in the mirabegron 50 and 100 mg groups similarly to patients in placebo group (2.8, 2.8 and 2.6%, respectively) wereas it was much more frequent among patients in the tolterodine ER 4 mg group (10.1%) (Khullar, Amarenco, et al., 2013). Another Phase III, randomized, parallel group, double-blind, placebo-controlled, multicenter trial by Nitti et al. assessed the safety of mirabegron (50 mg and 100mg). The overall proportion of patients with treatment-emergent AEs and the proportion with more commonly reported treatment-emergent AEs did not differ between the study groups with the exception of urinary tract infections, which were reported more commonly in both mirabegron groups. Two deaths not related to the study drug were reported (Nitti, Auerbach, et al., 2013). The tolerability of mirabegron for treating OAB was investigated in randomized, double-blind, parallel-Group, placebo- and active-controlled, multicenter study in Asia. The overall incidence of treatment emergent AEs was 33.9%, 28.7%, and 34.5% in the placebo, mirabegron 50mg and tolterodine ER 4mg groups. The most common treatment-emergent AEs (≥2% of patients) in the mirabegron 50mg group were dry mouth (4.9%), nasopharyngitis (2.5%), and constipation (2.2%). The incidence of these events was similar in the placebo group. Dry mouth occurred most frequently in the tolterodine ER 4mg group (8.1%). The incidence of serious treatment-emergent AEs was low. No drug-related serious treatment-emergent AEs were recorded in the mirabegron 50mg group. Most treatment-emergent AEs were mild or moderate in severity in all treatment groups. There was one death on day 44, 30 days after the last administration of placebo (Kuo et al., 2015). The efficacy and safety of mirabegron was also evaluated in a randomized, double-blind, phase IIIb, noninferiority study. The rate of treatment-emergent AEs was similar between mirabegron 50 mg (29.3%) and solifenacin 5 mg (30.2%). There was no difference in the rate of discontinuation due to AEs in the mirabegron 50 mg (1.4%) and solifenacin 5 mg (1.8%) groups. The majority of AEs were of mild or moderate severity with both treatments. Treatment-emergent AEs reported by ≥2% of patients in the mirabegron 50 mg and solifenacin 5 mg groups, respectively, were dry mouth (3.1% and 5.8%), constipation (2.2% and 2.5%) and headache (3.0% and 2.4%) (Batista et al., 2015). Table 2 summarizes the main AEs associated with the use of miranegron reported in phase III trials.

Cardiac Safety

β3-ARs are present in cardiac and vascular tissue and consequently mirabegron may affect cardiac function. A four-arm, parallel, two-way, double-blind and placebo- and active (moxifloxacin)-controlled crossover study assessed the cardiac safety in 352 healthy volunteers. No prolongation of the QT interval was observed in patients treated with mirabegron 50 or 100 mg, whereas, a prolongation of the QT interval was observed in females but not in males, at supratherapeutic dosage (200 mg). The heart rate (HR) raised in a dose-dependent manner: in females, the maximum mean HR increases were 8.53, 13.63, and 20.24 beats per min (bpm) for 50, 100 and 200 mg mirabegron treatments, occurring at 5, 4 and 5 h, respectively. In males, the corresponding HR increases were 5.46, 10.90, and 14.37 bpm, occurring at 4.5, 8 and 5 h, respectively (Malik et al., 2012). Clinical researches showed a mean increase in the HR during treatment, without higher incidence of cardiovascular AEs such as tachycardia and palpitations (Chapple, Amarenco, et al., 2013; Chapple, Dvorak, et al., 2013). A prespecified pooled analysis of three Phase III randomized, double-blind, placebo-controlled, 12-week studies (Herschorn et al., 2013; Khullar, Amarenco, et al., 2013; Nitti, Auerbach, et al., 2013) investigated the efficacy and safety of QD mirabegron (Nitti, Khullar, et al., 2013). This study demonstrated that there was a dose-dependent raise (0.6 - 2.3 bpm) from baseline to final visit in pulse rate (AM and PM measurements) in the mirabegron groups, but this was not associate with an increased incidence of cardiovascular AEs (Nitti, Khullar, et al., 2013). A recent systematic review aimed to provide a summary of cardiovascular effects of β 3-ARs agonists in clinical studies showing that cardiovascular safety of mirabegron appears to be acceptable at therapeutic doses and comparable with that of AM agents, currently first-line therapy for OAB(Rosa et al., 2015).

Discussion

OAB is estimated to affect >400 million people worldwide with a prevalence that increases with age, affecting approximately 15% aged ≥65 yr and 30–40% ≥75 yr(Irwin, Kopp, Agatep, Milsom, & Abrams, 2011). AMs agents have been the mainstay of OAB treatment (Leone Roberti Maggiore et al., 2012). However, improvements in the knowledge of OAB pathophysiology have identified three β-AR subtypes, β1, β2, and β3, in the bladder detrusor muscle and urothelium which has brought to the development of a new class of drugs for the treatment of OAB, β3-AR agonists. Mirabegron is the progenitor of β 3-AR agonists and it is currently marketed in all Western countries and Japan. Results from phase III studies have demonstrated the efficacy, safety and tolerability of mirabegron in treating patients with OAB; indeed, it reduces the number of urinary incontinence and micturition episodes, as well as the number of urgency and urgency incontinence episodes, and the mean volume voided (Table 1). In addition, improvement in OAB symptoms is associated with a good tolerability (Table 2). The risk of cardiovascular AEs is perhaps the major concerns to use mirabegron. However, a recent systematic review has shown that, at therapeutic doses, mirabegron appears to have an acceptable cardiovascular safety profile, comparable with that of AMs(Rosa et al., 2015). Future studies should focus on the assessment of the safety and tolerability of mirabegron in elderly patients, on the effects of mirabegron on cognitive function in the central nervous system and on the evaluation of the potential of the combination of mirabegron with AMs.

References

Aizawa, N., Homma, Y. & Igawa, Y. (2012). Effects of mirabegron, a novel beta3-adrenoceptor agonist, on primary bladder afferent activity and bladder microcontractions in rats compared with the effects of oxybutynin. *Eur Urol, 62*(6), 1165-1173. doi:10.1016/j.eururo.2012.08.056.

Andersson, K. E. (2009). Prospective pharmacologic therapies for the overactive bladder. *Ther Adv Urol, 1*(2), 71-83. doi:10.1177/1756287209103937.

Andersson, K. E. & Arner, A. (2004). Urinary bladder contraction and relaxation: physiology and pathophysiology. *Physiol Rev, 84*(3), 935-986. doi:10.1152/physrev.00038.2003.

Batista, J. E., Kolbl, H., Herschorn, S., Rechberger, T., Cambronero, J., Halaska, M. & group, B. s. (2015). The efficacy and safety of mirabegron compared with solifenacin in overactive bladder patients dissatisfied with previous antimuscarinic treatment due to lack of efficacy: results of a noninferiority, randomized, phase IIIb trial. *Ther Adv Urol, 7*(4), 167-179. doi:10.1177/1756287215589250.

Birder, L. A., Nealen, M. L., Kiss, S., de Groat, W. C., Caterina, M. J., Wang, E. & Kanai, A. J. (2002). Beta-adrenoceptor agonists stimulate endothelial nitric oxide synthase in rat urinary bladder urothelial cells. *J Neurosci*, *22*(18), 8063-8070. Retrieved from http://www.ncbi.nlm.nih.gov/ pubmed/12223560.

Chapple, C. R., Amarenco, G., Lopez Aramburu, M. A., Everaert, K., Liehne, J., Lucas, M. & Group, B. I. (2013). A proof-of-concept study: mirabegron, a new therapy for overactive bladder. *Neurourol Urodyn*, *32*(8), 1116-1122. doi:10.1002/nau.22373.

Chapple, C. R., Dvorak, V., Radziszewski, P., Van Kerrebroeck, P., Wyndaele, J. J., Bosman, B. & Dragon Investigator, G. (2013). A phase II dose-ranging study of mirabegron in patients with overactive bladder. *Int Urogynecol J*, *24*(9), 1447-1458. doi:10.1007/s00192-013-2042-x.

Chapple, C. R., Kaplan, S. A., Mitcheson, D., Klecka, J., Cummings, J., Drogendijk, T. & Martin, N. (2013). Randomized double-blind, active-controlled phase 3 study to assess 12-month safety and efficacy of mirabegron, a beta(3)-adrenoceptor agonist, in overactive bladder. *Eur Urol*, *63*(2), 296-305. doi:10.1016/j.eururo.2012.10.048.

Coyne, K. S., Sexton, C. C., Irwin, D. E., Kopp, Z. S., Kelleher, C. J. & Milsom, I. (2008). The impact of overactive bladder, incontinence and other lower urinary tract symptoms on quality of life, work productivity, sexuality and emotional well-being in men and women: results from the EPIC study. *BJU Int*, *101*(11), 1388-1395. doi:10.1111/j.1464-410X.2008.07601.x.

Edmondson, S. D., Zhu, C., Kar, N. F., Di Salvo, J., Nagabukuro, H., Sacre-Salem, B. & Weber, A. E. (2015). Discovery of Vibegron: A Potent and Selective Beta 3 Adrenergic Receptor Agonist for the Treatment of Overactive Bladder. *J Med Chem*. doi:10.1021/acs.jmedchem.5b01372.

Ellsworth, P. & Fantasia, J. (2015). Solabegron: a potential future addition to the beta-3 adrenoceptor agonist armamentarium for the management of overactive bladder. *Expert Opin Investig Drugs*, *24*(3), 413-419. doi:10.1517/13543784.2015.1001836.

Frazier, E. P., Peters, S. L., Braverman, A. S., Ruggieri, Sr. M. R. & Michel, M. C. (2008). Signal transduction underlying the control of urinary bladder smooth muscle tone by muscarinic receptors and beta-adrenoceptors. *Naunyn Schmiedebergs Arch Pharmacol*, *377*(4-6), 449-462. doi:10.1007/s00210-007-0208-0.

Gillespie, J. I., Palea, S., Guilloteau, V., Guerard, M., Lluel, P. & Korstanje, C. (2012). Modulation of non-voiding activity by the muscarinergic antagonist tolterodine and the beta(3)-adrenoceptor agonist mirabegron in conscious rats with partial outflow obstruction. *BJU Int*, *110*(2 Pt 2), E132-142. doi:10.1111/j.1464-410X.2012.11240.x.

Hatanaka, T., Ukai, M., Watanabe, M., Someya, A., Ohtake, A., Suzuki, M. & Kaku, S. (2013). Effect of mirabegron, a novel beta3-adrenoceptor agonist, on bladder function during storage phase in rats. *Naunyn Schmiedebergs Arch Pharmacol*, *386*(1), 71-78. doi:10.1007/s00210-012-0814-3.

Haylen, B. T., de Ridder, D., Freeman, R. M., Swift, S. E., Berghmans, B., Lee, J. & International Continence, S. (2010). An International Urogynecological Association (IUGA)/International Continence Society (ICS) joint report on the terminology for female pelvic floor dysfunction. *Neurourol Urodyn*, *29*(1), 4-20. doi:10.1002/nau.20798.

Herschorn, S., Barkin, J., Castro-Diaz, D., Frankel, J. M., Espuna-Pons, M., Gousse, A. E. & Van Kerrebroeck, P. (2013). A phase III, randomized, double-blind, parallel-group, placebo-controlled, multicentre study to assess the efficacy and safety of the beta(3) adrenoceptor agonist, mirabegron, in patients with symptoms of overactive bladder. *Urology*, *82*(2), 313-320. doi:10.1016/j.urology.2013.02.077.

Hristov, K. L., Cui, X., Brown, S. M., Liu, L., Kellett, W. F. & Petkov, G. V. (2008). Stimulation of beta3-adrenoceptors relaxes rat urinary bladder smooth muscle via activation of the large-conductance Ca2+-activated K+ channels. *Am J Physiol Cell Physiol*, *295*(5), C1344-1353. doi:10.1152/ajpcell.00001.2008.

Irwin, D. E., Kopp, Z. S., Agatep, B., Milsom, I. & Abrams, P. (2011). Worldwide prevalence estimates of lower urinary tract symptoms, overactive bladder, urinary incontinence and bladder outlet obstruction. *BJU Int*, *108*(7), 1132-1138. doi:10.1111/j.1464-410X.2010.09993.x.

Irwin, D. E., Milsom, I., Hunskaar, S., Reilly, K., Kopp, Z., Herschorn, S. &. Abrams, P. (2006). Population-based survey of urinary incontinence, overactive bladder, and other lower urinary tract symptoms in five countries: results of the EPIC study. *Eur Urol*, *50*(6), 1306-1314; discussion 1314-1305. doi:10.1016/j.eururo.2006.09.019.

Khullar, V., Amarenco, G., Angulo, J. C., Cambronero, J., Hoye, K., Milsom, I. & Chapple, C. (2013). Efficacy and tolerability of mirabegron, a beta(3)-adrenoceptor agonist, in patients with overactive bladder: results from a randomised European-Australian phase 3 trial. *Eur Urol*, *63*(2), 283-295. doi:10.1016/j.eururo.2012.10.016.

Khullar, V., Cambronero, J., Angulo, J. C., Wooning, M., Blauwet, M. B., Dorrepaal, C. & Martin, N. E. (2013). Efficacy of mirabegron in patients with and without prior antimuscarinic therapy for overactive bladder: a post hoc analysis of a randomized European-Australian Phase 3 trial. *BMC Urol*, *13*, 45. doi:10.1186/1471-2490-13-45.

Kuo, H. C., Lee, K. S., Na, Y., Sood, R., Nakaji, S., Kubota, Y. & Kuroishi, K. (2015). Results of a randomized, double-blind, parallel-group, placebo- and active-controlled, multicenter study of mirabegron, a beta3-adrenoceptor agonist, in patients with overactive bladder in Asia. *Neurourol Urodyn*, *34*(7), 685-692. doi:10.1002/nau.22645.

Leone Roberti Maggiore, U., Cardozo, L., Ferrero, S., Sileo, F., Cola, A., Del Deo, F. & Salvatore, S. (2014). Mirabegron in the treatment of overactive bladder. *Expert Opin Pharmacother*, *15*(6), 873-887. doi:10.1517/14656566.2014.898752.

Leone Roberti Maggiore, U., Salvatore, S., Alessandri, F., Remorgida, V., Origoni, M., Candiani, M., & Ferrero, S. (2012). Pharmacokinetics and toxicity of antimuscarinic drugs for overactive bladder treatment in females. *Expert Opin Drug Metab Toxicol*, *8*(11), 1387-1408. doi:10.1517/17425255.2012.714365.

Malik, M., van Gelderen, E. M., Lee, J. H., Kowalski, D. L., Yen, M., Goldwater, R. & Keirns, J. J. (2012). Proarrhythmic safety of repeat doses of mirabegron in healthy subjects: a randomized, double-blind, placebo-, and active-controlled thorough QT study. *Clin Pharmacol Ther*, *92*(6), 696-706. doi:10.1038/clpt.2012.181.

Michel, M. C. & Vrydag, W. (2006). Alpha1-, alpha2- and beta-adrenoceptors in the urinary bladder, urethra and prostate. *Br J Pharmacol*, *147 Suppl 2*, S88-119. doi:10.1038/sj.bjp.0706619.

Murakami, S., Chapple, C. R., Akino, H., Sellers, D. J. & Chess-Williams, R. (2007). The role of the urothelium in mediating bladder responses to isoprenaline. *BJU Int*, *99*(3), 669-673. doi:10.1111/j.1464-410X.2006.06679.x.

Nitti, V. W., Auerbach, S., Martin, N., Calhoun, A., Lee, M. & Herschorn, S. (2013). Results of a randomized phase III trial of mirabegron in patients with overactive bladder. *J Urol*, *189*(4), 1388-1395. doi:10.1016/j.juro.2012.10.017.

Nitti, V. W., Khullar, V., van Kerrebroeck, P., Herschorn, S., Cambronero, J., Angulo, J. C. & Martin, N. E. (2013). Mirabegron for the treatment of overactive bladder: a prespecified pooled efficacy analysis and pooled safety analysis of three randomised, double-blind, placebo-controlled, phase III studies. *Int J Clin Pract*, *67*(7), 619-632. doi:10.1111/ijcp.12194.

Ochodnicky, P., Uvelius, B., Andersson, K. E. & Michel, M. C. (2013). Autonomic nervous control of the urinary bladder. *Acta Physiol (Oxf)*, *207*(1), 16-33. doi:10.1111/apha.12010.

Otsuka, A., Shinbo, H., Hasebe, K., Matsumoto, R. & Ozono, S. (2008). Effects of a novel beta(3)-adrenoceptor agonist, AJ-9677, on relaxation of the detrusor muscle: an in vitro study. *Int J Urol*, *15*(12), 1072-1076. doi:10.1111/j.1442-2042.2008.02165.x.

Otsuka, A., Shinbo, H., Matsumoto, R., Kurita, Y. & Ozono, S. (2008). Expression and functional role of beta-adrenoceptors in the human urinary bladder urothelium. *Naunyn Schmiedebergs Arch Pharmacol*, *377*(4-6), 473-481. doi:10.1007/s00210-008-0274-y.

Otsuki, H., Kosaka, T., Nakamura, K., Mishima, J., Kuwahara, Y. & Tsukamoto, T. (2013). beta3-Adrenoceptor agonist mirabegron is effective for overactive bladder that is unresponsive to antimuscarinic treatment or is related to benign prostatic hyperplasia in men. *Int Urol Nephrol*, *45*(1), 53-60. doi:10.1007/s11255-012-0343-5.

Rosa, G. M., Ferrero, S., Nitti, V. W., Wagg, A., Saleem, T. & Chapple, C. R. (2015). Cardiovascular Safety of beta-adrenoceptor Agonists for the Treatment of Patients with Overactive Bladder Syndrome. *Eur Urol*. doi:10.1016/j.eururo.2015.09.007.

Sanford, M. (2013). Mirabegron: a review of its use in patients with overactive bladder syndrome. *Drugs*, *73*(11), 1213-1225. doi:10.1007/s40265-013-0086-3.

Takasu, T., Ukai, M., Sato, S., Matsui, T., Nagase, I., Maruyama, T. & Yamaguchi, O. (2007). Effect of (R)-2-(2-aminothiazol-4-yl)-4'-{2-[(2-hydroxy-2-phenylethyl)amino] ethyl} acetanilide (YM178), a novel selective beta3-adrenoceptor agonist, on bladder function. *J Pharmacol Exp Ther*, *321*(2), 642-647. doi:10.1124/jpet.106.115840.

Takemoto, J., Masumiya, H., Nunoki, K., Sato, T., Nakagawa, H., Ikeda, Y. & Yanagisawa, T. (2008). Potentiation of potassium currents by beta-adrenoceptor agonists in human urinary bladder smooth muscle cells: a possible electrical mechanism of relaxation. *Pharmacology*, *81*(3), 251-258. doi:10.1159/000114719.

Uchida, H., Shishido, K., Nomiya, M. & Yamaguchi, O. (2005). Involvement of cyclic AMP-dependent and -independent mechanisms in the relaxation of rat detrusor muscle via beta-adrenoceptors. *Eur J Pharmacol*, *518*(2-3), 195-202. doi:10.1016/j.ejphar.2005.06.029.

Vij, M. & Drake, M. J. (2015). Clinical use of the beta3 adrenoceptor agonist mirabegron in patients with overactive bladder syndrome. *Ther Adv Urol*, *7*(5), 241-248. doi:10.1177/1756287215591763

Wallukat, G. (2002). The beta-adrenergic receptors. *Herz*, *27*(7), 683-690. doi:10.1007/s00059-002-2434-z.

Wuest, M., Eichhorn, B., Grimm, M. O., Wirth, M. P., Ravens, U. & Kaumann, A. J. (2009). Catecholamines relax detrusor through beta 2-adrenoceptors in mouse and beta 3-adrenoceptors in man. *J Pharmacol Exp Ther*, *328*(1), 213-222. doi:10.1124/jpet.108.142562.

Yamaguchi, O. (2002). Beta3-adrenoceptors in human detrusor muscle. *Urology*, *59*(5 Suppl 1), 25-29. Retrieved from http://www.ncbi.nlm.nih.gov/pubmed/12007519.

Yamaguchi, O., Marui, E., Kakizaki, H., Homma, Y., Igawa, Y., Takeda, M. & Ohkawa, S. (2014). Phase III, randomised, double-blind, placebo-controlled study of the beta3-

adrenoceptor agonist mirabegron, 50 mg once daily, in Japanese patients with overactive bladder. BJU Int, 113(6), 951-960. doi:10.1111/bju.12649.

INDEX

A

acetylcholine (ACh), x, 4, 11, 48, 78, 84, 106, 107, 114, 127, 129, 130, 133, 134, 135, 137, 139, 142, 145, 149, 153, 155, 159
adenosine, xi, 79, 100, 128, 130, 131, 132, 135, 137, 139, 140, 141, 142, 143, 145, 146, 147, 149, 150, 151, 152, 153, 154, 155
adenosine deaminase, 133, 154
adenosine formation, 128, 130, 132, 135, 137, 155
adenosine level(s), 133, 135
adherence, viii, 2, 9, 19, 41, 47, 48, 53, 60, 61, 79, 88, 89, 145
ADP, xi, 128, 131, 132, 135, 136, 137, 139, 144, 147
adrenergic, viii, x, 2, 45, 73, 81, 95, 96, 101, 128, 129, 132, 140, 141, 158, 169
anticonvulsants, 98
antidepressants, 79, 98, 99, 158
ATP catabolism, 130, 137
ATP inactivation, 128, 137
ATP metabolism, 128
ATP release, xi, 118, 128, 129, 130, 132, 134, 135, 136, 137, 138, 139, 140, 141, 142, 143, 146, 153

B

benign prostatic hyperplasia, 16, 89, 104, 108, 120, 121, 129, 146, 163, 169
Biofeedback, 40, 55
bladder outflow obstruction (BOO), 100, 102, 107, 128, 129, 130, 131, 135, 136, 139
Botulinum Toxin, 11, 48, 91, 110
Botulinum toxin A, 15, 63, 139, 143
BPH, 80, 81, 89, 91, 106, 108, 129, 130, 131, 136, 139, 155

C

Cannabinoids, 104, 118
children, viii, ix, 35, 36, 37, 38, 39, 40, 41, 42, 43, 44, 45, 46, 47, 48, 49, 50, 51, 52, 53, 54, 55, 56, 57, 58, 60, 61, 62, 63, 64, 65, 66, 81, 90, 98, 113
connexin 43, 135
constipation, 3, 5, 8, 9, 37, 38, 40, 41, 46, 47, 52, 54, 55, 72, 76, 78, 79, 81, 165
Cox-Inhibitors, 107

D

detrusor, vii, ix, xi, 1, 2, 4, 7, 10, 11, 14, 18, 19, 36, 39, 43, 45, 46, 48, 50, 55, 56, 57, 58, 60, 61, 62, 63, 70, 73, 74, 76, 77, 78, 79, 80, 81, 82, 84, 85, 86, 90, 91, 92, 96, 100, 102, 104, 105, 106, 107, 108, 109, 110, 112, 113, 114, 115, 116, 117, 118, 119, 120, 121, 122, 127, 128, 129, 130, 131, 132, 133, 134, 135, 136, 137, 138, 139, 140, 141, 142, 143, 144, 145, 147, 153, 157, 158, 159, 162, 166, 169
detrusor contraction, xi, 2, 4, 7, 46, 50, 70, 73, 77, 78, 86, 108, 128, 130, 132, 133
detrusor overactivity (DO), 7, 14, 39, 43, 55, 58, 60, 62, 63, 70, 74, 77, 80, 90, 91, 96, 102, 112, 113, 116, 117, 118, 119, 121, 122, 130, 132, 136, 138, 140, 141, 142, 143, 144, 145, 153
Dual Therapy, 46, 66

E

ecto-5'-nucleotidase, 130, 131, 135, 137, 155
Elocalcitol, 108
epidemiology, viii, 21, 22, 23, 30, 33

F

fecal incontinence, 24, 37, 83
Fesoterodine, 43
frequency, vii, ix, 1, 2, 6, 10, 11, 12, 17, 23, 24, 25, 29, 36, 37, 38, 39, 41, 42, 43, 44, 45, 51, 52, 55, 69, 70, 71, 76, 78, 83, 85, 96, 105, 109, 111, 114, 115, 132, 134, 135, 139, 141, 153, 158, 159, 162, 163
Functional MRI, 88

G

GABA, 97, 98, 109, 112, 113, 121, 155, 156
Gabapentin, 98, 113

I

interstitial cystitis, xi, 92, 128, 129, 139, 144, 145, 146
Intravesical Instillations, 42

L

lamina propria, 134, 137, 147, 155
lower urinary tract symptoms, viii, 3, 18, 21, 22, 32, 33, 34, 38, 52, 58, 65, 71, 87, 89, 90, 112, 120, 131, 167, 168

M

Maxi-K, 110
micturition reflex, 4, 19, 96, 97, 99, 100, 101, 104, 109, 114, 116, 121, 138, 139, 143
Mirabegron, v, ix, xi, 10, 14, 17, 18, 36, 45, 58, 59, 66, 79, 89, 96, 112, 157, 158, 159, 160, 161, 163, 166, 168, 169
MOR, 101
mucosal bladder network, 100
muscarinic, ix, 4, 35, 43, 58, 73, 78, 79, 81, 96, 105, 115, 129, 132, 135, 139, 143, 146, 167
myofibroblast, 147

N

NANC, 128, 129
neurogenic bladder, xi, 6, 39, 43, 49, 50, 55, 57, 61, 62, 63, 107, 120, 127, 128, 129, 144
Neuromodulation, viii, 2, 12, 50, 82, 143
Nitric Oxid Donors, 107
nocturia, ix, 2, 8, 10, 11, 23, 25, 29, 36, 69, 70, 71, 72, 76, 78, 81, 96, 105, 113, 158, 164
Non-neuronal, 134
NTPDase, 132, 135, 137

O

Opioids, 101
Overactive bladder (OAB), i, iii, v, vii, viii, ix, x, xi, 1, 2, 3, 4, 5, 6, 7, 8, 9, 10, 11, 12, 13, 14, 20, 24, 25, 26, 27, 28, 29, 31, 35, 36, 37, 38, 39, 40, 41, 42, 43, 44, 45, 46, 47, 48, 49, 50, 51, 52, 53, 59, 60, 68, 69, 70, 71, 72, 74, 75, 76, 77, 78, 79, 81, 82, 83, 84, 85, 86, 87, 88, 95, 96, 97, 98, 99, 100, 101, 102, 103, 104, 105, 107, 108, 109, 110, 113, 114, 127, 128, 129, 135, 136, 137, 138, 139, 140, 157, 158, 159, 162, 163, 164, 165, 166
Oxybutynin, ix, 8, 9, 35, 40, 43, 53, 56, 79

P

P1, xi, 128, 132, 144
P2X, 100, 116, 128, 129, 131, 133, 134, 135, 137, 141, 142, 143, 144, 146, 147
P2Y, xi, 128, 131, 136, 141, 142, 144, 147
pannexin-1, x, 127, 134, 139, 146, 153
PDE-Inhibitors, 105
Pelvic floor disorders, viii, 21, 22
Percutaneous Tibial Nerve Stimulation (PTNS), 12, 16, 51, 82, 86
Persistence, 47, 60, 61, 88, 89
Potassium Channels Openers, 109
Propiverine, 45, 58, 81, 90
Purinergic Cascade, v, 127
purinergic tone, x, 127, 131, 132, 136, 137
Purines, 128

S

Sacral Neuromodulation, 15, 52, 90
sensory nerves, x, 127, 135, 136, 144
Serotoninergics, 99
Solifenacin, 10, 14, 20, 44, 57, 58, 67, 161
suburothelial nerve, xi, 102, 128, 134, 136, 137, 139, 140

T

tolterodine, ix, xi, 8, 9, 16, 35, 36, 43, 46, 47, 56, 57, 78, 80, 81, 82, 89, 90, 98, 101, 111, 113, 157, 162, 163, 164, 167
Topical Gel, 42
Transcutaneous Electrical Nerve Stimulation (TENS), 51, 64
Transdermal Patch, 42
transient receptor potential (TRP), 102, 117
Trospium, 44, 58
TRP, 102, 103, 104, 154
TRPV1, 74, 102, 103, 104, 117, 118, 136, 140

U

UDP, 132, 136, 139, 147, 152
umbrella cells, 133, 135, 137, 146, 147
urgency, vii, viii, ix, x, 1, 2, 3, 6, 7, 9, 10, 11, 12, 16, 23, 24, 27, 28, 29, 31, 32, 35, 36, 37, 38, 39, 40, 45, 56, 64, 69, 70, 71, 74, 76, 77, 78, 79, 83, 84, 85, 86, 96, 101, 102, 105, 107, 113, 127, 157, 158, 159, 160, 162, 163, 164, 166
urinary biomarker, 138
Urinary incontinence, 3, 8, 11, 13, 18, 20, 32, 33, 55, 63, 71
urothelium, xi, 4, 66, 74, 79, 100, 102, 104, 110, 111, 115, 117, 119, 123, 128, 133, 134, 135, 136, 137, 139, 140, 141, 142, 143, 145, 146, 153, 155, 158, 166, 168, 169
UTP, 136, 155

V

vesicle exocytosis, x, 127, 134
voiding diary, 6, 11, 38, 48

Γ

γ-aminobutyric acid, 97
γ-aminobutyric acid (GABA) receptors, 97

Μ

μ-opioid receptor (MOR), 101